Breast MRI

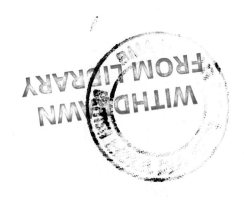

R. Edward Hendrick, PhD, FACR

Breast MRI

Fundamentals and Technical Aspects

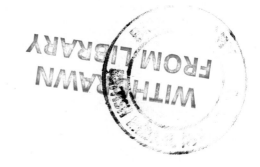

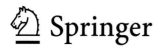 Springer

R. Edward Hendrick, PhD, FACR
Research Professor and Director, Breast Imaging Research (retired)
Lynn Sage Comprehensive Breast Center
Northwestern University's Feinberg School of Medicine
Northwestern Memorial Hospital
Chicago, IL
USA

Library of Congress Control Number: 2007932969

ISBN: 978-0-387-73506-1   e-ISBN: 978-0-387-73507-8

Printed on acid-free paper.

9 8 7 6 5 4 3 2 1

springer.com

This book is dedicated to my mother,
Enid Winifred Kimes Hendrick Thurston,
who has taught me so much about life,
and
to my wife,
Jean Rachelle Paquelet,
who makes every day worth living.

Foreword

Edward Hendrick has a unique position among physicists. Not only does he understand the physics of breast imaging, but he understands the fundamentals of breast cancer screening, detection, and diagnosis. I am fairly certain that most who read this text will be unaware that Dr. Hendrick played a major role in our understanding of breast cancer screening, particularly the benefit of screening women in their forties. He performed meta-analyses of the data from the randomized, controlled trials of screening and demonstrated a statistically significant benefit for screening women ages 40–49 when others were arguing incorrectly that there was no demonstrable benefit. His work permitted the rest of us to clarify the errors made by others in the interpretation of the data and it is in large measure due to Dr. Hendrick's efforts that life saving mammography screening is available for women in their forties.

Dr. Hendrick played a critical role in the development of quality standards for mammography, and guided the American College of Radiology Mammography Accreditation program and the effort to establish quality standards for mammography screening. He was a major force in trying to guide the FDA to understand the burden that unnecessary requirements placed on radiologists.

Dr. Hendrick is the Breast Imager's physicist. Recognizing the benefit of screening mammography, he has now turned his attention to the next major advance in breast evaluation – Magnetic Resonance Imaging (MRI). It seems somewhat strange to think of MRI as being a new "advance." Several of us were trying to apply MRI to the breast twenty years ago when it first became possible to use the technology for breast evaluation. We soon learned that without a contrast agent, the relaxation values of normal breast tissue and cancer were not sufficiently different and MRI lost favor until gadolinium became available. It is not clear why it has taken so long for breast MRI to come back, but my own belief is that MRI physicists found it easier to work with a more rigid structure like the brain and neurological system, and breast MRI had to wait for these applications to become robust before attention returned to the breast.

There is huge potential for MRI of the breast as we move into an era of renewed interest. For radiologists it is apparent that it is easier to "detect" a bright focus of enhancement against a black background (MRI) than it is to try to appreciate a lighter gray structure against a gray background (mammography). The huge expense of MRI is daunting when we think of applying it to screening, but costs can be reduced. Requiring the injection of a substance intravenously is also a limitation, but, as we have seen with the decision by the American Cancer Society to endorse MRI screening for high risk women, the opportunity to further reduce the death rate from the most feared of cancers among women will push the barriers back and more and more women will be having MR examinations. Having personally participated in the often heated debates about the merits of mammography screening, I am well aware of, and a strong supporter of, the importance of rigorous scientific validation for breast cancer screening tests. Unlike diagnostic evaluation where the anecdotal experience of the treating physicians may be the only way that decisions can be made and lives saved, screening involves "healthy" individuals who may be made "ill" by a false positive screening test. There are breast cancers that if left undetected would never be lethal, and there are breast cancers that have metastasized even before a new screening test can find them. If these are the cancers that a new screening study such as MRI finds, then there will be no benefit, and only "harm". It is for these reasons that I would strongly urge large randomized, controlled trials of MRI screening to prove a benefit. It has been argued that these would be prohibitively expensive. However, the gradual drift into MR screening of more and more women will be far more expensive, and the benefit will not be clear.

Regardless of how the use of breast MRI continues to evolve, it will continue to evolve and expand, and Breast Imaging radiologists need to understand breast MRI so that the information it provides can be integrated into the care of the patient along with the results from mammography and ultrasound and other tests as they are brought to bear on breast problems. I am personally grateful, and we should all be grateful that having helped us to understand x-ray physics and mammography, Dr. Hendrick has taken on MRI of the breast with equal energy, attention, and expertise. As he points out, breast MRI provides a major opportunity to increase our ability to detect early breast cancers, and this will likely translate into further reductions in the death rate from the most common cancer among women.

Thank you, Ed, for all of your important contributions.

Dan Kopans, MD, FACR
Professor of Radiology, Harvard Medical School
Founder and Senior Radiologist, Breast Imaging Division,
Massachusetts General Hospital
Boston, Massachusetts

Preface

From years of being both student and teacher, I've found that the best way to learn a new field is one-on-one, with an interested student, a willing teacher, and a pad of paper between them. As a result, the tone of this book is not that of a didactic classroom lecture, but an informal exchange between two colleagues. When you read each chapter, imagine that we are sitting side-by-side and that I am doing my best to explain the basics of magnetic resonance imaging (MRI) and the essentials of breast MRI to you. The figures and the occasional formula illustrate the essential concepts on the pad of paper between us.

An informal, one-on-one approach affords the opportunity to include a little history and provide a personal emphasis that is often difficult to communicate in the classroom. Therefore, do not be surprised by the occasional historical aside about developments in basic physics related to MRI, to the development of MRI, and breast MRI.

When I told Dr. Dan Kopans that I was writing a book to covey the basics of MRI to breast imagers, he had three words of advice: "keep it simple". I have tried to do that. Of course, Dan never keeps advice to just three words. He went on to say that the MRI physics explanations had to be simple enough that even he could understand them. At that point, I enlisted Dan, and a number of other practicing radiologists, to serve as reviewers of this book, to make sure the level and content are appropriate. In addition to Dr. Dan Kopans, I want to thank Dr. Jean R. Paquelet, Dr. Lora Barke, Dr. Eric Berns, and Dr. Richard Pacini for reading and commenting on each of the chapters in this book. Their efforts have made the task easier for you. Special thanks go to Dr. Frank Shellock for reviewing Chapter 12 on MRI safety and for providing the patient and personnel screening forms that are reprinted in the Appendix.

The one thing I ask of you as you start this book is that you give the story a chance to unfold. MRI is not a one-act play. It requires learning a number of fundamentals and then putting them all together before you can experience the breakthrough of understanding how MRI really works. I will try to minimize the unnecessary, extraneous facts, and will try to focus on the essentials that prepare you for that breakthrough.

One of the essentials of learning MRI is to equip yourself with models that convey a better intuitive feeling for how MRI actually works. This is certainly done in other texts, but this book places special emphasis on giving you pictorial models for the essential aspects of MRI. Hence, there will be more pictures and graphs that you probably want to take the time to look at, but each picture will be helpful in putting it all together to understand how MRI and breast MRI work.

My goal for this book is that when you finish the fundamentals, Chapters 1–7, you will understand how MRI works. At that point, you should have a clear understanding of why T2-weighted pulse sequences make cystic lesions bright without contrast and why T1-weighted imaging makes lesions bright with contrast. Moreover, you should be beginning to arm yourself with the tools you need to understand the intricacies of MR pulse sequences. If you already know all this, then skip to Chapter 8 for the start of breast MRI. My goal with the second part of the book is that by the time you get to Chapter 11, you will have a good idea of how breast MRI works and how you can best perform breast MRI in your own practice, including the selection of breast protocols. By the end of Chapter 11, you should know the differences between good and bad breast MRI and how you can maximize image quality with your current equipment.

Chapter 12 is on MR safety, with an emphasis on breast imaging. Chapter 13 focuses on newer techniques that may help improve the sensitivity and specificity of breast MRI. This section describes some of the new techniques being developed that might make breast MRI (and possibly MRS) that rare examination that has both high sensitivity and high specificity for breast cancer.

Finally, I would appreciate your feedback on this book. I'm sure that even after careful review and editing, it won't be free of errors or perfectly clear to everyone who reads it. If you see ways that I can correct or improve the book, please let me know by e-mail at: edward.hendrick@gmail.com. If you like certain aspects of the book, I would appreciate hearing about that, too. Both forms of feedback complete the one-on-one student-teacher relationship, where neither person is entirely student or entirely teacher, and both benefit from the experience. I sincerely hope that you do.

Chicago, Illinois   R. Edward Hendrick, PhD, FACR

Contents

Chapter 1
Fundamentals of Magnetic Resonance Imaging

Magnetic resonance imaging (MRI) combines some of the most interesting principles of physics and some of today's most sophisticated technology to make medical images of amazing clarity and surprisingly high diagnostic accuracy.[1-4] MRI today is more revolutionary than x-ray imaging was a century ago. Twenty-five years ago, when MRI was first introduced to clinical practice, its richness of applications to medical imaging could not have been imagined. It quickly was demonstrated that MRI is useful in diagnosing diseases in the brain and spine. Today, MRI provides not only exquisite anatomic detail and contrast but also provides functional information that can help characterize disease. We now use MRI routinely to assess blood flow, to quantify diffusion within cells, and to localize thought processes in the human brain. The richness of MRI is continuing to unfold.

Breast imaging is one more example of the unexpected versatility of MRI. Emerging data comparing MRI to mammography, ultrasound, single photon emission computed tomography (SPECT), and positron emission tomography (PET) indicate that MRI is more sensitive than any other medical test in detecting breast cancer and is more accurate in characterizing extent of disease.[5-13] Newer results suggest that functional MRI and MR spectroscopy (MRS) applied to enhancing breast lesions may help increase specificity for detecting breast cancer.

To the radiologist, understanding MRI can seem insurmountable. In 1990, Dr. Anne Osborne, Dr. Manny Kanal, and I wrote a basic MR physics article that began: "For the radiologist, the crux of medical imaging is what makes black things black and white things white."[14] This is still true nearly two decades later. Understanding the basis of image contrast in mammography is relatively easy: the greater the attenuation of x-rays in a denser region of the breast, such as a cancer, the fewer the number of x-rays reaching the film, and the lighter the area of the processed film under that denser region. The lack of such simple rules for what makes a lesion black or white makes MRI more difficult to interpret. For example, a cystic breast lesion will be dark on non-fat-suppressed T1-weighted MR images (Figure 1.1A), brighter, but slightly darker than fibroglandular tissues, on fat-suppressed T1-weighted images (Figure 1.1B), and bright on T2-weighted or spin-density weighted images (Figure 1.1C and D). Other lesions, such as cystic breast lesions containing blood, can reverse their appearance, appearing bright on T1-weighted images and dark on

R.E. Hendrick (ed.), *Breast MRI: Fundamentals and Technical Aspects.*
© Springer 2008

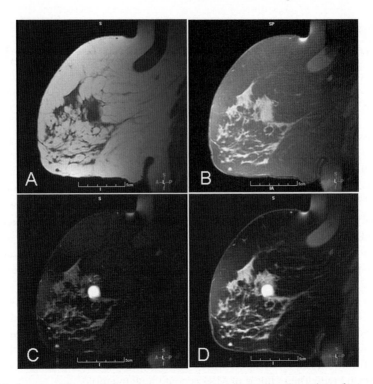

Fig. 1.1 Images of the same slice of the same volunteer illustrating the variety of appearances of fat, normal fibroglandular tissue, and cysts in the breast. (A) T1-weighted image without fat-suppression. Fat is the brightest tissue in this image, while the circular cyst in the center of the breast and fibroglandular tissue are dark. (B) Identical T1-weighted image with fat-suppression. Here, fibroglandular tissue and cyst are isointense and light gray, while fat is darker. (C) T2-weighted image with fat-suppression. Here the circular cyst is bright, fibroglandular tissues dark gray, and fat dark. (D) Spin-density weighted image with fat-suppression. Here, fibroglandular tissues are brighter than in C, but still not as bright as cystic fluid. Fat is dark, but not uniform.

T2–weighted images. The explanation of a lesion's brightness on an MR image depends not only on inherent tissue properties but also on MRI technique: the pulse sequence and its timing parameters can bestow completely different appearances to the same tissue.

This book is aimed at making MRI in general, and breast MRI in particular, comprehensible. Its primary goal is to make sure that you understand why black things are black and white things are white on breast MRI. Understanding that requires reviewing a few basic principles of MR physics. Those principles include the magnetic properties of nuclei that create tissue magnetization (the "nuclear" part), the collective effects of nuclei placed in a strong magnetic field (the "magnetic" part), and the interactions of nuclei with radio waves that explain tissue excitation and signal measurement (the "resonance" part). The relaxation properties of nuclei are discussed in Chapter 2; these explain T1-, T2-, T2*- and spin-density-weighting, the primary sources of tissue contrast in MRI. The equipment design and pulse sequences that permit extraction of an MR signal from the human body are discussed in Chapters 3–6. Chapter 7 is devoted to signal, contrast, and noise issues in MRI. Chapter 8 describes MRI contrast agents. Chapters 9 and 10 are devoted to breast MR image acquisition and post-processing protocols. Chapter 11 describes artifacts in breast MRI. Chapter 12 describes MR safety, and Chapter 13 summarizes some of the new technical developments in breast MRI.

This book is aimed at making breast MRI accessible to breast imagers who may have shied away from the physics of MRI in training. If you persist through the first few chapters, you will learn how MRI works and, more important, you should begin to develop intuition about MRI techniques and their application to breast imaging.

Breast MRI is a rich and exciting field. I hope this book helps you understand how MRI works and how to obtain breast MRI exams of exquisite quality, with high sensitivity to breast cancer. We begin with some basics: properties of the atom and its constituents.

Subatomic Particles

Three subatomic particles comprise atoms: the proton, the neutron, and the electron. Of these three, the electron is the simplest. It is a point-like, infinitesimal particle with the smallest measured unit of negative charge (-1.6×10^{-19} Coulombs) and the smallest measured unit of quantized spin ($h/(4\pi)$, where h is Planck's constant (h = 6.626×10^{-34} Joule-seconds, which is the ratio of the energy of a photon to its frequency; particles having this smallest unit of quantized spin are referred to as spin-½ particles). By point-like and infinitesimal, physicists mean that the electron has no structure. You can strike it with another particle that has as much energy as possible and thereby approach it as closely as possible, and it still interacts as a point-like structure.

The proton has exactly the same magnitude of charge as the electron, but of opposite sign ($+1.6 \times 10^{-19}$ Coulombs). The proton also has exactly the same amount of quantized spin as the electron ($h/(4\pi)$) making it, like the electron, a spin-½ particle. But that is where the resemblance between electron and proton ends. The proton is 1836 times more massive than the electron, is not an infinitesimal, point-like particle, but has a structure something like that of a fuzzy tennis ball, with a charge radius of about 0.8–0.9×10^{-15} m (0.8–0.9 femtometers). In addition to interacting through electromagnetic forces, the proton exerts strong nuclear forces on other protons and on neutrons. It is these strong nuclear forces that cause protons and neutrons to bind together to form the nuclei of atoms, in spite of the electrical repulsion that pushes protons apart.

The neutron, like the proton, is a spin-½, strongly interacting particle, meaning that it binds with other protons and neutrons in the nuclei of atoms. It has almost the same mass as the proton, about 1837 times the mass of the electron but is electrically neutral, so it does not attract or repel electrons or protons through electrostatic forces. The neutron has about the same radius as the proton and is

Figure 1.2 Schematic of the electron (e⁻), proton (p⁺), and neutron (n⁰).

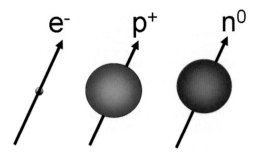

Table 1.1 Properties of atomic constituents

Particle	Electron	Proton	Neutron
Charge:	-1.6×10^{-19}C	$+1.6 \times 10^{-19}$C	0
Mass:	1 emu	1836 emu	1837 emu
Spin:	$\frac{1}{2}\, h/(2\pi)$	$\frac{1}{2}\, h/(2\pi)$	$\frac{1}{2}\, h/(2\pi)$
Magnetic Dipole Moment:	$1836\,\mu_N$	$2.79\,\mu_N$	$-1.91\,\mu_N$

Note: C = Coulomb
emu = electronic mass unit, 1 emu = 9.1×10^{-31} kilograms
h = Planck's constant, h = 6.626×10^{-34} Joule-seconds
μ_N = one nuclear magneton

attracted to protons through strong nuclear forces. These strong nuclear forces bind protons and neutrons together as stable atomic nuclei. Except for hydrogen, the number of neutrons must equal or exceed the number of protons to form a stable atomic nucleus.

Figure 1.2 and Table 1.1 summarize the basic properties of these 3 atomic constituents.

The Atom

Every atom is made up of electrons, protons, and neutrons, with the exception of the lightest and most abundant atom in the universe, hydrogen. The hydrogen atom consists of only one proton and one electron (Figure 1.3A). The proton and electron are bound together through electrostatic forces, the attraction of oppositely charged particles. The effective radius of the hydrogen atom is about 0.25×10^{-10} meters or one-quarter of an Angstrom (1 Angstrom = 10^{-10} meters), so its size is about 30,000 times larger than the charge radius of the proton alone. The outer boundary of the hydrogen atom is defined by the cloud of the single, rapidly moving electron that ranges around the nucleus. In fact, both electron and proton are in orbit around their collective center of mass, but since the proton is 1836 times more massive than the electron, the electron ranges 1836 times more widely than the proton. Thus, it is almost correct to picture the hydrogen atom as a fixed proton nucleus with an electron moving rapidly and ranging widely about it (Figure 1.3A). This picture is the Bohr model of the hydrogen atom.

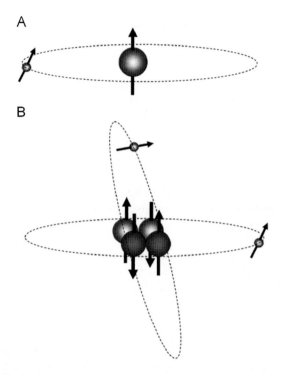

A

B

Figure 1.3 (A) The hydrogen atom consisting of one proton and one electron. (B) The helium atom consisting of two protons, two neutrons, and two electrons.

The second lightest atom is helium. Its nucleus consists of two protons and two neutrons (Figure 1.3B). Why does the most stable version of helium include two neutrons in its nucleus, rather than just two protons alone? It's because electrostatic forces cause the two protons alone to repel one another. The two neutrons provide an adequate amount of strong nuclear binding force to glue the helium nucleus together in spite of the electrostatic repulsion of the two protons. And because the helium nucleus has two electrostatic units of positive charge from the two protons, the helium atom is completed by two electrons ranging about the nucleus. The effective radius of the helium atom, set by the size of the electron cloud, is about 65% larger than that of the hydrogen atom. Helium is four times more massive than hydrogen, due to having 4 nucleons (protons or neutrons) in its nucleus, compared to 1 nucleon for hydrogen.

As you move up the atomic chart, from element number 2 (helium) to element number 3 (lithium), the atom gains one proton and one electron (for a total of 3 each), and two neutrons (for a total of 4). The extra neutron provides more strong binding force, making the lithium nucleus more stable. As you continue stepping up the atomic chart from element to element, each atom gains one proton, one electron, and one neutron until you get to element number 6 (carbon), whose nucleus is most stable with 6 neutrons. The number of electrons, along with their configuration (that is, how many electrons comprise the outer electron shell), determines each atom's chemical properties, while the number of nuclear constituents determines each atom's nuclear properties.

Magnetic Dipole Moments

The fundamental property that enables magnetic resonance imaging (MRI) is that charged, spinning particles, such as the proton, have a magnetic dipole moment. A large-scale (macroscopic) example of a magnetic dipole is a bar magnet, which has a north and a south magnetic pole, hence the term "dipole." Everyone knows that if you put a bar magnet in a strong, externally applied magnetic field, it will be forced to align its north-south axis along the direction of the magnetic field.

Another way that you could make a macroscopic magnetic dipole would be to take a sphere, such as a basketball, and place static electric charge on its surface, say, by rubbing it with cat fur. When the charged sphere is stationary, it can experience electrical forces, but not magnetic forces. When you spin the charged basketball on your finger, it becomes a magnetic dipole, like a bar magnet, with its magnetic north-south axis pointing along the axis about which the basketball is spinning (Figure 1.4). When placed in an externally applied magnetic field, the spinning, charged sphere will experience a twisting force, or torque, that acts to align the axis of rotation so that it points along the direction of the magnetic field, just as for a bar magnet. We all know that if you exert enough twisting force, you can orient a bar magnet (or the spinning basketball) at any angle you wish relative to the externally applied magnetic field, but it requires energy to do so.

Magnetic dipoles such as a bar magnet or a spinning, charged basketball are referred to as macroscopic objects because they are made up of so many particles or atoms that they obey the laws of classical physics. Macroscopic objects can have any amount of mass, charge, and angular momentum (spin).

Protons and electrons, on the other hand, are "quantized" particles. They obey the laws of quantum physics and can have only one discrete mass, one discrete charge, and one discrete spin. As a result of having discrete amounts of mass, charge, and spin, quantum particles such as the electron and proton have discrete magnetic dipole moments.

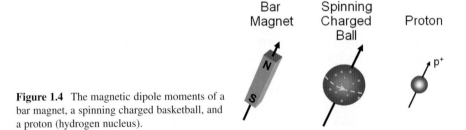

Figure 1.4 The magnetic dipole moments of a bar magnet, a spinning charged basketball, and a proton (hydrogen nucleus).

Another difference between macroscopic objects and quantized particles is the way their magnetic dipoles can align with an externally applied magnetic field. A bar magnet or spinning, charged basketball can have any orientation relative to an external magnetic field, although it requires externally applied energy to twist them away from alignment with the static magnetic field. The magnetic moment of a proton or electron, however, can align with an externally applied magnetic field in only two ways: up, meaning that the magnetic dipole moment of the particle points along the magnetic field lines, or down, meaning that the dipole moment of the particle points opposite the magnetic field lines. These two orientations have slightly different energy levels: it takes more energy for a dipole to point down than up. This energy difference between up and down orientations of the magnetic dipole equals the energy of electromagnetic waves that must be supplied to excite magnetic dipoles within tissue, which determines the resonant frequency of the dipole.

How strong are the magnetic dipole moments of the electron and proton? The Dirac model, developed in 1928, assumed the electron to be a quantized, point-like particle and predicted that the magnetic dipole moment of the electron is:

$$\mu_e = \frac{q_e h}{4\pi m_e}, \text{(the Bohr magneton)} \tag{1.1}$$

that is, the magnetic dipole moment of the electron is directly proportional to its charge (q_e) and spin ($h/(4\pi)$), and is inversely proportional to its mass (m_e). The magnetic dipole moment of the electron is the most accurately measured quantity in science, and amazingly, the theoretical prediction of the Dirac model agrees with the experimentally measured magnetic dipole moment of the electron precisely, to about 8 significant figures. The success of the Dirac model in correctly predicting the measured magnetic dipole moment of the electron provided strong evidence not only that the quantum theory of the electron was correct, but also that Dirac's assumption about the nature of the electron was correct: the electron indeed is a point-like fundamental particle.

What happens when you apply the same theoretical model to the proton, substituting the mass of the proton for that of the electron? The model fails miserably, underestimating the measured magnetic dipole moment of the proton by a factor of nearly 3. The Dirac model applied to the proton predicts that the magnetic dipole moment of the proton should be:

$$\mu_N = \frac{q_p h}{4\pi m_p}, \tag{1.2}$$

a quantity called the nuclear magneton, since the mass of the proton replaces the mass of the electron in the formula. The nuclear magneton is 1836 times smaller than the Bohr magneton, since the mass of the proton is 1836 times greater than that of the electron, while they have the same magnitude of charge and spin. When nuclear physicists carefully measured the magnetic dipole moment of the proton in the 1930s, it was found to be 2.79 times larger than that predicted by the theoretical model: $\mu_p = 2.79\,\mu_N$. This large discrepancy between theory and experiment puzzled physicists for decades and led physicists to conclude that, unlike the electron, the proton is not a point-like fundamental particle, but a complex particle. We now believe that the proton is not a fundamental particle at all, but is composed of smaller, more fundamental constituents: quarks. More will be said about quarks in the discussion of the neutron.

The magnetic dipole moment of the electron is 658 times stronger than the magnetic dipole moment of the proton. This is because the proton has 1836 times more mass than the electron, making the proton's magnetic moment a factor of 1836 less, and the proton is 2.79 times more magnetic than expected because of its more complex quark composition (1836/2.79 = 658). Given that the hydrogen atom consists of one proton and one electron and given that the magnetic dipole moment of the electron is 658 times stronger than the magnetic dipole moment of the proton, why is the proton the source of signal in MRI, rather than the electron? The answer is that the electromagnetic waves needed to excite hydrogen nuclei occur in the right energy range (radio waves) to penetrate tissue; the electromagnetic waves that excite the electron's magnetic moment are 658 times more energetic, placing them in the microwave part of the electromagnetic spectrum. Microwaves matching the electron's transition energy penetrate only a few centimeters of tissue before being absorbed. This effect is demonstrated when you heat a bowl of soup in a microwave oven: the soup heats primarily at its edges because most of the microwave energy is absorbed by the first few centimeters of water. The same effect makes electron spin resonance (ESR) unsuitable for studying disease in the human body due to its high energy deposition in surface tissues. Researchers do use ESR, also called electron paramagnetic resonance (EPR), to study properties of matter, but the bioeffects of the electromagnetic radiation needed to excite electron "spins" make ESR far less acceptable than MRI for revealing diseases in humans.

The magnetic dipole moment of the electron is useful in MRI, not as a source of signal, but in a different role. Atoms with several unpaired outer shell electrons, such as the rare earth element gadolinium, make excellent magnetic resonance contrast agents. When placed in a strong, externally applied magnetic field, the magnetic dipoles of the unpaired outer shell electrons in gadolinium align, creating strong, non-uniform magnetic fields in the vicinity of the gadolinium atom. Such materials are termed "paramagnetic": they have magnetic effects only when placed in a strong, externally applied magnetic field. Paramagnetism is used to advantage in contrast-enhanced MRI, where chelated forms of gadolinium (non-chelated gadolinium is toxic) are injected into the human body to shorten the tissue relaxation times of hydrogen nuclei near gadolinium. This is discussed in greater detail in Chapters 2 and 8.

A brief historical note: the method developed to measure the magnetic dipole moments of nuclei to high accuracy was developed by I.I. Rabi in the late 1930s and was called "nuclear magnetic resonance."[15] Rabi's idea was to use radio waves of just the right frequency to flip nuclear magnetic dipole moments from one orientation to another; that is, to produce a "resonance" between the radio wave and atomic nuclei. This ability to use radio waves to flip nuclear magnetic moments led to very precise measurements of their dipole moments and won I.I. Rabi the 1944 Nobel Prize in physics. I.I. Rabi went on to train several generations of research physicists in nuclear and atomic physics. One of his graduate students, Polykarp Kusch, won the 1955 Nobel prize in physics for measuring the magnetic dipole moment of the electron more precisely than ever before using magnetic resonance techniques. This measurement shed light on the fundamental nature of the electron and motivated the development of quantum electrodynamics.

During World War II, two physicists, Felix Bloch and Edward Purcell, worked with Rabi and a team of physicists at the Radiation Lab at MIT to speed the development of radar. In 1946, after the war, their two groups independently demonstrated that the nuclear magnetic resonance techniques developed by Rabi could be applied to the collective magnetization of materials, including human tissues.[16,17] Bloch of Stanford and Purcell of Harvard shared the 1952 Nobel prize in physics for their development of the powerful analytic techniques of nuclear magnetic resonance (NMR).

Based on classical physics, the neutron, being chargeless, should not have a magnetic dipole moment at all. Physicists were astonished when the measured magnetic dipole moment of the neutron was not zero, but was found to be nearly as large in magnitude as that of the proton, but opposite in sign: $\mu_n = -1.91\,\mu_N$. How could a chargeless particle have a magnetic dipole moment? If the neutron were a point-like, uncharged particle, it couldn't. The explanation for the neutron having a magnetic dipole moment is that, like the proton, the neutron is not a point-like particle. Although chargeless, the neutron is composed of three fractionally charged, spin-½ particles, called quarks. While quarks have never been found in free space, the anomalous magnetic dipole moments of both the proton and neutron, along with their charges, masses, and spins, are explained by the quark model, in which the proton, neutron, and all other strongly interacting particles, are composed of quarks.

Nuclear Magnetic Moments

The magnetic dipole moments of all nuclei are explained by the magnetic moments of the proton and neutron and by the number of protons and neutrons making up each nucleus. When protons occur in pairs or neutrons occur in pairs in a nucleus, they pair up like two bar magnets and cancel the effect of each other's magnetic dipole moments outside the nucleus. Thus, only nuclei with an unpaired proton, an unpaired neutron, or both, have a net magnetic dipole moment.

The first atom on the atomic chart, hydrogen, has the simplest nucleus: a single, unpaired proton (Figure 1.3A). Its nucleus has the strongest nuclear magnetic dipole moment of any atom due to its large magnetic dipole moment (that of a single proton) and its relatively small mass (also that of a single proton) compared to other atomic nuclei.

The second nucleus on the atomic chart, the helium nucleus, consists of two protons and two neutrons (Figure 1.3B). The two protons in the helium nucleus pair up exactly to cancel their net magnetic effects; and the two neutrons, which have

Table 1.2 Nuclei with non-zero magnetic dipole moments occurring in the human body, their isotopic abundance, gyromagnetic ratios, and relative sensitivities in NMR

Nucleus	Symbol	Isotopic Abundance	Gyromagnetic Ratio (MHz/T)	Relative Sensitivity
Hydrogen-1	^{1}H	99.98%	42.6	1.0
Carbon-13	^{13}C	1.11%	10.7	0.016
Nitrogen-14	^{14}N	99.63%	3.1	0.001
Fluorine-19	^{19}F	100%	40.4	0.83
Sodium-23	^{23}Na	100%	11.3	0.093
Phosphorus-31	^{31}P	100%	17.2	0.066

Note: 98.89% of naturally occurring carbon occurs as carbon-12, which has no nuclear magnetic dipole moment. 1.11% is carbon-13, and 0.0000000001% is carbon-14.

different magnetic moments than the proton, also pair up exactly to cancel their magnetic effects. Thus, the helium nucleus has no net magnetic dipole moment. Due to this pairing of protons and neutrons, most atomic nuclei have no magnetic dipole moment and are, therefore, not suitable for NMR or MRI.

The most stable isotope of nitrogen, nitrogen-14, has seven protons and seven neutrons in its nucleus. Six of the seven protons pair up and six of the seven neutrons pair up, leaving one unpaired proton and one unpaired neutron. Because these two particles have different magnetic dipole moments, the unpaired proton and unpaired neutron do not cancel one another, so the nitrogen nucleus has a magnetic dipole moment that is less than the magnetic dipole strength of either the proton or neutron. This illustrates that nuclei with both an unpaired proton and an unpaired neutron still have a net magnetic dipole moment.

Table 1.2 lists nuclei occurring in the human body that have magnetic dipole moments and, thus, are suitable for NMR. Most, other than hydrogen, occur in such small quantities that they are difficult to detect *in vivo*. But a few, such as carbon-13, sodium-23, and phosphorus-31 occur in adequate quantities to be measurable in NMR experiments. Hydrogen occurs in adequate quantities not only to be detectable in NMR, but to be amenable to MRI.

Tissue Magnetization

The collective effect of huge numbers of hydrogen nuclei produces a net tissue magnetization when the human body is placed in a strong magnetic field. The reason for having a strong magnetic field in MRI systems is to create a measurable amount of tissue magnetization from the hydrogen nuclei in the human body. A cubic millimeter of tissue contains approximately 10^{19} hydrogen atoms, mostly in water molecules (H_2O) and in fat molecules (mostly CH_2). Not all of these hydrogen nuclei contribute to the MR signal. As mentioned before, when placed in an externally applied magnetic field, hydrogen nuclei, because they are spin-½ particles, have only two possible orientations: they align either with (up) or against the external magnetic field (down) (Figure 1.5). If these two orientations occurred in precisely equal amounts, there

Figure 1.5 A slight imbalance of the number of hydrogen dipoles aligned with the static magnetic field, B_0, over and above those pointing opposite B_0, produces the net magnetization from a voxel of tissue (M_0). The imbalance occurs because the energy of dipoles oriented along B_0 is slightly lower (by an energy $E_0 = \Delta E$) than the energy of dipoles oriented opposite to B_0.

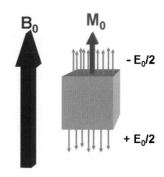

would be no net tissue magnetization; if that were the case, we would not be able to generate an NMR signal from tissue. Fortunately, the two possible orientations of the magnetic dipole moments of hydrogen nuclei occur in slightly different amounts because the two different orientations have slightly different energy states. Magnetic dipoles aligned <u>with</u> the externally applied magnetic field have a slightly lower energy than those that are aligned <u>against</u> the magnetic field. The difference in the energy of the two states depends only on the nucleus's magnetic dipole strength, μ, and the strength of the externally applied magnetic field, B_0:

$$\Delta E = \mu B_0. \qquad (1.3)$$

This energy difference is a key quantity in MRI. Using a wave description, an electromagnetic wave supplying exactly this energy difference can cause the magnetic dipole moment of the nucleus to "flip" from its lower energy state to its higher energy state, thereby "exciting" the nucleus. Using a quantum description of the same phenomenon, a photon with precisely the right energy can strike a nucleus and flip its magnetic dipole from its lower to higher energy state. This resonance phenomenon was the trick that Rabi used to make precise measurements of the magnetic dipole moments of nuclei. The electromagnetic wave frequency that achieves this energy transition is the "resonant" or "Larmor" frequency. It depends only on the nuclear constituent you want to excite and the external magnetic field strength applied to the tissue sample:

$$\Delta E = h\nu_0 = h\omega_0 /(2\pi) = \mu B_0, \qquad (1.4)$$

where ν_0 is the Larmor frequency in units of Hertz or cycles per second (1 Hertz (Hz) = $1/s$ = s^{-1}), ω_0 is the Larmor frequency in units of radians per second (2π radians = 1 cycle), μ is the magnetic moment of the nucleus or particle of interest, and B_0 is the magnetic field strength in which the nucleus resides. At typical B_0 values for MRI, this energy difference is very small. For B_0 = 1.5 T, and for hydrogen nuclei ($\mu = \mu_p$), $\Delta E = 2.64 \times 10^{-7}$ electron-volts (eV). In comparison, the ionization energy of the hydrogen atom, the energy binding the electron to the proton, is 13.7 eV. Thus, the energy needed to flip a hydrogen nuclear dipole from its lower energy state to its higher energy state is 52 million times less than the energy causing ionization of hydrogen atoms. This explains why the radiofrequency (RF) waves used to excite nuclei in MRI are non-ionizing.

The Larmor frequency for the hydrogen nucleus is given by the Larmor equation:

$$\omega_0 = \gamma_p B_0. \tag{1.5}$$

From Eq. (1.4), we get that $\gamma_p = 2\pi\mu_p/h$; γ_p is the gyromagnetic ratio of the proton. The gyromagnetic ratio of a particle or nucleus is the ratio of its magnetic dipole moment (μ) to its spin angular momentum, which is given in units of $h/(2\pi)$. As written in Eq (1.5), ω_0 is in units of radians/second and γ_p is in units of radians/sec/T (radians per second per Tesla). For the proton, $\gamma_p = 2.68 \times 10^8$ radians/second/Tesla. It is more common to specify the Larmor frequency in cycles/second or MHz (millions of cycles per second) and the gyromagnetic ratio in units of megaHertz per Tesla (MHz/T). Thus, even though the Larmor equation is written as in Eq (1.5), the Larmor frequency is more often specified as $v_0 = \omega_0/(2\pi)$ (that is, in units of MHz) and the gyromagnetic ratio is specified as $\gamma_p/(2\pi)$ (that is, in units of MHz/Tesla). Table 1.2 gives gyromagnetic ratios (in units of MHz/T) for the few types of nuclei that have non-zero magnetic dipole moments and occur in the human body.

Eq. (1.5) is the Larmor equation, which is the most important equation in MRI. It tells us the precise frequency of electromagnetic radiation that must be sent into tissue to excite hydrogen nuclei, and it tells us the electronic frequency we must "listen to" to measure the MRI signal emitted from the human body. For example, using hydrogen nuclei as the source of MR signal at 1.5 T, the resonant frequency is:

$$v_0 = \omega_0/(2\pi) = \gamma_p/(2\pi) B_0 = (42.6 \, \text{MHz/T})(1.5 \, \text{T}) = 63.9 \, \text{MHz}. \tag{1.6}$$

The Larmor frequency of hydrogen at 1.5 T is 63.9 MHz.[1]

From a physics standpoint, something important happens when you go from a single magnetic dipole of a hydrogen nucleus to the collective effects of 10^{19} hydrogen nuclear dipoles in a cubic millimeter of tissue. You go from a quantum description to a classical description. There is an entire field of physics, statistical mechanics, devoted to describing this transition from quantum physics to classical physics. The one thing we need from statistical mechanics is the Boltzmann equation, which describes the imbalance of hydrogen dipoles in a macroscopic ensemble of dipoles (all the hydrogen nuclei contained in a voxel of tissue) when placed in a strong magnetic field. It says that in a voxel of tissue, the difference in the numbers of hydrogen nuclei in the two different energy states (up and down) is determined by the ratio of the energy difference between the two magnetic dipole energy states and the thermal energy of tissue. While electromagnetic interactions between hydrogen dipoles and their surroundings are responsible for dipoles making the energy transition from higher to lower energy states, it is the rate of tumbling of molecules, which is determined by their temperature, that determines how readily the surroundings take up this excess energy and equalize the two energy states. The thermal energy of tissue is determined entirely by its temperature: the hotter the tissue, the more thermal interactions tend to equalize

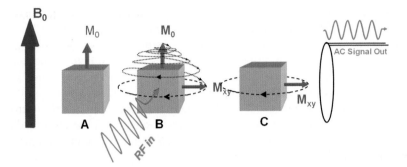

Figure 1.6 (A) When placed in a sufficiently strong static magnetic field, magnetization M_0 is induced in a voxel of tissue. (B) An RF pulse applied at the correct (Larmor) frequency and for the correct duration flips the magnetization away from the direction of B_0, the longitudinal direction, and into the transverse plane (perpendicular to B_0) where the precessing magnetization can be measured. (C) Once flipped away from B_0, the transverse magnetization precesses around an axis parallel to B_0. This precession of transverse magnetization at a fixed, known frequency (the Larmor frequency) aids in its measurement. The precessing magnetization causes a changing magnetic flux to link the nearby receiver coil, thereby inducing a current in the receiver coil that oscillates at the Larmor frequency. The amplitude of oscillating current measured at the Larmor frequency is the MR signal strength. A-C together summarize the basic NMR experiment.

the number of nuclei in each energy state. This population difference is described precisely by the Boltzmann equation.

At an externally applied magnetic field strength of 1.5 Tesla and at the temperature of the human body (about 310° Kelvin), the Boltzmann equation says that about 5 more hydrogen nuclei per million are aligned <u>with</u> the magnetic field (B_0) than are aligned <u>opposite</u> to B_0 (Figure 1.5). The collective effect of this imbalance in orientation of hydrogen nuclei produces the net magnetization of human tissue (Figure 1.6A). An imbalance of 5 per million nuclei seems small, but because there are so many hydrogen nuclei per unit volume, there is a net magnetization of about $5 \times 10^{13} \mu_p$ from each cubic millimeter of tissue placed in a 1.5 T MR scanner. If you used a magnet with a field strength of 3.0 T, this would double the imbalance in nuclei from 5 per million to 10 per million pointing along B_0 that are not cancelled by those pointing opposite B_0. This would double the tissue magnetization. If you turn off the magnet (not recommended) or remove the patient from the bore of the magnet (a better idea), the tissue magnetization disappears (or almost so), as there is not a magnetic field (other than the earth's magnetic field) to cause magnetic dipoles to align and create a net magnetization in tissue.

Magnetic Fields

To put the magnetic fields of modern MRI scanners in perspective, the earth's magnetic field is about ½ gauss at the earth's surface, and 1 gauss is 1/10,000th Tesla (T) (10,000 gauss = 1 T). A 1.5 T scanner has a magnetic field strength about

30,000 times stronger than the earth's magnetic field, and, therefore, the tissue magnetization in the human body is about 30,000 times greater in a 1.5 T scanner than outside the scanner on the surface of the earth. Physicists have tried taking images of the human body using only the earth's magnetic field as the uniform magnetic field source, with limited success, due to the much weaker signal available. Since tissue magnetization and, consequently, measurable MR signal, is linearly proportional to the magnetic field strength, there has been a push to stronger and stronger magnets to improve the signal, and signal-to-noise ratio (SNR), in MRI. This is the driving force behind the effort to build MRI units with magnetic field strengths of 3.0 T, 4.0 T, and beyond.

Precession and Magnetic Resonance

The challenge in MRI is to measure tissue magnetization in the presence of the strong magnetic field that was applied to create tissue magnetization in the first place. It is like trying to find a needle in a haystack. The trick used in NMR and MRI to measure tissue magnetization is twofold: (1) to rotate the tissue magnetization out of the direction of the static magnetic field (called the longitudinal direction) and into the plane perpendicular to B_0 (called the transverse plane), where it can be more easily measured (see Figure 1.6B), and (2) to take advantage of the fact that once rotated out of the direction of B_0, the magnetization precesses about an axis parallel to B_0. The typical macroscopic example of precession is the motion of a spinning top when not precisely upright. The top's axis of spin sweeps out a circle, keeping a fixed angle relative to the vertical. Tissue magnetization behaves similarly when rotated out of the direction of B_0. The magnetization precesses about B_0 with a fixed precessional frequency (Figure 1.6C). This precessional frequency is given by the Larmor equation, Eq (1.5) or Eq. (1.6) above.

Thus, in a 1.5 T scanner, hydrogen precesses at a fixed frequency of 63.9 MHz. This fixed precessional frequency means that the tissue magnetization, once rotated into the transverse plane, is frequency-encoded at this specific frequency, making it far easier to measure. As we shall see later, by modifying the magnetic field as a function of location along a particular axis (ie, applying a magnetic field gradient), we can modify the precessional frequency as a function of position to help localize the source of MR signal.

Tissue Excitation

So how is tissue magnetization pointing along the static magnetic field B_0 rotated (or tipped) into the transverse plane? By applying a radiofrequency (RF) pulse that precisely matches the Larmor frequency of the nuclei of interest. To excite hydrogen nuclei in tissue in a 1.5 T scanner, a radiofrequency wave oscillating at 63.9 MHz is applied. This radiofrequency corresponds to a photon energy that exactly equals the energy needed to cause the hydrogen dipole to flip from pointing along B_0 (up) to pointing opposite B_0 (down). This is the trick that I.I. Rabi used to measure precisely the magnetic dipole moments of nuclei. As in Rabi's experiments, the RF transmitters in MR scanners are tuned very precisely in frequency, with a narrow range of frequencies of about 100 Hertz (Hz) around the center frequency. Hence, the RF pulse is said to have a "narrow bandwidth", a narrow range of frequencies. In MR scanners the applied RF pulse cannot be physically limited to just a single voxel, or to just a small region of the body; it is applied to all tissues in the center of the magnet. For breast or body imaging, RF pulses are usually applied using large RF transmitter coils that are located just inside the large bore of the magnet. In some other parts of the anatomy, such as the head, the head coil itself is used as both the RF transmitter and receiver coil.

In addition to needing to get the frequency of the RF pulse just right, the strength and duration of the RF pulse determine how much tipping of tissue magnetization occurs (the "flip angle"). The longitudinal magnetization can be flipped by any desired angle by adjusting both the strength and duration of the applied RF pulse. In most MR scanners, the duration is fixed and the strength of the RF pulse is varied to flip tissue magnetization from a few degrees relative to B_0 up to $180°$ from the longitudinal direction. The maximum signal is measured when the longitudinal magnetization is tipped fully into the transverse plane: a flip angle of exactly $90°$. Once tissue magnetization is tipped into the transverse plane so that it can be measured, the RF transmit pulse is turned off so that signal measurement can begin without interference from the much stronger transmitted RF pulse, which is at the same Larmor frequency.

Measuring the Magnetic Resonance Signal

Once tipped into the transverse plane, the tissue magnetization from the imbalance of magnetic dipoles precesses about B_0. In a reasonably short amount of time (on the order of tenths of seconds), the transverse magnetization decays away. The mechanisms of decay will be discussed in Chapter 2. Hence, in the first tenth of a second or so, while there is still a reasonable amount of signal precessing in the transverse plane, the signal must be measured.

Measuring precessing transverse magnetization is done by making use of one of the basic principles of electromagnetism: Faraday's law of induction. Faraday's law of induction states that a changing magnetic field (or changing magnetic flux) induces an electrical current in a nearby loop of wire. In the case of precessing transverse magnetization, the magnetic field is created by the collective effect of hydrogen nuclear magnetic dipoles; the change in magnetic flux linking a loop of wire is due to those dipoles precessing in phase nearby (Figure 1.6C). Faraday's law describes the changing electrical current in a loop of wire (in this case, the RF receiver coil) placed near a changing magnetic field (here, the precessing magnetic dipoles in the body). Since the dipoles are precessing at 63.9 MHz in a 1.5 T scanner, the current induced in the radiofrequency receiver coil is an alternating current with a frequency of 63.9 MHz, a radio frequency just below the FM radio band. This "frequency-encoding" makes the MR signal more easily measurable.

In breast imaging, the RF receiver coil is a specialized breast coil. In the early days of breast imaging, most RF receiver coils were unilateral, but today most are bilateral. Most modern breast coils have far more elaborate designs than single loops of wire. They are, however, precisely tuned to generate peak electrical signal (i.e., to resonate) at the RF frequency of hydrogen at the particular field strength of the scanner. Thus, it is not possible to take the same breast coil designed for a 1.5 T scanner and use it on a 3.0 T scanner.

As we will discuss and illustrate in Chapter 7, breast coils are designed to receive signal from the breasts, axilla, and chest wall, but not from the entire upper torso. This is because the larger the sensitive volume of the receiver coil, the more unwanted noise is measured, interfering with the signal from the breasts that you would like to measure. Thus, body coils are almost never used for breast imaging, because the noise measured in the larger sensitive volume of the body coil would be excessive compared to the noise measured in a more limited volume breast coil.

The Basic Nuclear Magnetic Resonance Experiment

We can summarize what we have covered so far by demonstrating the basic nuclear magnetic resonance (NMR) experiment, illustrated in Figure 1.6. NMR is distinct from MRI in that it does not require localizing the source of signal. A tissue sample is placed in the sensitive volume of the NMR system, and signal is received from the entire sample. When outside the magnet, tissue magnetization is zero, since magnetic dipole moments of hydrogen nuclei in tissue are randomly oriented. When placed in the strong magnetic field of the NMR system, tissue magnetization points along B_0 but is not easily measured when along B_0. To measure tissue magnetization, an RF pulse at just the right frequency to excite hydrogen nuclei, the Larmor frequency, is applied with just the right strength and duration to flip tissue magnetization into the transverse plane, where it can be measured. Then, the RF pulse is turned off and the electronic "listening" begins by measuring the frequency-encoded signal coming from a radio wave receiver coil placed near the tissue of interest. The receiver coil's signal is proportional to the strength of signal coming collectively from the hydrogen nuclei precessing in the tissue sample.

In contrast, MRI measures the signal from excited tissues but goes on to localize the MR signal from each voxel in a tissue sample. Chapter 3 will take us from NMR to MRI. There we discuss how signal is measured in each voxel in the human body.

Chapter Take-home Points

- Atomic nuclei with either an odd number of protons or an odd number of neutrons have nuclear magnetic dipole moments.

- The signal in MRI results from the magnetic dipole moments of hydrogen nuclei.
- A strong magnetic field is needed to align hydrogen nuclear magnetic dipole moments preferentially along the magnetic field, the longitudinal direction.
- The precessional or Larmor frequency is determined by the magnetic field strength and the nucleus of interest.
- Radio-frequency electromagnetic waves applied at the Larmor frequency are used to flip the collective magnetization of tissue into the transverse plane where it can be measured.
- The precession of magnetic dipole moments around the direction of the magnetic field at the Larmor frequency causes tissue magnetization to induce an alternating electric current in a nearby receiver coil, enabling signal measurement.

References

1. Haacke EM, Brown RW, Thompson MR, et.al. Magnetic Resonance Imaging: Physical Principles and Sequence Design. New York: John Wiley & Sons, 1999.
2. Hendrick RE. Physics and technical aspects of breast MRI. In "Categorical Course in Diagnostic Radiology Physics: Advances in Breast Imaging–Physics, Technology, and Clinical Applications." Oak Brook, IL: RSNA Publications, 2004, p. 259–278.
3. Stark DD, Bradley WG, eds. Magnetic Resonance Imaging, 3rd Edition. New York: C.V. Mosby Publishing Co, 1999, especially Ch 1–14.
4. Markisz JA, Aquilia MG. Technical magnetic resonance imaging. Stamford, CT: Appleton & Lange, 1999.
5. Morris EA, Liberman L. Breast MRI: Diagnosis and Intervention. New York: Springer, 2005.
6. Warren R, Coulthard A, eds. Breast MRI in practice. London: Martin Dunitz, 2002.
7. Fischer U. Practical MR Mammography. Stuttgart: Thieme Publishing Co, 2004.
8. Heywang-Kobrunner SH, Dershaw DD, Schreer I. Diagnostic Breast Imaging. Stuttgart, New York: Thieme Publishing Co., 2001.
9. Morris EA. Breast cancer imaging with MRI. Radiol Clin North Am 2002; 40: 443–466.
10. Orel SG, Schnall MD. MR imaging of the breast for the detection, diagnosis, and staging of breast cancer. Radiology 2001; 220: 13–30
11. Schnall MD. Breast imaging technology: Application of magnetic resonance imaging to early detection of breast cancer. Breast Cancer Res. 2001, **3:** 17–21
12. Weinreb JC, Newstead G. MR imaging of the breast. Radiology 1995; 196: 593–610.
13. Kuhl CF, ed. Breast MR imaging. Magnetic Resonance Imaging Clinics. London: Elsivier Saunders, 2006; 14: 293–430.
14. Hendrick RE, Osborn A, Kanal E. Basic MRI physics. In Kressel H, Modic M, Murphy W. Syllabus: Special Course - MR 1990. Chicago: RSNA Publications, 1990, p. 7–30.
15. Rabi, I. I., Zacharias, J. R., Millman, S. and Kusch, P. A new method of measuring nuclear magnetic moment. Physical Review 1938; 53, 318–323.
16. Purcell EM, Torrey HC, Pound RV. Resonance absorption by nuclear magnetic moments in a solid. Phys. Rev. 1946; **69**, 37–38.
17. Bloch F, Hansen WW, Packard M. Nuclear induction. Phys. Rev. 1946; 69, 127.

Chapter 2
Tissue Relaxation

Nuclear Magnetic Resonance

At this point, we have referred to MR in two different ways: nuclear magnetic resonance (NMR) and magnetic resonance imaging (MRI). NMR is the analytical technique of exciting and obtaining MR signal from an entire sample, breaking the measured signal into its individual frequency components to identify different molecules containing the nucleus of interest, but not separating the signal by location within the sample. In contrast, MRI is the technique of separating a sample or region of tissue into individual volume elements (voxels) and producing images based on the total signal from the nucleus of interest in each voxel. The techniques of dividing tissue into voxels to produce MR images will be discussed in Chapter 3. This chapter describes tissue relaxation times that provide the contrast seen in MR images. Relaxation times are strictly MR-based parameters that describe the re-growth of longitudinal magnetization (T1) and loss of transverse magnetization (T2) after a radiofrequency (RF) pulse flips magnetization out of alignment with the externally applied static magnetic field, B_0.

In 1952, Bloch and Purcell were awarded the Nobel Prize in physics for independently demonstrating that NMR could be performed on liquids and solids.[1,2] Based on their work, equipment to perform quantitative NMR was developed and refined. An NMR spectrometer consists of a strong magnet, a radiofrequency (RF) transmitter coil tuned to the resonant frequency of the nucleus of interest, and a RF receiver coil tuned to the same frequency. NMR spectrometers are not designed to separate the sample into individual voxels but simply to measure the collective signal from a single sample. NMR systems require a highly homogeneous magnetic field over the entire sample so that all nuclei of a particular type in the sample have the same resonant frequency except for inherent small differences in resonant frequencies caused by slightly different nuclear shielding occurring due to different molecular structure.

For example, hydrogen nuclei in water resonate at a Larmor frequency that is higher by 3.4 parts per million (ppm) than hydrogen nuclei in fat. This is due to the slightly different molecular environment of the hydrogen nuclei in H_2O compared to that in CH_2. At 1.5 T, 3.4 ppm amounts to a frequency shift of 214 Hz in resonant

R.E. Hendrick (ed.), *Breast MRI: Fundamentals and Technical Aspects.*
© Springer 2008

frequency. This is quite small compared to the differences in resonant frequency of different nuclei, shown in Table 1.2, which are MHz or tens of MHz. The nucleus with resonant frequency closest to that of hydrogen is fluorine-19, which has a gyromagnetic ratio of 40.4 MHz/T. At 1.5 T, F-19 resonates at a frequency of 60.6 Megahertz ($1.5\,T^*40.4\,MHz/T$) compared to a resonant frequency of 63.9 MHz for hydrogen, a difference of 3.3 MHz. The frequency shift between hydrogen in fat and hydrogen in water of 214 Hz is extremely small compared to the difference of 3,300,000 Hz between resonant frequencies of hydrogen and fluorine.

Most NMR spectrometers have small bore sizes that accommodate only small samples, because it is easier and less expensive to build a magnet with a uniform magnetic field over a small volume. Thus, typical spectrometer bore sizes are 10 cm or less. NMR spectrometers usually lack the magnetic gradients necessary to separate the sample into individual voxels.

In addition to using NMR as analytic tools to determine the chemical constituents of materials, by the early 1970s, researchers were beginning to measure NMR relaxation parameters of excised tissue samples. In so doing, they learned that tissue relaxation times differ between normal and diseased tissues. In 1971, Damadian demonstrated that the MR relaxation times, specifically the T1/T2 ratios of tissues, could be used to distinguish cancers from normal tissues.[3]

To a physicist, one of the remarkable aspects of MRI is that the signal coming from a hydrogen nucleus, which has a size of about 10^{-15} meters (m), is sensitive to macroscopic disease in tissue. Most nuclear phenomena tell us only about the nucleus itself or, occasionally, about atomic structure, but are shielded from differences in tissues that occur at the size scale of macromolecules within cells. The reason that the magnetic properties of hydrogen nuclei can tell us something about disease is that the relaxation times T1 and T2 of hydrogen nuclei depend on their macromolecular environments. Therefore, while the magnetic dipole moments of hydrogen nuclei are the probes, these probes are sensitive to differences in their macromolecular environments through their relaxation times. Thus, signals coming from hydrogen nuclei are affected by phenomena that occur on the much larger size scale, that of macromolecules within cells, which are of submicron to micron sizes (10^{-8} to 10^{-6} meters). Moreover, while the quantity of hydrogen within soft tissues might vary up to a few percent, T1 and T2 in different soft tissues can vary by up to 100%, making relaxation times more sensitive sources of contrast than hydrogen density alone.[4] This is one of the underlying reasons that MRI is exquisitely sensitive to disease.

The NMR experiment described at the end of Chapter 1 indicated that the maximum measurable MR signal occurs just after tissue magnetization is rotated into the transverse plane, perpendicular to B_0, by a 90° RF pulse. Two separate phenomena take place after a 90° pulse is applied. One phenomenon is the recovery of the longitudinal magnetization, described by the time constant T1 and called spin-lattice relaxation, T1 relaxation, or T1-recovery. The other phenomenon is the decay of transverse magnetization, the magnetization that is flipped into the transverse plane, which is described by the time constant T2 or T2* and is called spin-spin relaxation or T2-decay. We will describe each of these phenomena separately.

T1 Relaxation

T1-relaxation or T1-recovery describes the recovery of longitudinal magnetization along the direction of the static magnetic field, B_0, just after applying an RF pulse.[4] Recall that there are two energy states the hydrogen nucleus can occupy in the presence of an externally applied magnetic field: up, the lower energy state where the magnetic dipole moment points along B_0, or down, the higher energy state where the magnetic dipole points opposite B_0. Thinking of tissue magnetization as a collection of hydrogen dipoles, after a 90° RF pulse there is an equal population of hydrogen dipoles in the lower energy and higher energy states. T1-relaxation describes the recovery of longitudinal magnetization due to thermal interactions between excited, higher energy hydrogen nuclei (spins) and nearby, large macromolecules within the sample (the lattice). These interactions decrease the number of higher energy state (down-oriented) dipoles and increase the number of lower energy (up-oriented) hydrogen nuclear dipoles. As these energy transitions take place, the strength of tissue magnetization pointing along B_0 increases. Because T1 recovery involves interactions between spins and the larger surrounding lattice, it is sometimes referred to as "spin-lattice" relaxation.

This phenomenon of recovery of longitudinal magnetization is described by the relaxation time T1. The thermal interactions that cause T1-recovery occur primarily when tissues contain large macromolecules that have appropriate energy states to absorb the exact amount of energy to allow hydrogen nuclei to go from their excited, higher-energy state to their lower-energy state. The amount of energy released by the hydrogen nucleus equals the energy absorbed by the macromolecule.

As described in Chapter 1, the amount of energy released by the hydrogen dipole undergoing this transition from higher to lower energy states is determined by the magnetic field strength and by the nuclear type undergoing this transition, which in MRI is hydrogen. The required energy transfer is given by the Larmor equation (Eq (1.3) or Eq. (1.4)):

$$\Delta E = h\nu = h\omega_0 / (2\pi) = \mu_p B_0, \qquad (2.1)$$

where h is Planck's constant, ν is the frequency in units of cycles per second (1/s or s^{-1}), ω_0 is the Larmor frequency in units of radians per second, μ_p is the magnetic moment of the proton, and B_0 is the magnetic field strength in which the proton resides.

The rate at which this spin-lattice energy transfer takes place is one minus an exponential, reflecting the fact that the longitudinal magnetization starts out as zero just after a 90° pulse and recovers quickly at first, since there are a large number of higher energy dipoles. As time progresses and more dipoles flip to their lower energy state along B_0, recovery slows because there are fewer hydrogen dipoles available in the excited, higher energy state to make the energy transition (Figure 2.1). The equation that describes the strength of longitudinal magnetization, $M_z(t)$, at a time t after the application of a 90° pulse is:

$$M_z(t) = M_0 (1 - e^{-t/T1}), \qquad (2.2)$$

Figure 2.1 Illustration of the population change as T1-relaxation occurs in a voxel of tissue. Over time, fewer and fewer hydrogen dipoles are in the higher-energy state (down) and the number of energy transitions from higher to lower energy (up) states is fewer, slowing the rate of recovery of longitudinal magnetization. T1 is defined as the time after a 90° pulse needed for the longitudinal magnetization to recover to $(1-e^{-1})$ or 63% of M_0, the longitudinal magnetization achieved with infinite TR.

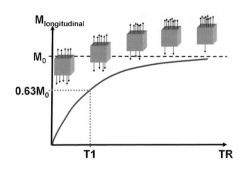

where M_0 is the maximum longitudinal magnetization occurring in the sample at that magnetic field strength and t is the time since the 90° pulse. T1 is defined as the time it takes after a 90° pulse for the longitudinal magnetization to recover to $M_0(1-e^{-1}) = M_0(1-(1/(2.713))) = 0.63M_0$; that is, to 63% of its maximum possible strength. Mathematically, it takes an infinite amount of time for the longitudinal magnetization to fully recover to M_0, the magnetization it had before the 90° pulse was applied. In practical terms, however, the longitudinal magnetization is 95% recovered along B_0 after a time interval equal to 3T1, 99% recovered after 5T1, and 99.9% recovered after 7T1.

Tissues with more macromolecules of the correct size to enable these thermal interactions have shorter T1 values, indicating that the energy exchange between hydrogen nuclei and macromolecules occurs more rapidly. Tissues with very dilute concentrations of macromolecules, such as cerebrospinal and cystic fluids, have long T1-values, on the order of several seconds, because energy transfer occurs more slowly. In the breast, T1 values are shortest for fat (about 250 ms at 1.5 T), intermediate for fibroglandular tissues (about 700 ms at 1.5 T), higher for most lesions, including cancers (800 ms to 1 second at 1.5 T), and highest for non-bloody cystic fluids (about 3 seconds at 1.5 T). The reason that T1 is higher for most breast lesions, including cancers, than for normal fibroglandular tissues is that lesions tend to have higher water concentrations, and therefore fewer macromolecules per unit volume, than normal breast tissues. The exceptions to this rule are lesions with high fat content, such as lipomas, or lesions with a high fibrous content, both of which have shorter T1 values than normal fibroglandular tissues.

The primary effect of administering gadolinium chelates, such as Gd-DTPA, is to shorten the T1 relaxation times of hydrogen nuclei.[5] Gd-chelates, like other macromolecules, act as energy sponges, absorbing the energy needed for the hydrogen nuclei to transition from their excited to unexcited states. Hence, when Gd-chelate molecules are present in adequate numbers, T1 is shortened. Since Gd-chelates are selectively taken up by lesions, especially cancerous lesions that have recruited more vessels and capillaries to support tumor growth, the T1 relaxation times of lesions are shortened from 800 to 1000 ms to 200 to 400 ms on the first pass of Gd-chelates, making the recovery of longitudinal magnetization faster in enhancing lesions than in all other breast tissues except fat. The fact that enhancing lesions have similar T1-values to fat is why enhancing lesions often are isointense with fat on non–fat-suppressed T1-weighted images.

T2 Relaxation

If the transverse magnetization is measured just after a 90° pulse, the measured signal oscillates at the Larmor frequency and decreases quickly over time, as shown in Figure 2.2. The main reason transverse magnetization is lost is that the magnetic dipoles of hydrogen nuclei begin to dephase because different hydrogen nuclei have subtly different magnetic field environments and therefore precess at slightly different rates (Figure 2.3). This difference in precessional frequencies means that the transverse magnetization decreases in magnitude over time. The dephasing of the measurable MR signal, the transverse magnetization, is described by T2 or T2*, depending on how the transverse signal is formed before being measured.

Without distinguishing between T2 and T2* yet, T2-type decay describes the exponential loss of transverse magnetization immediately after a 90° pulse. T2 is the parameter that describes how quickly the magnitude of the transverse magnetization decreases over time. The shorter T2, the more rapidly transverse magnetization decreases. The transverse magnetization, $M_{xy}(t)$, at a time t after a 90° RF pulse is described by the equation:

$$M_{xy}(t) = M_{xy} e^{-t/T2}, \tag{2.3}$$

where M_{xy} is the transverse magnetization immediately after a 90° pulse, at t=0. The magnitude of measured transverse magnetization is observed to have an exponential rate of decrease (Figure 2.3). The parameter T2 in the above equation is

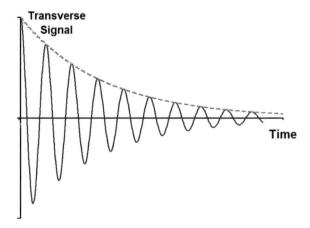

Figure 2.2 Measured transverse magnetization oscillates at the Larmor frequency and quickly decreases in magnitude due to T2 or T2* decay.

Figure 2.3 The dephasing of hydrogen dipoles flipped into the transverse plane over time and is responsible for T2 (or T2*) decay. T2 (or T2*) is defined as the time needed for the transverse magnetization to decrease to 1/e (or 37%) of the signal strength in the transverse plane just after a 90° pulse.

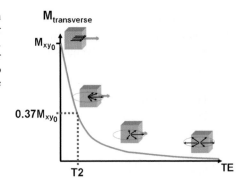

defined as the time it takes for the signal to decrease to 1/e or to 37% of the original signal strength it had just after the 90° pulse. Hence, tissues with shorter T2-values have a more rapid loss of transverse magnetization. In the breast, fat and normal fibroglandular tissues have the shortest T2 values (60 to 80 ms). Most breast lesions, including cancers, have slightly longer T2 values (80 to 100 ms), and cystic fluids have the longest T2-values (several hundred ms).

Mathematically, it takes an infinite amount of time for transverse magnetization to completely disappear, but after 3T2 the transverse magnetization is at 5%, and after 5T2 it is at 1% of its original strength.

For a given tissue, T2 is always shorter than T1 because the rate at which transverse magnetization decreases is faster than the rate at which longitudinal magnetization recovers along B_0. This is because T1-recovery is only one of several reasons that the measurable transverse signal decreases after a 90° pulse. If T1-recovery were the only reason for signal loss, then T2 would equal T1 and only one decay parameter would be needed in NMR or MRI. Because there are other, more dominant sources of transverse magnetization loss, the transverse signal decreases more rapidly than the longitudinal magnetization recovers. Hence, two separate NMR parameters are needed, T1 and T2, with T2 shorter than T1, usually by a factor of 5 to 10.

The dephasing of magnetic dipoles making up the tissue magnetization from a sample or voxel is similar to a grade-school ballet ensemble performing Swan Lake. The dipoles (dancers) start out pointing in the same direction as they precess (turn) in unison, but as more rotations take place, they start pointing in different directions due to their slightly different rates of precession (turning). In Swan Lake, the ensemble turns once every few seconds, but it takes only a few turns for inexperienced dancers to point in different directions. In hydrogen nuclei at 1.5 T, magnetic dipoles precess 64,000 times every millisecond, so it takes only subtly different magnetic field environments for the dipoles to point in slightly different directions after a few milliseconds. This dephasing decreases the measurable amount of transverse magnetization and is responsible for T2-decay.

In T2-decay, one hydrogen dipole (a "spin") creates a non-uniform magnetic environment for other hydrogen dipoles (other "spins") nearby. Therefore, these subtle magnetic interactions that are the main cause of T2-decay are called "spin-spin" interactions. This type of dephasing is referred to as "true T2 dephasing," because it results from the inherent molecular environment, which changes rapidly in time, and cannot be reversed by gradient or RF pulse manipulations. These true T2 dephasing effects are excellent indicators of disease. It is these dephasing effects that MRI depends on to distinguish one tissue from another in T2-weighted imaging.

The role that macromolecules play in T2 relaxation is different than the role they play in T1-recovery. In pure water, where there are few or no macromolecules, there are plenty of hydrogen dipoles to affect the magnetic environments of other hydrogen dipoles, but the rate at which water molecules are moving is so rapid that each hydrogen dipole "sees" or experiences a relatively uniform magnetic environment. Thus, T2 is relatively long in pure water. As more macromolecules are added to water, the rate of motion of water molecules is slowed. This slowing means that the average amount of time that a hydrogen nucleus spends in contact with other molecules is longer. This increases the non-uniformity in the magnetic environment experienced by each hydrogen dipole, making dephasing occur more rapidly and thus making T2 shorter.

This effect is responsible for the subtly different magnetic environments of hydrogen nuclear dipoles and the resulting T2 differences between normal and diseased tissues. Diseased tissues typically are more edematous than normal tissues and therefore have lower concentrations of macromolecules. Therefore, T2 in diseased tissues is typically longer because hydrogen nuclei move more rapidly and the magnetic environment seen by each hydrogen nucleus is more uniform.

Gadolinium-based paramagnetic contrast agents shorten T2 as well as T1, since adding Gd-chelates has a similar effect to adding macromolecules to tissues. The primary reason that T1-weighted imaging, rather than T2-weighted imaging, is used with Gd-based contrast agents is that T1 is much longer than T2 in unenhanced tissues; as a result, the fractional change in T1 due to contrast agent uptake is greater than the fractional change in T2.[5] Thus, T1-weighted imaging shows a bigger effect of the contrast agent than T2-weighted imaging. In addition, we will see later that T1-weighted imaging can be done more rapidly than T2-weighted imaging. Finally, we will also see later that Gd-chelates act as a positive contrast agent on T1, making lesions that take up Gd-chelates brighter, but act as a negative contrast agent on T2. The convention in MRI is that higher signal is depicted as brighter in the MR image. Gd-chelates shorten T1 and T2. Shortening T1 causes signal to be higher on T1-weighted images, making lesions taking up gadolinium to be brighter. Shortening T2 causes signal to be lower on T2-weighted images, making lesions that take up gadolinium darker. There is a viewer preference for searching for bright enhancing areas rather than darker, suppressed areas on a heterogeneous background such as the breast, so positive contrast is preferred.

Distinguishing T2 and T2*

There is another cause of transverse magnetization dephasing beyond true T2-effects: namely, non-uniform magnetic fields across the sample or voxel of tissue.[6] These magnetic field inhmogeneities are usually caused by external factors and thus are not useful indicators of disease. Magnetic field inhomogeneities may be due to a non-uniform primary magnetic field (B_0), intentional applications of magnetic gradients that are needed to resolve the sample into voxels, and magnetic non-uniformities due to the presence of metallic objects or differences in magnetic susceptibility (the ability of tissues to maintain a magnetic field) in the tissue itself. T2* includes all of these causes of transverse magnetization dephasing. T2* is the dephasing parameter that applies to "free-induction decay," the decay occurring when the transverse magnetization is measured just after a 90° pulse, without any attempt to "rephase" it, as shown in Figure 2.2. Thus, the simple NMR experiment described at the end of Chapter 1 is a free-induction decay experiment, and $T2^*$ governs the decay of the magnitude of measured transverse magnetization in that experiment according to Equation 2.3, with $T2^*$ replacing T2. $T2^*$ is shorter than T2 because it includes magnetic field inhomogeneities as a way to decrease transverse magnetization:

$$1/T2^* = 1/T2 + \gamma \pi \Delta B_0 \qquad (2.4)$$

where γ is the gyromagnetic ratio and ΔB_0 is the magnetic field inhomogeneity across a voxel, including all possible causes. In Eq. 2.4, since $1/T2^*$ is made larger by the additional term due to magnetic field inhomogeneities (ΔB_0), $T2^*$ is smaller than T2. In extremely homogeneous magnetic fields, $T2^*$ values are approximately equal to T2 values. In voxels with magnetic inhomogeneities due to either non-uniform magnetic fields or magnetic susceptibility inhomogeneities, $T2^*$ will be shorter than T2. Even being in a different location in the MR scanner, away from isocenter, can lower $T2^*$, but not T2. Figure 2.4 illustrates the difference between T2 and $T2^*$ decay.

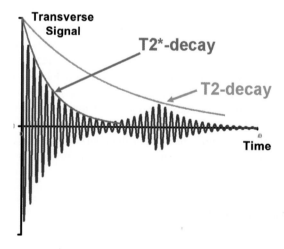

Figure 2.4 Illustration of the difference between $T2^*$ and T2. T2 describes the decay between initial transverse magnetization and the peak magnetization formed by a spin-echo. $T2^*$ describes the decay due to true T2 relaxation plus magnetic field non-uniformities across the sample or voxel.

T2 describes the dephasing of transverse magnetization when a spin-echo is formed. A spin-echo is formed by applying a 180° RF pulse halfway between the 90° pulse and peak signal measurement (Figure 2.5). Prior to the 90° pulse, some dipoles precess faster than others due to both irreversible effects (true T2 decay) and reversible effects (such as non-uniform magnetic fields across the sample or voxel). The effect of the 180° pulse is to exchange the orientation of the faster precessing hydrogen dipoles with that of slower precessing hydrogen dipoles. The 180° pulse flips the faster precessing dipoles into the position of slower precessing dipoles, and vice versa (Figure 2.6). The beauty of a spin-echo is that it eliminates almost all sources of T2 dephasing other than true T2 effects; that is, spin-echo pulse sequences eliminate reversible dephasing effects, such as static magnetic field non-uniformities, gradient non-uniformities, and magnetic susceptibility effects. Hence T2 is greater than T2*, as shown in Figure 2.4. Thus, T2-weighted spin-echo imaging is more robust than free-induction decay in that it yields the greatest measured signal for a given delay time. T2-weighted spin-echo imaging is also more useful diagnostically because it focuses on true T2-decay effects that reflect inherent tissue differences rather than including system effects such as magnetic field, gradient, or magnetic susceptibility differences.

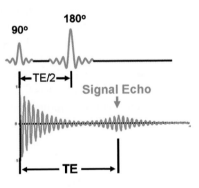

Figure 2.5 Formation of a spin-echo by applying a 180° pulse halfway between the 90° pulse and signal measurement. The 90° pulse flips longitudinal magnetization into the transverse plane, where it can be measured. The application of a 180° pulse forms the signal echo and eliminates the dephasing effects of magnetic field uniformities.

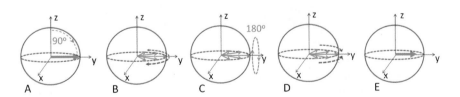

Figure 2.6 (A) After a 90° pulse, hydrogen magnetic dipoles are precessing in-phase. These diagrams are in the "rotating frame" where dipoles precessing at exactly the Larmor frequency are pointing along the y-axis. (B) After a short time, faster precessing dipoles have advanced in phase relative to more slowly precessing dipoles. (C) A 180° pulse is applied to the sample. This causes the magnetization vectors of faster precessing dipoles to be rotated to the orientation of slower dipoles, and vice versa. (D) Over the next brief interval, reversible effects are rephrased. (E) An equal time after the 180° pulse, maximum signal is rephrased in the transverse plane.

The Physical Basis of Relaxation Times

This section summarizes the effects of tissue properties on T1 and T2 relaxation times. Pure water, CSF, or clear cystic fluids have the longest T1 and T2 values. T1 values in these fluids are long (a few seconds) because there are few macromolecules to absorb energy from excited hydrogen magnetic dipoles and allow them to transition to lower energy states (Figure 2.7A). T2 in these fluids are long, but not as long as T1, because the rapidly moving water molecules create a relatively uniform magnetic environment for all hydrogen nuclei, so there is slow dephasing of hydrogen magnetic dipoles after a 90° RF pulse.

Normal fibroglandular tissues have shorter T1 and T2 values than water or cystic fluid. T1 is shorter among normal breast tissues because there are sufficient numbers of macromolecules to absorb the energy of excited hydrogen nuclei and permit them to transition to the lower energy states (Figure 2.7B). T2 is shorter in fibroglandular tissues than in pure water, CSF, or cystic fluid because the higher concentration of macromolecules in normal breast tissue slows the motion of water molecules, causing them to experience greater magnetic field non-uniformities and therefore dephase more rapidly.

Breast cancers have T1 and T2 values somewhat higher than those of normal fibroglandular tissues because they are typically edematous, with lower concentrations of macromolecules than fibroglandular tissues (Figure 2.7C). Therefore, their T1 and T2 values are slightly longer than those of fibroglandular tissues but not nearly as long as CSF or cystic fluids.

Water molecules locked in a crystalline or lattice structure (Figure 2.7D) tend to have longer T1 values because the exchange of energy between hydrogen nuclei and macromolecules is limited, but shorter T2 values than in A-C because of the large magnetic field inhomogeneities maintained by the lattice structure.

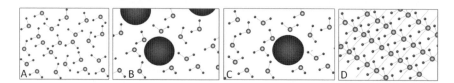

Figure 2.7 (A) Distilled water consisting of randomly organized water molecules. A moving picture would show individual water molecules moving so rapidly that each hydrogen dipole would see a uniform magnetic field environment, causing T1 and T2 to be very long. (B) Water with macromolecules typical of a normal cell. The macromolecules slow down water molecules in their vicinity, undergoing thermal collisions to take up energy from excited hydrogen dipoles, shortening T1, and providing magnetic field non-uniformities, which shortens T2. (C) Dilute macromolecules, typical of a cancer or benign lesion. Here, T1 and T2 are shortened by the mechanisms described in (B), but to a lesser extent due to the lower concentration of macromolecules. (D) In a solid or semi-solid lattice, water molecules are locked more rigidly in place within the lattice, making T1 longer due to fewer possible energy transfers from spins to the lattice, but T2 very short due to magnetic inhomogeneities caused by the lattice.

Fat has the shortest T1 values in the breast because of the presence of a sufficient number of macromolecules to enable the rapid transition of hydrogen nuclei in CH_2 from the excited higher energy state to the lower energy state. T2 values of hydrogen in fat are similar to, or slightly longer than, those in fibroglandular tissues primarily because the motion of hydrogen in CH_2 is similar to the motion of hydrogen in H_2O in fibroglandular tissues, so T2 dephasing effects are similar.

The rule that cysts have longer T1 and T2 values is broken by bloody cysts. Blood, like Gd-chelates, is a paramagnetic agent, due to unpaired electrons in iron ions in hemoglobin. As a result, blood-filled cysts have shorter T1 and T2 values than normal cystic fluid and can even have shorter T1 and T2 values than normal breast tissues, making blood-filled cysts appear brighter than fibroglandular tissues on T1-weighted images and darker than fibroglandular tissues on T2-weighted images.

These basic concepts are responsible for the contrast observed in MRI of the breast. To understand how T1 and T2 contribute to image contrast, we need to describe how MR pulse sequences manifest T1 and T2 contrast, which is described in detail in Chapter 4 and beyond.

Chapter Take-home Points

- Longitudinal and transverse relaxation times are determined largely by the macromolecular environment of hydrogen nuclei.
- The more macromolecules of the correct size, the shorter T1.
- The more slowly water molecules move and the longer they spend in the vicinity of larger molecules, the shorter T2 and $T2^*$.
- Diseased tissues tend to have longer T1 and T2 values, and higher spin-densities, than normal tissues.
- The uptake of Gd-chelates in tissues causes T1, and to a lesser extent T2, to shorten dramatically; this makes lesions with Gd-chelate uptake bright on T1-weighted sequences because tissues with shorter T1 values have higher signal.

References

1. Bloch F, Hansen WW. Packard ME. Nuclear induction. *Phys Rev*. 1946; 69: 127–129.
2. Purcell EM, Torrey HC, Pound RV. Resonance absorption by nuclear magnetic moments in a solid. *Phys Rev*. 1946; 69: 37–38.
3. Damadian R. Tumor detection by nuclear magnetic resonance. Science 1971; 171: 1151–1153.
4. Gore JC, Kennan RP. Physical and physiological basis of magnetic relaxation. In Stark DD, Bradley WG, eds. Magnetic Resonance Imaging, 3rd Edition. New York: C.V. Mosby Publishing Co, 1999; Vol 1, pp 33–42.
5. Hendrick RE, Haacke EM. Basic physics of MR contrast agents and maximization of image contrast. J. Magn. Reson. Imaging 1993; 3: 137–148.
6. Padhani AR. Contrast agent dynamics in breast MRI. In Warren R, Coulthard A, eds. Breast MRI in practice. London: Martin Dunitz, 2002. p. 43–52.

Chapter 3
Spatial Resolution in Magnetic Resonance Imaging

In 1973, Dr. Paul C. Lauterbur published his seminal article on using magnetic field gradients to resolve the sources of nuclear magnetic resonance (NMR) signals into pixels or voxels.[1] Most physicists at the time believed this to be impossible, due to the general principle that spatial resolution is limited by the wavelength of the electromagnetic radiation used as a probe. At a magnetic field strength of 1 Tesla, the wavelength of electromagnetic radiation that excites hydrogen nuclei is 7 meters (3×10^8 meters/second/(42.6×10^6 1/seconds) = 7.04 meters), which would make studying details in the human body impossible. Lauterbur correctly recognized and demonstrated that this limitation, while applying to scattering experiments, was cleverly overcome by using magnetic field gradients to localize signals in NMR. He called his new technique "zeugmatography". Until the early 1980s, most researchers favored the name "NMR imaging". The "nuclear" in NMR imaging was dropped when whole-body scanners became clinically available in the early 1980s. This was done to avoid adverse reactions from the public about potential association with "nuclear" imaging and its associated radiation effects. Paul Lauterbur shared the 2003 Nobel Prize in medicine for his invention of MRI.

MRI describes the process of exciting and measuring MR signals while dividing the tissue sample into individual voxels. MRI systems require several basic elements to accomplish this: a magnet that produces a strong, uniform magnetic field, radiofrequency (RF) transmitter coils, RF receiver coils, and magnetic gradients.[1-3] Each of these components is described briefly in this section.

Basic Components of a Magnetic Resonance Imaging System

Magnets

Strong magnetic fields suitable for whole-body scanning are producing using a superconducting solenoidal magnet.[3] The main magnetic field produced by this magnet, B_0, is responsible for inducing a measurable magnetization in tissue. Permanent and resistive magnets can produce magnetic fields up to 0.4 Tesla, but those are typically inadequate for good breast imaging. Only superconducting solenoidal magnets can produce magnet fields above 0.5 Tesla, so we restrict our discussion to that magnet design. These magnets consist of a series of 4 to 8 solenoidal rings, each carrying a large amount of current to produce a large magnetic field within the ring. A single current-carrying circular ring produces a magnetic field that is perpendicular to the plane of the ring and completely uniform within the plane of the ring itself (Figure 3.1). Away from the plane of the ring, however, the magnetic field is not uniform. By using several different rings in a solenoidal design, as shown in Figure 3.2, the magnetic field can be made approximately uniform in all three dimensions (x and y in the plane of the ring, and z perpendicular to the plane of each ring) over a reasonable volume. To accommodate the entire human body, magnets need a minimum bore size of 50 to 60 cm, which means that the solenoidal rings must have a diameter greater than 50 to 60 cm. Solenoidal magnets are designed so that the most homogeneous region is in the very center of the magnet, the isocenter (the spheroid in Figure 3.2). To do body and breast imaging, the magnetic field must be uniform over a volume surrounding the isocenter that is 30 to 40 cm in diameter.

The main magnetic fields are produced by superconducting coils. These coils are made of large copper rings into which are imbedded loops of niobium-titanium, a soft metal that carries current without electrical resistance when cooled to temperatures below 15° K above absolute zero (0°K). At normal atmospheric pressure, helium is a liquid below 4.2°K and a gas above 4.2°K. Thus, as long as the composite solenoidal coils are bathed in liquid helium, the niobium-titanium strands are superconducting, carrying current without electrical resistance and without the resulting heat produced when electric current flows through a resistive circuit. Only when the temperature rises above 15°K would electrical current flow through the copper coil and then it would do so with resistance. Below the boiling point of helium, currents in MR magnets can be maintained for years without recharging. Superconducting, solenoidal magnets can produce magnetic field strengths up to

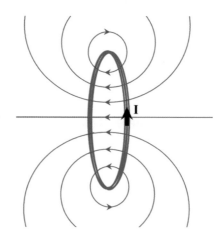

Figure 3.1 The magnetic field produced by a single, current-carrying loop. Lines of constant magnetic field are shown in blue. Note that the magnetic field is uniform in the plane of the loop, but not on either side of that plane.

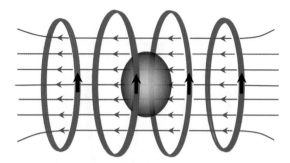

Figure 3.2 To produce a magnetic field uniform over a volume, a number of current-carrying loops are lined up to form a solenoidal arrangement. The three-dimensional region of highest homogeneity is at the center of the loop configuration, shown by the spheroid at the center of the magnet.

10 T; MRI systems approved for clinical use by the U.S. Food and Drug Administration (FDA) have magnetic field strengths up to 3.0 T.

In addition to the main magnets, additional coils placed in MR scanners help shim the magnet; that is, they make the magnetic field in a volume around the isocenter as uniform as possible. Minor adjustments in electrical currents in these shim coils make minor adjustments in the magnetic field strength at the center of the magnet to compensate for slight non-uniformities in the main magnetic field and to correct for magnetic field non-uniformities caused by construction and objects outside the magnet. Magnetic field shimming is done by the service engineer at installation and at preventive maintenance. Some MR systems also permit shimming on a patient-by-patient basis by the technologist to correct for non-uniformities due to the patient and the specialized receiver coils that are placed in the bore of the magnet. Separate circuits control the shim coils, and re-shimming the magnet by adjusting the current flowing in those coils can increase magnetic field uniformity across the sensitive volume of the anatomical region being imaged.

With good shimming, the typical 1.5 Tesla magnet will be uniform to within 1 part per million (ppm) over a 30 to 40 cm volume at the isocenter of the MR scanner. This means that the magnetic field everywhere in that volume of 30 to 40 cm diameter will be within 1.5±0.00000075 T, a total difference of 0.0000015 T over the volume. A magnetic field homogeneity of 1 ppm is adequate to distinguish between hydrogen in water and hydrogen in fat, a difference of 3.4 ppm, across the entire volume. This high degree of uniformity enables chemically selective fat suppression because the frequency shift across the sensitive volume of the scanner, caused by non-uniform magnetic fields, is considerably less than the frequency shift between hydrogen in water and hydrogen in fat.

Radiofrequency Transmitter Coils

RF transmitter coils are used to excite nuclei; that is, to flip the magnetization in tissue away from the direction of B_0 so that it can be measured. As described in Chapter 1, RF transmitter coils must be capable of transmitting at the Larmor

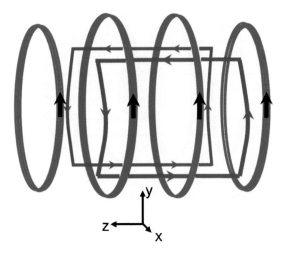

Figure 3.3 Radio-frequency (RF) transmitter coils (blue) are typically located just inside the main magnet coils to produce uniform RF pulses over the central volume of the MR system.

frequency of hydrogen in the magnet (63.9 MHz at 1.5 T) and must be precisely controlled in terms of duration and amplitude to produce the desired flip angle. RF transmitter coils are typically large coils built into the bore of the magnet inside the superconducting coil rings (Figure 3.3). Just as it is important to have a uniform main magnetic field, it is important to have uniform transmitted RF fields so that the RF signal strength and the resulting flip angle will be similar across the entire excited volume of tissue. Larger transmitter coils generally produce more uniform RF fields and therefore more uniform flip angles.

Radiofrequency Receiver Coils

RF receiver coils measure the signal emitted from excited tissue. RF receiver coils must be tuned to receive maximum signal at the Larmor frequency; that is, the coils and their associated electronics are built to "resonate" at the Larmor frequency, which depends on the scanner's magnetic field strength. Thus, a RF receiver coil suitable for imaging hydrogen at 1.5 T must be tuned to resonate at 63.9 MHz. Receiver coils tuned for imaging at 1.5 T are not suitable for imaging at any other magnetic field strength, nor are they suitable for obtaining spectroscopy signals at 1.5 T from nuclei other than hydrogen. For breast and many other applications, such as head, spine, and extremities, RF receiver coils are of limited volume so that they receive signal only from tissues of interest (Figure 3.4). This is because increasing the sensitive volume of the receiver coil increases the noise measured by the receiver coil, assuming some additional tissue is present in the larger sensitive volume. On the other hand, increasing the volume of the receiver coil does nothing to improve signal strength, since the signal comes only from the restricted slice or volume targeted by the pulse sequence. Thus, receiver coils that are best in terms of maximizing signal-to-noise ratio (SNR) are those that just fit the anatomy of interest, without including additional tissue. For the breast, an ideal receiver coil would be a set of loops just large enough to accommodate both breasts, the axilla and chest wall. Since patients and their breast sizes vary markedly, ideally sites would have a series of properly tuned coils of varying sizes that just fit each breast size or a coil with a sensitive volume that would adjust to the size of each patient. Most breast coils are single-sized and tend to accommodate larger breasts, at the expense of decreased SNR for smaller breasts. To ensure that they include all breast tissue, larger breast coils also include signal from tissues outside the breast including the chest and heart. The more unwanted tissue included, the worse the SNR for breast tissues. In Chapter 13, a new commercially-available coil design that adjusts to each patient is described.

Magnetic Gradients

Magnetic gradients are sets of current-carrying coils that produce magnetic fields that change their strength linearly as a function of position and can be switched rapidly on and off. MRI systems have three separate gradient systems. Each gradient produces a magnetic field that points in the same direction as the main magnetic field, B_o, (along the z-axis) but varies its magnetic field strength linearly with one of the three spatial dimensions: x, y, or z (Figure 3.5).

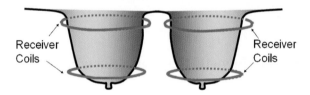

Figure 3.4   Schematic of a simple bilateral breast coil consisting of two parallel loops surrounding each breast.

Figure 3.5   Magnetic field gradients in the x-, y-, and z-directions. All produce magnetic field vectors that point along the main magnetic field, B_o, which points along the z-axis. The x-gradient produces a magnetic field that varies linearly along the x-axis, the y-gradient produces a magnetic field that varies linearly along the y-direction, and the z-gradient produces a magnetic field that varies linearly along the z-direction.

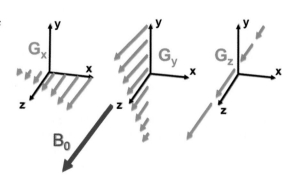

To form images, magnetic gradients must be switched on and off rapidly. The time it takes for the gradient to reach its maximum strength is called the gradient rise-time. A major improvement in MR systems in recent years has been the production of magnetic gradients with higher maximum gradient strengths (up to 30–50 milliTesla per meter, mT/m) and shorter rise times (down to 200 microseconds, μs). Shorter rise times mean that shorter TR (pulse sequence repetition time) and TE (echo delay time) values can be used, which in turn means that pulse sequences can be performed more rapidly. Decreasing TR decreases total imaging time, especially in the 3D gradient-echo imaging used for contrast-enhanced breast MRI. Decreasing TE means that more heavily T1-weighted imaging can be performed, increasing T1-weighted contrast among tissues.

The intermittent audible noise generated in MR systems during scanning is due to the magnetic gradient coils experiencing torques due to opposing gradient coils (coils on opposite sides of the scanner from one another carrying currents in opposite directions). As gradient coils are turned on and off, one gradient coil induces a changing magnetic flux through an opposing coil. This causes each gradient coil to experience a repelling force and a turning force or torque. These forces and torques are transmitted to the coil supports in the bore of the magnet. The audible noise they make is due to the coils flexing against the coil supports. MR patients are often required to wear earplugs or headphones to reduce their noise exposure from pulsed gradients. An experienced operator can tell what kind of pulse sequence is being performed by listening to the frequency and strength of the gradient pulses from outside the scan room. A recent improvement in MR system design is to better isolate gradient coils and damp the forces and torques they experience so that the noise they generate is reduced.

Slice Selection in Magnetic Resonance Imaging

In a perfectly uniform static magnetic field, B_0, the precessional frequencies of all hydrogen nuclei in water are identical. When a magnetic gradient is turned on in addition to the static magnetic field, the precessional frequencies of hydrogen nuclei change linearly with position. For example, when the z-gradient is turned on, the magnetic field increases linearly with location along the z-axis (Figure 3.6). As a result, the precessional frequencies of hydrogen nuclei are higher toward the head of the patient than the foot (assuming the head is out). This provides a way to distinguish the location of MR signals along the z-direction by measuring the strength of signals emitted at different precessional frequencies.

Another way to distinguish location is to turn on a magnetic field gradient during tissue excitation. For example, if the z-gradient is turned on while a narrowband RF excitation pulse is being sent into the patient, only a narrow band of tissues will be excited (Figure 3.7A). This is how single-slice excitation is performed. The slice selected with the z-gradient turned on extends uniformly through the patient in x- and y-directions and is perpendicular to the z-direction, yielding a transaxial slice. The

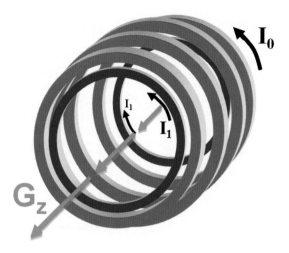

Figure 3.6 A more detailed description of the z-gradient. When turned on in a positive sense, the z-gradient produces a magnetic field that is stronger near the head of the patient (out) than the feet and varies linearly in strength in between. This is achieved by two parallel loops (in addition to the main loops each carrying a current I_0 to produce the main magnetic field B_0), each carrying current I_1 in opposite directions. The loop near the patient's head carries current in the same direction as the main magnetic field coils, so the field produced by this coil adds to B_0. The gradient loop near the patient's feet (farther into the scanner) carries current in the opposite direction to the main magnetic field coils, producing a field that subtracts from B_0. The net result is the z-gradient shown by the red arrows.

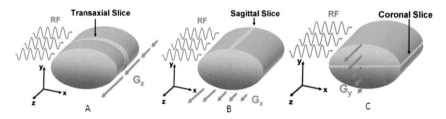

Figure 3.7 (A) Slice-selection in the transaxial plane is achieved by turning on the z-gradient while a narrow-band RF pulse is sent into the patient. The center frequency of the RF pulse is chosen to match the Larmor frequency of the desired slice location. (B) Slice-selection in the sagittal plane is achieved by turning on the x-gradient while a narrow-band RF pulse is sent into the patient. (C) Slice-selection in the coronal plane is achieved by turning on the y-gradient while a narrow-band RF pulse is sent into the patient.

location of the slice can be determined by the match between the magnetic field strength at a particular location along the z-axis (with the z-gradient turned on) and the particular RF frequency transmitted into the patient. A higher RF frequency would excite a slice farther toward the head of the patient with a positive z-gradient applied.

This process of sending in a narrowband RF pulse in the presence of a magnetic gradient is called "selective excitation".[4] If we assign the x-direction as left-to-right relative to the patient lying in the scanner, turning on the x-gradient during excitation

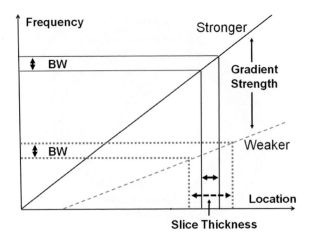

Figure 3.8 The bandwidth of the RF pulse and the strength of the slice-select magnetic gradient determine the resulting slice thickness.

with a narrowband RF pulse would selectively excite a sagittal slice (Figure 3.7B). The y-direction would then be vertical, in the anterior-to-posterior direction relative to the patient. Thus, turning on a y-gradient during excitation would selectively excite a coronal slice (Figure 3.7C).

In slice selection, the thickness of the excited slice depends on two factors: the strength of the applied magnetic gradient and the bandwidth of the RF pulse sent into the patient. A narrower slice can be selected by using a stronger gradient or by narrowing the frequency range or "bandwidth" of the RF pulse (Figure 3.8). In 2D imaging, slices typically have a thickness between 1 and 10 mm. In 3D imaging, instead of exciting a narrow slice of tissue, a thicker slab of tissue, typically 15 to 40 cm is excited, which uses a wider bandwidth RF pulse or a weaker magnetic gradient applied as the RF pulse is sent into the patient.

Magnetic Resonance Imaging Pulse Sequence

The MRI pulse sequence is the series of RF pulses, gradient manipulations, and signal collections that permit collection of an image or set of images.[5] The typical way the body is resolved into voxels in MRI is to use magnetic gradients in all three directions, applying each gradient at different times during the pulse sequence. For example, in 2D transaxial imaging, the z-gradient is turned on during slice excitation to excite a single slice perpendicular to the z-axis. Then the z-gradient is turned off. A short time later, during signal measurement, a gradient is turned on briefly in one of the two in-plane directions (x or y), say, the x-direction. This gradient is termed the frequency-encoding or "read" gradient, since it alters the precessional frequency along the x-direction while the signal is being read out from the excited slice. By measuring the signal emitted from the entire excited slice over multiple time points while the frequency-encoding gradient is turned on, the signal can be broken into its different frequency components. This is done by taking the discrete one-dimensional Fourier transform of the time-encoded signals to get frequency-encoded signals. The number of time points at which signal is measured equals the number of frequency bands into which the slice is divided, which is typically 256 or 512. This divides the slice into 256 or 512 different frequency components. Because the x-gradient creates a one-to-one correspondence between resonant frequency and location, this divides the slice into 256 or 512 strips at different locations along the x-axis (Figure 3.9). Because the 256 or 512 signal measurements at slightly different time points are collected quickly during signal measurement (over a fraction of a millisecond to a few milliseconds), there is little or no additional time delay for collecting signals at more time points and therefore resolving the signal into more frequency bands along the x-direction. The electronics of the RF receiver system simply need to be fast enough to accommodate this more rapid rate of data acquisition.

Resolving the individual strips that are divided along the x-axis, but extend unresolved along the y-axis, into individual voxels involves the use of a phase-encoding gradient applied along the y-axis (the y-gradient). This phase-encoding gradient is applied sometime between signal excitation (when the z-gradient is turned on) and signal measurement (when the x-gradient is turned on). Without applying a y-gradient, all dipoles located along each strip (selected as described above) precess in phase. With the application of a y-gradient for a brief interval (typically, less than a millisecond) between excitation and signal measurement, dipoles at different y-locations are given a different phase, as shown in Figure 3.10. By different "phase," we mean that hydrogen dipoles farther along the y-axis have intentionally been made to precess faster for a brief interval while the y-gradient was turned on; therefore their dipole axes point in different directions than dipoles at other locations on the y-axis. If this were done only once, it would alter the total signal measured from each strip but would not permit resolution of each strip into voxels. By repeating the pulse sequence many times, each time with a different amount of phase-encoding by applying a slightly different phase-encoding gradient strength, the measured signal can be resolved into voxels. The number of times the pulse sequence is repeated, each time with a different amount of phase-encoding, determines the number of voxels that can be resolved in the

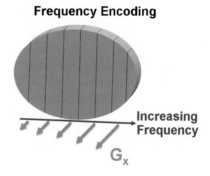

Frequency Encoding

Increasing Frequency

G_x

Figure 3.9 Turning on the x-gradient while measuring signal from a selected transaxial slice divides the measured signals into those precessing at different frequencies. Each different frequency corresponds to a different location along the x-axis.

No y-gradient applied **Weak y-gradient applied**

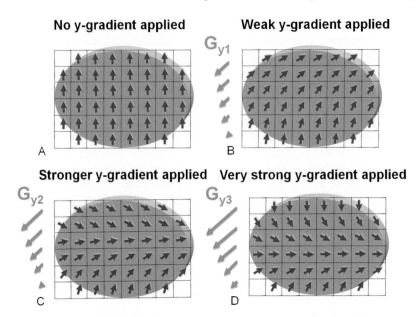

A   B

Stronger y-gradient applied   Very strong y-gradient applied

C   D

Figure 3.10 Brief application of the y-gradient sometime between signal excitation and signal measurement alters the phase of magnetic dipoles along the y-direction. (A) No y-gradient leaves all voxels along the y-direction in the same phase. (B) A very weak y-gradient causes voxels farther along the y-axis to have a slightly greater phase-shift than those near y = 0. (C) A stronger y-gradient causes voxels farther along the y-axis to have greater phase-shift relative to those near y = 0. (D) A very strong y-gradient causes even greater phase shift. By acquiring a number of distinct phase-encoding views (equal to the number of pixels in the y-direction), each with the same frequency-encoding applied during signal measurement, sufficient data are acquired to reconstruct the image by 2-dimensional Fourier transform (2DFT).

phase-encoding direction. For example, if the pulse sequence is repeated 256 times, each time with a uniquely different phase-encoding gradient strength, then the slice can be resolved into 256 different voxels in the phase-encoding direction. On each repetition of the pulse sequence, the same slice would be selected using the z-gradient and signal would be frequency-encoded in the same way by turning on the same x-gradient during signal measurement. The only thing that would change from one repetition to the next is that a different amount of phase-encoding (y-gradient strength) would be applied. Since increasing the number of pulse sequence repetitions used to form an image increases the total imaging time, there is a time penalty for improving spatial resolution in the phase-encoding direction: resolving the image into 512 voxels along the phase-encoding direction takes twice as long as resolving the image into 256 voxels along the phase-encoding direction.

The procedure above describes how single-slice 2D MRI is performed. To acquire transaxial slices, the z-gradient is the slice-select gradient, which is turned on as the excitation pulse is sent into the body. Then phase-encoding and frequency-encoding gradients are the gradients perpendicular to the z-axis, the x- and y-gradients. If the x-axis were chosen to be the frequency-encoding gradient, then the y-axis would be the phase-encoding gradient, and vice-versa. The choice of frequency-encoding and phase-encoding directions is important, because motion artifacts and image wrap occur primarily along the phase-encoding direction. This is illustrated in Chapter 9.

The reason that motion propagates primarily in the phase-encoding, rather than frequency-encoding, direction is that the time between different phase-encoding views is much longer than the time interval between different frequency-encoding views (at the same phase-encoding). Without going into the details of the pulse sequence at this point, if TR is the duration of the basic pulse sequence, then TR is the time that separates signal measurement from the first phase-encoding view to the second, the second phase encoding view from the third, etc. TR can range from several milliseconds to several seconds, depending on the pulse sequence used. In 2D imaging, it is typically hundreds of milliseconds in T1-weighted imaging and several seconds in T2-weighted imaging. For example, if TR is set at 500 ms, then there is half a second between collection of each different phase-encoding view. On the other hand, the interval between different time-point signal measurements during signal collection is very short, typically a fraction of a millisecond, since 256 or 512 different signal measurements must be acquired within the period of signal measurement for each pulse sequence, which is usually only a few milliseconds. If 512 signal measurements are taken during a 5 millisecond signal measurement interval, then each time-point measurement is separated by only 0.01 ms (5 ms/512). Thus, the time interval between each different phase-encoding view is 50000 times longer (500 ms/0.01 ms) than the interval between each different frequency-encoding view, so there is a much longer interval for motion and mis-registration to occur between different phase-encoding views than between different frequency-encoding views. This is the underlying reason that motion artifact ghosting propagates mainly in the phase-encoding direction.

Forming a Magnetic Resonance Image

The point of MRI is to collect enough data to form an image. In this example, we will be concerned with collecting enough data to form an image of a single slice. If the single slice is a transaxial slice (perpendicular to the z-axis), then the in-plane directions are along the x- and y-axes. To construct a complete image, we want to know the signal value in each pixel of the x-y grid, shown in Figure 3.11A. This x-y grid is in two-dimensional position-space, with x marking the location of discrete pixels along the horizontal axis and y marking the location of discrete pixels along the vertical axis. We can specify any particular pixel by a giving pair of x-y coordinates. The image consists of the signal strength at each discrete x-y location in this two-dimensional position-space.

Voxel Size

Spatial dimensions of voxels are determined by the slice thickness (Δz) and the field-of-view and matrix in each in-plane direction. The in-plane pixel size of each voxel is

$$\Delta x = L_x/N_x \text{ and } \Delta y = L_y/N_y \tag{3.1}$$

where L_x and L_y are the FOVs in the x- and y-directions, and N_x and N_y are the number of matrix elements in x- and y-directions. The voxel size is Δx by Δy by Δz, and the voxel volume is the product of these three factors. For example, an acquisition with a square 20 cm FOV, 256 frequency-encoding steps, and 192 phase encoding steps, and a 3 mm slice thickness would have a voxel size of Δx = 200 mm/256 = 0.78 mm by Δy = 200 mm/192 = 1.04 mm by Δz = 3 mm, assuming frequency-encoding is along the x-direction, phase-encoding in along y, and slice-selection is along z. The volume of each voxel in this acquisition would be (0.78 mm)(1.04 mm)(3 mm) = 2.44 mm³.

k-Space

The two-dimensional Fourier transform of an image in position space is an "image" (a matrix of signal strengths) in "frequency-space"(Figure 3.11B).[3] Here, "frequency" means spatial-frequency. The spatial frequency axes are k_x and k_y. Just as position is measured along the x-axis, spatial frequency along the x-direction is measured by k_x. Since position (x, y) is measured in units of length (meters), spatial frequencies k_x and k_y are measured in units of 1/(length) (or oscillations per unit length). $k_x = 0$ is zero spatial frequency, a constant in the x-direction. $k_y = 0$ is a constant in the y-direction. Therefore, for a particular image, the signal strength at the point $k_x = 0$ and $k_y = 0$ (in spatial frequency space) specifies how much of the image is a constant in both x- and y-directions, not varying from pixel to pixel; that is, how much of the image is a constant across x and y. The signal strength at $k_x = 1$ and $k_y = 0$ tells us how much of the image is composed of a spatial frequency component that oscillates at a rate of 1 oscillation per meter in the x-direction and is uniform in y.

In MRI, image data are actually acquired by collecting signal strength data in frequency space (k_x and k_y) or "k-space" and then taking its discrete two-dimensional Fourier transform (2DFT) to get the image in position space (x and y). The signal measurements that occur in 2D imaging can be thought of as filling out signal strength data in k-space (Figure 3.11B). Assuming that the y-gradient is the phase-encoding gradient, each different phase-encoding view provides a single line of data at a fixed y-location. Each individual frequency-encoding view (signal measurement) provides a single point along the x-direction, with the x-gradient being the frequency-encoding gradient. This k-space picture depicts how image data is collected in spatial-frequency space. If 256 × 256 data points are collected

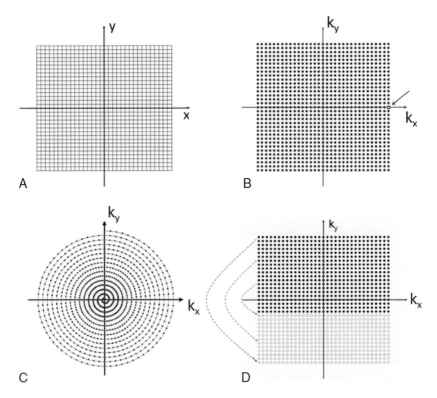

Figure 3.11 (A) A planar image is a grid of pixels representing signal values in two dimensions, x and y. (B) The two-dimensional Fourier transform (2DFT) of signal values in position space (x and y) is the set of signal values at discrete values of spatial frequency, k_x and k_y. Data collection for an MR image can be thought of as collecting adequate data to fill the grid in k-space (k_x and k_y). The image in position space is constructed by taking the 2DFT of the k-space signal data. The highest spatial frequency that can be recorded with a pixelated image such as A occurs when the signal changes from maximum to minimum (white to black), and vice versa, from one pixel to the next. This maximum spatial frequency (or Nyquist limit) in the x-direction, and zero spatial frequency in y, since the image is not changing intensity as a function of y, is shown as the open circle (arrow) in B (k_x = maximum, $k_y = 0$). (C). Spiral imaging collects k-space data in an expanding helical pattern which concentrates collected data toward the center of k-space, where image contrast information is collected, with less dense data collection toward the edges, where higher spatial frequency (sharp edge) data are collected. (D) Half-Fourier imaging assumes that signal values for negative values of k_y (open circles) are identical to their corresponding positive values of k_y (solid circles). This "phase symmetry" assumption, as shown by the curved arrows for three lines of data, can reduce the number of collected phase-encoding views by nearly 50%, thereby reducing total image acquisition time by nearly a factor of two. As shown here, some data on either side of $k_y = 0$ are collected to improve image contrast and reduce artifacts in half-Fourier images.

in spatial-frequency space by performing 256 different phase-encoding views and, within each phase encoding view, by measuring signal at 256 different time points, then the resultant image will be a 256 × 256 image in position space, with 256 pixels in each in-plane (x and y) direction. To form a complete image, all the points in frequency space must be measured, out to some maximum spatial frequency in k_x

and k_y. The maximum spatial frequencies (k_x and k_y) at which image data are collected determines the maximum spatial frequencies (in line pairs per unit length) that are contained in the resultant image (the Nyquist frequencies in x- and y-directions). The highest spatial frequency that can be represented in a digital image, the Nyquist frequency, occurs when image signal oscillates from white to black and back again from pixel to adjacent pixel across the entire image. For example, with 256 matrix elements collected in each in-plane direction and with a square 20 cm FOV, each pixel is 0.78 mm in x- and y-directions. The highest spatial frequency that could be captured with these spatial parameters is $1/(2(0.78 \, mm)) = 0.64$ line pairs per millimeter.

While conventional 2DFT imaging collects a rectangle of data in k-space, as shown in Figure 3.11B, other schemes for data collection can be used, some of which can speed image acquisition. For example, spiral imaging collects data in a spiral pattern in k-space, as shown in Figure 3.11C.[6,7] This has the advantage of concentrating data collection at the center of k-space (where the most important contrast information in the image is collected), while sampling the higher spatial-frequency components (where more information about image detail is collected), which are farther from the center of k-space, less frequently. This approach can be used to speed image acquisition.

Another way to speed image acquisition is to sample only half or slightly more than half of k-space and to assume that the unsampled, negative frequency signals are identical to the sampled, positive frequency components. This is the idea behind half-Fourier imaging, which speeds data acquisition by nearly a factor of two by collecting only the positive frequency phase-encoding views and assuming that the unmeasured negative-frequency phase-encoding views are identical to the measured positive-frequency phase-encoding views, matching signal strength frequency by frequency (Figure 3.11D).[7,8] It saves little or no time to invoke this sort of phase symmetry in the frequency-encoding direction, because there is little or no time penalty for collecting more frequency-encoding views. Data collection symmetry is almost always applied in the phase-encoding direction to reduce total imaging time by requiring fewer phase-encoding views.

In Chapters 4-6, we combine the concepts from Chapters 1 through 3 to describe in detail how MRI pulse sequences are performed and how details of the pulse sequence affect image contrast and imaging time.

Chapter Take-home Points

- High-field MRI systems use superconducting solenoidal magnets to produce highly uniform magnetic fields over the body.
- Radiofrequency transmitter and receiver coils are required to excite tissue and to measure the signal emitted from tissue.
- Magnetic gradients applied in three orthogonal directions are used to localize the sources of signal in MR images.

- The MRI pulse sequence describes the RF pulses sent into the patient, the gradient manipulations, and the signal measurements taken by the MRI system to produce an MR image.
- k-space is a convenient way to describe data collection in MRI.

References

1. Lauterbur PC. Image formation by induced local interactions: examples employing nuclear magnetic resonance," Nature 1973; *242*: 190–191.
2. Hendrick RE, Osborn A, Kanal E. Basic MRI physics. In Kressel H, Modic M, Murphy W. Syllabus: Special Course - MR 1990. RSNA Publications, Chicago, IL, 1990, pp. 7–30.
3. Matwiyoff NA, Brooks WM. Instrumentation. In Magnetic Resonance Imaging, 3rd Edition. Eds DD Stark and WG Bradley. St. Louis: Mosby Publishing Co., 1999. Volume 1, Ch. 2, p. 15–32.
4. Wood ML, Wehrli FW (1999) Principles of magnetic resonance imaging. In Magnetic Resonance Imaging, 3rd Edition. Eds DD Stark and WG Bradley. St. Louis: Mosby Publishing Co., 1999. Volume 1, Ch. 1, p. 1–14.
5. Hendrick RE. Image contrast and noise. In Stark DD, Bradley WG. Magnetic Resonance Imaging, 3rd Edition. St. Louis: Mosby Publishing Co., 1999, Vol 1, Ch 4, 43–68.
6. Sachs TS, Meyer CH, Hu BS, et. al. Real-time motion detection in spiral MRI using navigators. Magn Reson Med. 1994; 32: 639–45.
7. Frahm J, Haenicke W. Rapid scan techniques. In Stark DD, Bradley WG. Magnetic Resonance Imaging, 3rd Edition. St. Louis: Mosby Publishing Co., 1999, Vol 1, Ch 6, 87–124.
8. Perman WH, Heiberg EV, Herrmann VM. Half-Fourier, three-dimensional technique for dynamic contrast-enhanced MR imaging of both breasts and axillae: initial characterization of breast lesions. Radiology 1996; 200: 263–269.

Chapter 4
The Spin-echo Pulse Sequence

The pulse sequence in MRI describes the series of RF pulses, gradient manipulations, and signal measurements that permit collection of sufficient data to form an image or set of images.[1] The pulse sequence diagram is like an orchestral score. Time proceeds linearly from left to right. Instead of orchestrating different instruments, the MRI pulse sequence diagram (Figure 4.1) describes the different operations that must occur to generate and collect image data: RF pulses, gradient manipulations, and signal measurement.

The top line in the pulse sequence diagram describes RF pulses sent into the patient. The next three lines describe the slice-select, phase-encoding, and frequency-encoding magnetic gradients. The bottom line illustrates the signal measured to obtain an MR image. Not shown in a pulse sequence diagram is the static magnetic field, B_0, since it is always on and constant. Also not shown in the pulse sequence diagram are the details of signal measurement within the measurement interval or sampling interval, T_s. During the interval T_s, a fixed number of signal measurements (e.g., 256 or 512) are acquired at evenly spaced time points. Individual time samples are not shown since this level of detail would unnecessarily complicate the diagram. This sampling is discussed later in this chapter.

Spin-echo Pulse Sequence Diagram

Different pulse sequences are best distinguished by the details of their pulse sequence diagrams. We begin by describing the pulse sequence diagram for one of the earliest and most versatile imaging pulse sequences, spin-echo imaging. The spin-echo pulse sequence was adapted from MR spectroscopy techniques by adding gradient manipulations to provide a robust pulse sequence for imaging.[2] The "spin-echo" itself describes the way the signal is formed for measurement. As described briefly in Chapter 2, maximum signal is measured after performing a 90° RF pulse, then measuring the magnetization precessing in the transverse plane. Rather than immediately measuring the signal just after a 90° pulse, in spin-echo imaging a brief time interval (TE/2) is included to let transverse magnetization dephase. Then a 180° pulse is applied. The effect of this 180° pulse is to invert all magnetization about a particular

R.E. Hendrick (ed.), *Breast MRI: Fundamentals and Technical Aspects.*
© Springer 2008

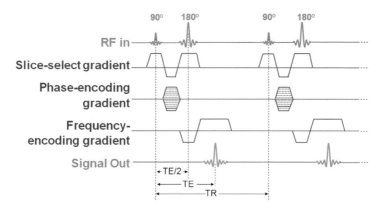

Figure 4.1 The spin-echo pulse sequence. Time flows from left to right. The top line shows RF pulses sent into the patient. The second line shows the slice-select gradient. The third line shows the phase-encoding gradient. The fourth line shows the frequency-encoding or read gradient. The bottom line shows the signal generated from tissue. (From Hendrick RE. (1) Adapted with permission from Elsevier).

axis. As a result of the 180° pulse, the faster precessing magnetic dipoles in the transverse plane are flipped 180°, putting them in the position of the slower precessing dipoles in the transverse plane, and vice versa (Figure 4.2). An equal amount of time after the 180° inversion pulse (TE/2), a spin-echo is formed (at time TE after the initial 90° pulse). Thus, TE is the "echo time": the time after the initial 90° pulse at which peak signal strength is measured.

This spin-echo approach is more suitable for imaging than the approach of measuring the signal immediately after a 90° RF pulse, which is called the "free-induction decay" approach.[3] In free-induction decay, the signal fades rapidly after the 90° pulse, since no signal echo is formed, so it is important to measure the signal as quickly after the 90° pulse as possible. The spin-echo approach puts a time gap between the 90° pulse and peak echo signal. This gives the spin-echo approach several advantages. First, the spin-echo approach allows time between the 90° pulse and signal measurement to perform the gradient manipulations needed to separate the selected slice into individual voxels, while free-induction decay does not. Second, in free-induction decay the lack of a time gap between the RF pulse sent into the patient and signal measurement means that the received RF signal can be contaminated by the transmitted RF pulse, an effect called "ring-through." Spin-echo imaging avoids ring-through by intentionally putting a time gap between the transmitted RF pulse and the signal received from the patient, without significant loss of signal as would occur in free-induction decay. Third, the spin-echo approach is more resilient than free-induction decay to signal loss due to magnetic susceptibility effects and B_0 non-uniformities.

We will describe each component of the spin-echo pulse sequence while referring to the spin-echo pulse sequence diagram (Figure 4.1). The top line demonstrates the RF pulses sent into the patient by the RF transmitter coil. The basic spin-echo pulse

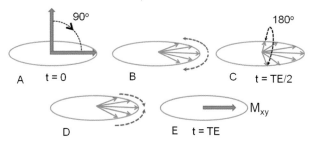

Figure 4.2 Schematic diagram illustrating the formation of a spin-echo. (A) A 90° pulse flips all longitudinal magnetization, which points along B_0, into the transverse plane, which is perpendicular to B_0, so that it can be measured. (B) During the interval TE/2, the transverse magnetization dephases due to different hydrogen nuclear dipoles in the sample or voxel experiencing slightly different magnetic field environments. Those hydrogen magnetic dipoles sitting in a slightly higher magnetic field precess faster than the Larmor (center) frequency; those dipoles sitting in a slightly weaker magnetic field precess slower than the Larmor frequency. The result of different precessional rates is that the transverse magnetization dephases as time progresses. (C) At the time TE/2, a 180° pulse is applied, which re-orients the faster precessing dipoles to point in the direction that slower dipoles pointed prior to the 180° pulse, and vice versa. (D) During the interval TE/2 after the 180° pulse, because the magnetic field environment is largely unchanged (other than microscopic irreversible "true T2 effects"), the faster precessing dipoles tend to catch up and the slower precessing dipoles tend to fall back. (E) At a time TE after the 90° pulse, a spin-echo occurs due to the rephasing of transverse magnetization. The peak transverse signal at the time TE is less than the transverse signal just after the 90° pulse due to "true T2" relaxation effects. Signal is measured just before, during, and just after this peak echo signal.

sequence consists of a 90° pulse, followed by a 180° pulse. The time between the 90° and 180° pulses is TE/2, where TE is the time from the 90° pulse to peak spin-echo signal. The time between the first repetition of the basic pulse sequence and the next repetition of the 90° – 180° pulse pair is TR, the pulse sequence repetition time. This pair of pulses is repeated enough times (e.g., 192, 256, 384, or 512) to achieve adequate spatial resolution in the phase-encoding direction, as described in Chapter 3 and in more detail later in this chapter.

The second line in Figure 4.1 describes the slice-select gradient, which is the z-gradient in transaxial imaging, the x-gradient in sagittal imaging, and the y-gradient in coronal imaging. As can be seen in the figure, the slice select gradient is ramped up just before applying each RF pulse, is kept constant during the each RF pulse, and is ramped down after each pulse. The purpose of the slice select gradient is to ensure that the RF pulse excites only a narrow slice of tissue at the desired location, that is, to make the RF pulse "slice-selective". This is done by using a narrow-band RF pulse that is specific to the resonant frequency of the slice of interest. When the slice-select gradient is shown to be constant in the pulse sequence diagram (non-zero and flat), it indicates that a magnetic field gradient is applied that changes the magnetic field linearly along the direction perpendicular to the selected slice so that resonant frequencies change linearly with position along the gradient direction, as shown in Figure 3.7A. The slice-select gradient is manipulated in exactly the same way on each repetition of the basic spin-echo pulse sequence.

The third line in Figure 4.1 describes the phase-encoding gradient. The purpose of the phase-encoding gradient is to apply a different amount of phase encoding on each repetition of the spin-echo sequence so that a series of collected spin-echo signals can be used to form a two-dimensional image. This different amount of phase encoding on each repetition of the pulse sequence is accomplished by turning on the phase-encoding gradient for the same brief duration, but with a different strength, on each repetition of the spin-echo sequence, as indicated by the dotted lines at different vertical heights for the phase-encoding gradient. The phase-encoding gradient is applied sometime between signal excitation and signal measurement. This provides the phase difference in each repeated signal collection that permits resolving each frequency-encoded strip into individual voxels in the phase-encoding direction, as described in Chapter 3.

The fourth line in Figure 4.1 describes the frequency-encoding gradient. As indicated in the figure, the frequency encoding gradient is turned on during signal measurement to separate the selected slice into strips, producing signals at different frequencies during signal measurement. This allows the different strips to be separated along the frequency-encoding direction during signal measurement. Because the application of any gradient causes dephasing of the transverse magnetization within the excited slice, turning on the frequency encoding gradient in only one direction would decrease the signal that is being measured. To counteract this signal decrease, the frequency-encoding gradient is turned on in the opposite direction prior to signal measurement. This leads to peak signal at the time TE due to the combined effects of a spin-echo (due to the 180° pulse) and a gradient echo (due to reversal of the frequency-encoding gradient). The frequency-encoding gradient is manipulated in exactly the same way on each repetition of the spin-echo pulse sequence.

The fifth line in the spin-echo pulse sequence diagram illustrates the signal emitted by tissue in the excited slice. The peak echo signal occurs at time TE after the 90° pulse. The bottom line on the pulse sequence diagram illustrates the period of signal measurement. During a brief time interval, T_s, evenly spaced signal measurements are taken at slightly different time points. The sampling interval T_s is centered on the spin-echo signal peak (Figure 4.3). In that way, the

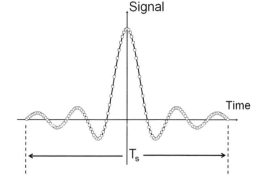

Figure 4.3 Detail of signal measurement showing that N signal measurements (typically with N = 256 or 512) evenly spaced in time are taken symmetrically about the peak signal of the spin-echo.

required number of measurements (e.g., 256 or 512) can be obtained to provide adequate spatial resolution (256 or 512 pixels, respectively) in the frequency-encoding direction.

Signal Dependence on TR and TE in Spin-echo Imaging

Figure 4.4 illustrates the behavior of longitudinal and transverse magnetization from a single voxel at each stage in the spin-echo pulse sequence. Prior to the 90° pulse, the longitudinal magnetization is M_0, the maximum possible longitudinal magnetization. The 90° pulse flips the entire amount of longitudinal

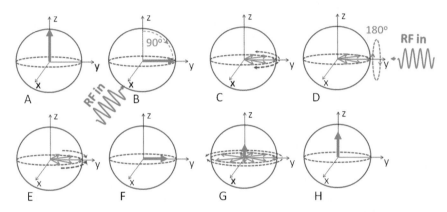

Figure 4.4 The behavior of longitudinal and transverse magnetization from a single voxel at each stage in the spin-echo pulse sequence. (A) Prior to the 90° pulse, the longitudinal magnetization points along the direction of the static magnetic field, B_0. (B) The 90° pulse applied along the x-axis flips all longitudinal magnetization into the transverse plane, where it precesses at the Larmor frequency. So just after the 90° pulse, longitudinal magnetization is zero and transverse magnetization equals the longitudinal magnetization just before the 90° pulse. (C). During the interval TE/2, hydrogen nuclear dipoles diphase due to both irreversible "true T2" relaxation effects and reversible effects such as a magnetic gradient across the sample or voxel. The net effect is dephasing of the transverse magnetization and loss of measurable signal strength. (D) At the time TE/2, a 180° pulse is applied around the y-axis, which flips faster precessing dipoles into the orientation of slower precessing dipoles, and vice versa. (E). During the interval TE/2 following the 180° pulse, reversible transverse magnetization dephasing effects are rephrased, while irreversible true T2 dephasing effects continue. (F) At time TE after the 90° pulse, peak echo signal occurs. Signal is measured during this peak. (G) After a time several times T2, the transverse magnetization has completely dephased and the measurable signal is zero. At the same time, longitudinal magnetization begins to slowly regrow. (H) At a time comparable to T1 later, the longitudinal magnetization has regrown to about two-thirds of its maximum possible value. At a time TR after the initial 90° pulse, the next repetition of the pulse sequence begins with a 90° pulse that flips the recovered longitudinal magnetization into the transverse plane. It is through this mechanism that the TR setting determines the amount of T1-weighting in subsequent repetitions of the sequence. (From Hendrick RE. (1) Adapted with permission from Elsevier).

magnetization, M_0 into the transverse plane, where it can be measured. During the interval TE/2, there is irreversible dephasing of the transverse magnetization due to true T2 decay, and there is reversible dephasing due to magnetic field non-uniformities across the voxel (see Chapter 2). At time TE/2, the 180° pulse is applied, which flips the faster precessing dipoles into the position of the slower precessing dipoles, and vice versa. In the remaining interval TE/2, the faster precessing dipoles catch up, while the slower precessing dipoles fall back. This forms the spin-echo. Irreversible T2 decay decreases the transverse magnetization during the interval TE between the 90° pulse and peak signal measurement, as described by the formula:

$$M_{xy}(TE) = M_0 \, e^{-TE/T2} \tag{4.1}$$

and as shown in Figure 2.6 with t = TE. Equation 4.1 indicates that TE controls the amount of T2 decay in spin-echo imaging. The longer TE, the more time there is for true T2 decay to decrease the signal between the 90° pulse and signal measurement, so the smaller the signal that will be measured.

After signal measurement, and in fact after the 180° pulse, longitudinal magnetization recovers along the direction of B_0. The time TR-(TE/2), which is nearly equal to TR, since TE is usually much smaller than TR, governs the amount of T1 recovery that occurs prior to the next 90° pulse, which starts the next repetition of the spin-echo sequence. The interval TR governs how much longitudinal magnetization has recovered and is flipped into the transverse plane by the next 90° pulse. Thus, the selection of TR governs how much T1 recovery is permitted prior to the next repetition of the pulse sequence. On the next repetition, and on each subsequent repetition of the spin-echo sequence, the signal measured in the spin-echo pulse sequence is governed by both T1 and T2 according to the approximate formula:

$$M_{SE}(TR, TE) = M_0(1 - e^{-TR/T1})e^{-TE/T2} \tag{4.2}$$

This formula indicates that TR controls the amount of T1-weighting, while TE controls the amount of T2-weighting, in the spin-echo pulse sequence. In addition, the amount of hydrogen spin-density in a given voxel influences the strength of M_0, so the full dependence of signal strength from a pixel is often written:

$$S_{SE}(TR, TE) = N[H](1 - e^{-TR/T1})e^{-TE/T2}, \tag{4.3}$$

where S_{SE}(TR, TE) is the signal from a given voxel, and N[H] is the hydrogen spin density in that voxel. TR and TE are the user-selectable parameters in spin-echo imaging, which apply to every voxel in the image. T1, T2, and N[H] are the inherent tissue parameters of a given voxel, which determine signal strength from that voxel. Differences between T1, T2, and N[H] from voxel to voxel are the sources of tissue contrast in spin-echo imaging.

Contrast in Spin-echo Imaging

To illustrate contrast in spin-echo imaging, consider a simple example: the contrast between a cyst and normal breast tissue. As stated in Chapter 2, at 1.5 T, normal fibroglandular breast tissue might have tissue parameters of T1 = 700 ms, T2 = 70 ms, and N[H] = 1.0 (N[H] is specified on a relative scale). At the same magnetic field strength, a cyst might have T1 = 3000 ms (3 s), T2 = 300 ms, and N[H] = 1.1; that is, T1, T2, and N[H] are all significantly higher in the cyst than in normal breast tissues, due to the higher water content and therefore fewer macromolecules per unit volume in a cyst than in normal fibroglandular tissue. As you can see, there are larger differences between cystic fluid and normal tissues in T1 and T2 than in N[H].

We will use this example to illustrate the effect of the user-selectable parameters, TR and TE, on contrast in spin-echo imaging.[1] Figure 4.5 illustrates the differences in signal strength between normal fibroglandular tissue and a cyst for the full range of TR and TE values, based on Equation 4.3. The TR dependence is shown by the T1-factor, $(1-e^{-TR/T1})$, which is plotted for normal fibroglandular tissues (blue) and cystic fluid (red) in Figure 4.5A. The longer T1 value of cystic fluid means that it takes longer for the longitudinal magnetization to recover in cystic fluid than in normal fibroglandular tissue. If signal could be measured isolating just this T1 effect (which it cannot), then on the next repetition of the spin-echo pulse sequence, fibroglandular tissues would have higher signal (and thus be brighter) than a cyst.

Figure 4.5B shows the combined effects of the spin-density and T1-factors multiplied together: while the shorter T1 value of fibroglandular tissue tends to make the fibroglandular tissue brighter than a cyst, the lower spin-density of fibroglandular tissue works in the opposite direction to the T1-factor, tending to make fibroglandular tissue slightly darker than a cyst. Which factor dominates, N[H] or the T1-factor, depends on the amount of T1-weighting that is selected, which in turn depends on the user-selectable parameter TR. If a shorter TR value (comparable to the T1-values of the two tissues) is selected, the T1-factor dominates, making fibroglandular tissue brighter than the cyst. If a very long TR value is chosen, then the T1-effect is minimized and the spin-density factor dominates, making the cyst slightly brighter than fibroglandular tissue. No pulse sequence exists that can measure the T1-factor alone, the spin-density factor alone, or just the product of those two factors.

Figure 4.5C shows the combined effects of all three factors (N[H], the T1-factor, and the T2-factor) in Equation 4.3 at a particular, relatively short TR value (500 ms) for a range of TE values from 0 to 120 ms. The inset graph shows that T2 decay occurs more quickly for fibroglandular tissue than for cyst, due to fibroglandular tissue's shorter T2 value. As a result, like hydrogen spin-density, T2 works in the opposite direction to T1-contrast: T1 effects tend to cause fibroglandular tissue to have higher signal (be brighter) than cyst, while both spin-density and T2 effects tend to make fibroglandular tissues darker than cysts. To optimize T1-weighted spin-echo imaging, pulse sequence parameters must be chosen that maximize T1-contrast and

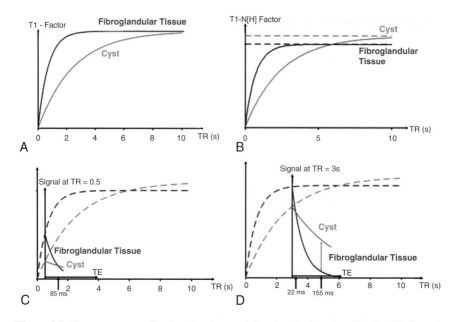

Figure 4.5 The components affecting signal strength in spin-echo imaging. (A). The T1-factor in SE imaging depends on the user-selectable parameter TR and the inherent tissue T1. Because the T1 of fibroglandular tissue is shorter than that of cyst, the T1-factor of fibroglandular tissue is greater than that of cyst for every TR value, but T1 contrast between the two tissues decreases for long TR values (B). The combination of spin-density (N[H]) and T1-factors in SE imaging. Generally, tissues with longer T1 values have higher spin densities, as is the case for cyst compared to fibroglandular tissue. Note that for short TR values (where T1 contrast is manifested), the spin-density-factor works against the T1-factor, reducing contrast between the two tissues (C). The combination of all three factors (N[H], T1, and T2) affecting signal strength in SE imaging, where a fixed TR value of 500 ms has been assumed. Note that the T2-factors work against the T1-factors, reducing the contrast between fibroglandular tissue and cyst. The T2-factors depend on TE, and as TE increases, T1W contrast decreases. In SE imaging, T1W contrast is achieved by having a TR comparable to or less than that of the shorter T1 values of the tissues of interest, with TE as short as possible (D). The combination of all three factors (N[H], T1, and T2) affecting signal strength in SE imaging, where a fixed TR value of 3 s (3000 ms) has been assumed. Here, with a sufficiently long TE value (greater than 22 ms), cyst is brighter than fibroglandular tissue. With longer TE values, the T2-factor and spin-density-factor work in concert to make cyst brighter, while the T1-factor works in the opposite direction. To emphasize T2-weighting, TE values greater than 60 ms are used, with longer TR values (greater than 3 seconds) to minimize T1W. (From Hendrick RE. (1) Adapted with permission from Elsevier).

minimize T2-contrast effects. This is done by selecting a relatively short TR value to maximize T1-contrast, and by selecting as short a TE value as possible to minimize T2-contrast. No choice of TR or TE can cancel spin-density weighting, which is always present and tends to work against T1-contrast.

Figure 1.1 shows an example of spin-echo imaging in a breast with normal fibroglandular tissues and a cyst. Figure 1.1 A and B were acquired with TR = 500 ms, TE = 20 ms with and without fat-saturation. Both are T1W, corresponding to the schematic diagram in Figure 4.5C with a TE of 20 ms, making fibroglandular tissue slightly brighter than cyst.

Figure 4.5D shows the combined effects of all three factors in Equation 4.3 for a longer TR value (3000 ms) for a range of TE values from 0 to 150 ms. This longer TR value tends to decrease the effect of T1-contrast. The inset graph shows that T2 decay occurs more quickly for fibroglandular tissue than for cyst, due to the shorter T2 for fibroglandular tissue. As a result, for TE values greater than 22 ms, spin-density and T2-contrast dominates to make cyst brighter than fibroglandular tissue. Normal T2-weighted spin-echo pulse sequences have TR = 2.5 to 3 s and TE = 80–120 ms, where cysts would be very bright relative to all other tissues in the breast due to their elevated spin density and T2 values, as shown by the separation of solid curves for cyst and fibroglandular tissue in Figure 4.5D.

Figure 1.1C shows an example of fibroglandular tissues and cyst in a spin-echo image with relatively long TR = 3 ms and TE = 80 ms. As predicted by Figure 4.5D, at these TR and TE values cyst is considerably brighter than fibroglandular tissues primarily because of the T2 differences of the two tissues, which are emphasized with longer TE values. When TE is made shorter to minimize T2 effects and TR is kept long to minimize T1 effects, hydrogen spin-density weighted images occur, as in Figure 1.1D. In this example, cyst is still brighter than fibroglandular tissue for spin-density weighted imaging at long TR and very short TE due to the higher spin-density of cyst relative to fibroglandular tissue.

This example shows a few general principles of contrast in spin-echo imaging. Spin-density and T2-weighting tend to work with one another; that is, higher spin density values make tissues brighter and higher T2 values make tissues brighter. On the other hand, both spin-density and T2-contrast tend to work in the opposite direction to T1-weighted contrast: spin-density and T2 differences make longer-T2 tissues such as cysts brighter, while T1 differences make shorter-T1 tissues such as fat and fibroglandular tissues brighter. Which effect dominates depends on the specific selection of TR and TE. In general, T1-weighting dominates at shorter TR and very short TE values. T2-weighting dominates at longer TR and longer TE values. Spin-density effects can be highlighted by choosing a very long TR to minimize T1-weighting and by choosing a very short TE to minimize T2-weighting. Table 4.1 summarizes these effects.

Table 4.1 Selection of TR and TE for contrast weighting in spin-echo imaging

Contrast Weighting	TR Setting	TE Setting
T1	Comparable to T1s of tissues (300–600 ms)	As short as possible (< 10–15 ms)
T2	Long (> 2–3 s)	Comparable to T2s of tissues (60–120 ms)
N[H]	Long (> 2–3 s)	As short as possible (< 10–15 ms)

Source: Hendrick RE. (1) Adapted with permission from Elsevier.

Acquisition Times in Spin-echo Imaging

The time to acquire a single-slice spin echo image is determined by three factors: TR, the number of phase encoding steps (N_{pe}), and the number of excitations (N_{ex}), which is more precisely defined as the number of times each phase-encoding view is acquired. In early MRI at lower field strength, it was often necessary to make N_{ex} greater than 1 to obtain adequate SNR in spin-echo images. At 1.5 T with modern MR systems, $N_{ex} = 1$ is typically chosen. Nonetheless, the time required to collect the data sufficient for a single-slice spin-echo image is:

$$T_{total} = (TR)(N_{pe})(N_{ex}) \qquad (4.4)$$

For example, in T1-weighted spin-echo imaging with TR = 500 ms, 256 phase-encoding steps, and one excitation per phase-encoding step ($N_{ex} = 1$),

$$T_{total} = (TR)(N_{pe})(N_{ex}) = (0.5s)(256)(1) = 128s = 2.1 \, minutes.$$

In T2-weighted spin-echo imaging with TR = 3 s, 256 phase-encoding steps, and $N_{ex} = 1$,

$$T_{total} = (TR)(N_{pe})(N_{ex}) = (3.0s)(256)(1) = 768s = 12.8 \, minutes,$$

which is long for a single pulse sequence scan. Patient motion is a likely, unwanted complication of scans longer than a few minutes.

Multi-slice Imaging

MRI would be unfeasible if it required 2–12 minutes to acquire a single-slice image acquisition. An early breakthrough in the clinical application of MRI was the development of multi-slice imaging, which enables the acquisition of many slices in approximately the same time as required for a single-slice acquisition.[4] Multi-slice MRI is achieved by multiplexing the excitation and signal collection process so that many nearly contiguous slices are excited and measured during the dead-time after excitation and collection of signal from the first slice. Figure 4.6 illustrates this multiplexing technique. During the interval TR, a series of slices are excited, taking advantage of the fact that that TR is much longer than TE in spin-echo imaging (because T1 is much longer than T2 in tissue), and taking advantage of slice-selective excitation. While waiting for the recovery of longitudinal magnetization after signal measurement in the first excited slice, other slices at nearby locations can be excited and their signal measured. Each specific slice is excited once every TR, each time with a different degree of phase-encoding, but many slices are excited during each TR interval. Thus, signal collection is multiplexed in multi-slice imaging.

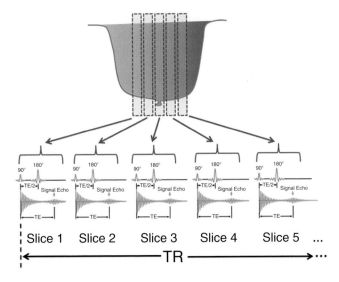

Figure 4.6 Illustration of the multiplexing technique that permits a number of parallel slices to be obtained in the same amount of time required for a single slice. Because TR is much longer than TE in spin-echo imaging, during the time after signal measurement that longitudinal magnetization is recovering in slice 1, a number of additional slices can undergo excitation and signal measurement. Since the 90° and 180° pulses applied are slice selective, they act only on a single specific slice at a time. This permits each previously excited slice to recover undisturbed while other slices are undergoing excitation and signal measurement.

There is a limit on how many slices can be acquired within a given TR, which is set by the time required to excite and collect the echo from each slice: $TE + T_c$. TE is the echo delay time, the time from 90° pulse to peak echo signal, and T_c is the time from peak echo until signal acquisition ends, which is usually only a few milliseconds in spin-echo acquisitions. The maximum number of slices that can be acquired during the interval TR is:

$$N_{Slices}(max) = TR/(TE+T_c),\qquad(4.5)$$

as illustrated in Figure 4.6. For example, in T1-weighted spin-echo imaging with TR = 500 ms, and TE = 15 ms, T_c = 5 ms, the maximum number of slices would be:

$$N_{Slices}(max) = TR/(TE+T_c) = (500\,ms)/(15\,ms+5\,ms) = 25\,slices.$$

In T2-weighted spin-echo imaging, with TR = 2500 ms, TE = 80 ms, and Tc = 5 ms, the maximum number of slices would be:

$$N_{Slices}(max) = TR/(TE+T_c) = (2500\,ms)/(80\,ms+5\,ms) = 29\,slices.$$

Software on modern MR scanners automatically performs this calculation based on details of the specific pulse sequence and reports the maximum number of slices for a given TR or the minimum TR for the prescribed number of slices.

Chapter Take-home Points

- The spin-echo pulse sequence consists of a $90°$ pulse followed by a $180°$ pulse followed an equal time later by signal collection.
- The two user selectable delay times in spin-echo imaging are the sequence repetition time, TR, and the echo time, TE.
- TR controls the T1-weighting, while TE controls the T2-weighting of the spin-echo pulse sequence.
- T1-weighted SE images are achieved with TR set near the T1 values of tissues of interest, with very short TE values to minimize T2-weighting.
- T2-weighted SE images are achieved by setting TR very long to minimize T1-weighting and setting TE near the T2 values of tissues of interest.
- Spin-density-weighted SE images are achieved by setting TR long and TE very short.
- Total scan time is 2D spin-echo imaging is determined by the product of TR, the number of phase-encoding steps (N_{pe}), and the number of excitations per phase-encoding step (N_{ex}).
- In multislice SE, many slices are collected in the same scan time as a single slice. The maximum number of slices is determined by TR and TE, the longer TR and the shorter TE, the more slices that can be acquired.

References

1. Hendrick RE (1999) Image contrast and noise. In Stark DD, Bradley WG (eds). Magnetic Resonance Imaging, 3rd Edition St. Louis: Mosby Publishing Co. Volume 1, pp 43–68.
2. Hahn EL (1950) Spin echoes. Physical Review 80: 580.
3. Haacke EM, Brown RW, Thompson MR, et.al. (1999) Magnetic Resonance Imaging: Physical Principles and Sequence Design. New York: John Wiley & Sons, especially Ch 8, p 118–129.
4. Crooks L, Hoenninger J, Arakawa M, et.al. High resolution magnetic resonance imaging: technical concepts and their implementation. Radiology 1984; 150; 163–171.

Chapter 5
Gradient Echo Sequences and 3D Imaging

Gradient-echo imaging was introduced in 1985 by Frahm and Haase as a way to speed image acquisition.[1–5] The gradient echo pulse sequence is simpler than the spin-echo sequence and can be performed more rapidly, enabling a variety of tasks, including real-time MRI, flow imaging[3,4], and 3D or volume imaging.[5] There are two primary differences between spin-echo and gradient echo imaging. In spin-echo imaging, a 90° pulse is used on each repetition of the pulse sequence to flip all longitudinal magnetization into the transverse plane. In gradient-echo imaging, a smaller flip angle is used to leave some longitudinal magnetization undisturbed.[6,7] For example, if a 30° flip angle is used (Figure 5.1), then half of the longitudinal magnetization ($M_0 \sin 30°$) is flipped into the transverse plane where it can contribute to measurable signal. On the other hand, 87% of the longitudinal magnetization ($M_0 \cos 30°$) remains along the direction of B_0, so little time is needed to let the longitudinal magnetization recover along B_0 before beginning the next repetition of the pulse sequence in gradient-echo imaging. This means that TR, the time between successive repetitions of the pulse sequence, can be made much shorter, which reduces total imaging time.

The second difference is that while spin-echo imaging uses a 180° pulse to form a spin echo, gradient-echo imaging uses gradient reversal to form a gradient echo.[7] In fact, if a 180° pulse were used in conjunction with a partial flip angle, it would be counterproductive, because a 180° flip angle would take all remaining longitudinal magnetization and flip it in the direction opposite to B_0. If this were done, even longer delay times (TR) would be needed to permit longitudinal magnetization to recover. A gradient echo leaves the longitudinal magnetization undisturbed so that a large fraction of the full longitudinal magnetization, M_0, is immediately available for the next repetition of the pulse sequence.

The gradient-echo concept was discussed briefly in Chapter 4, where it was pointed out that the spin-echo sequence reforms signal at the "echo" by performing both a spin-echo (due to the 180° pulse) and a gradient-echo (due to reversal of the frequency-encoding gradient). In gradient-echo imaging, only the reversal of the frequency-encoding gradient is used to form a signal echo, as shown in Figure 5.2. This has the advantage of leaving the remaining longitudinal magnetization undisturbed but has the disadvantage of making the measured signal somewhat less robust than in spin-echo imaging. Spin-echo imaging is relatively immune to the effects of static

R.E. Hendrick (ed.), *Breast MRI: Fundamentals and Technical Aspects.*
© Springer 2008

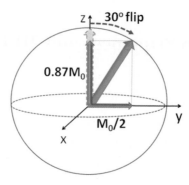

Figure 5.1 Schematic of the magnetization vector after a 30° pulse. If the longitudinal magnetization is M_0 before the RF pulse (dotted vertical arrow), then after a 30° pulse, the component of magnetization in the transverse plane is $M_0\sin(30°) = M_0/2$, while the component of magnetization remaining in the longitudinal direction is $M_0\cos(30°) = 0.87\,M_0$. This amount of longitudinal magnetization is left undisturbed and grows during echo formation and signal measurement, so that little or no additional time is needed to permit recovery of longitudinal magnetization before the next repetition of the pulse sequence in gradient-echo imaging.

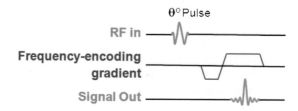

Figure 5.2 Schematic of reversal of the frequency-encoding gradient to form a "gradient echo". The frequency-encoding gradient is applied first in one direction (here negatively), which dephases transverse magnetization, then in the opposite direction (here positively), which rephrases transverse magnetization. Peak echo signal occurs when the area under the positive gradient lobe matches the area in the previously applied negative gradient lobe.

magnetic field inhomogeneities and magnetic susceptibility artifacts because of the 180° pulse, while these magnetic non-uniformities degrade the signal in gradient-echo imaging. Figure 5.3 illustrates the difference between a T1-weighted spin-echo image and a T1-weighted gradient echo image of a normal breast.

The Gradient-echo Pulse Sequence Diagram

The pulse sequence diagram for gradient-echo imaging is shown in Figure 5.4. As in the spin-echo diagram, the top line represents RF pulses sent into the patient. In gradient-echo imaging, the 90° pulse has been replaced by a θ-degree pulse, where

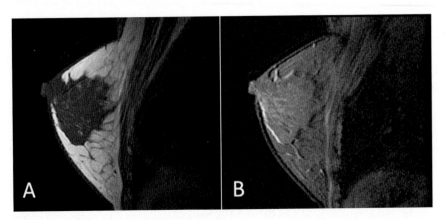

Figure 5.3 (A) T1-weighted spin-echo image (TR = 300 ms, TE = 9 ms) of a normal breast. (B) T1-weighted gradient-echo image (TR = 200 ms, TE = 9.3 ms, flip angle = 20°) of a normal breast. Both images had the same spatial parameters: 256 × 256 matrix, 3 mm slice thickness, and were acquired without fat-suppression. The artifacts at the interfaces of fat and water are chemical shift artifacts, described in Chapter 11 and further illustrated in Figure 11.8.

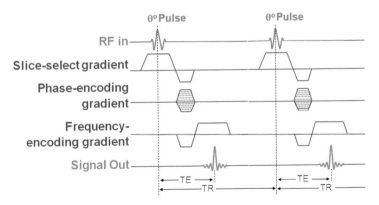

Figure 5.4 The 2D (planar) gradient-echo pulse sequence diagram. As with previous pulse-sequence diagrams, time flows from left to right. The top line shows RF pulses sent into the patient, which in the case of gradient-echo imaging is an evenly spaced series of θ° pulses, with time TR between each pair of θ° RF pulses. The next three lines show the slice-select, phase-encoding, and frequency-encoding gradients, respectively. The bottom line shows signal echoes and signal measurement symmetrically spaced around each signal echo at time TE. (From Hendrick RE. (7) Adapted with permission from Elsevier).

θ is an angle between 0° and 90°. The 180° pulse is completely absent in gradient-echo imaging.

The next three lines in Figure 5.4 show that the gradient manipulations in gradient-echo imaging are nearly identical to those in spin-echo imaging. Slice-selection, phase-encoding, and frequency-encoding are all performed in the same way as in spin-echo imaging. With the absence of a 180° pulse, it is reversal of the frequency-encoding gradient that reforms the signal echo shown on the bottom line of the diagram. It is not necessary to reverse the frequency-encoding gradient at exactly TE/2. The maximum signal echo forms when the area under the positive lobe of the frequency encoding gradient equals the area under the negative lobe that precedes it. The point at which negative and positive lobes are equal defines the center of the gradient-echo, and signal is measured at time TE for a sampling time T_s. Multiple repetitions of the basic gradient-echo pulse sequence are required, each with a different amount of phase encoding, to provide adequate data to reconstruct a gradient-echo image. As in spin-echo imaging, TR is the time between the start of each succeeding repetition of the gradient-echo pulse sequence.

The behavior of longitudinal and transverse magnetization in a gradient-echo pulse sequence is shown in Figure 5.5, where a flip angle of 30° is assumed. The first 30° pulse results in $M_0\sin(30°) = M_0/2$ being flipped into the transverse plane, while $M_0\cos(30°) = 0.87\,M_0$ remains along the longitudinal direction just after the 30° pulse. In the short interval TR, slightly more longitudinal magnetization recovers so that on the next repetition of the 30° pulse, the longitudinal magnetization is between $0.87\,M_0$ and M_0. After a few repetitions of the gradient-echo sequence, the longitudinal magnetization attains an equilibrium or "steady-state" level that is constant on each subsequent repetition of the pulse sequence. As a result, there is a fixed influence of T1 on the gradient-echo signal, since a fixed amount of longitudinal magnetization is flipped into the transverse plane each time the basic pulse sequence is repeated.

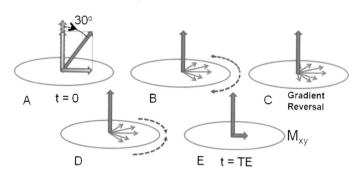

Figure 5.5 The behavior of longitudinal and transverse magnetization in a gradient-echo pulse sequence where $\theta = 30°$. (A) At $t = 0$, the 30° pulse flips half the longitudinal magnetization into the transverse plane, leaving 87% of the longitudinal magnetization along the direction of B_0. (B) During the interval between t=0 and gradient reversal, the transverse magnetization dephases due to T2* relaxation (true T2 plus any magnetic field inhomogeneities within a voxel) plus the effects of applied gradients. (C) Gradient reversal occurs. Note that gradient reversal leaves longitudinal magnetization undisturbed. (D) during the subsequent interval, dephasing due to the effects of applied gradients is reversed, while other T2* dephasing effects continue. (E) At $t = TE$, peak echo signal occurs due to gradient reversal. Note that longitudinal magnetization has regrown slightly from $t = 0$ and is ready for another $\theta = 30°$ pulse without need for a long TR to get recovery of the longitudinal magnetization. (From Hendrick RE. (7) Adapted with permission from Elsevier).

Peak gradient-echo signal occurs at the time TE but depends on a different T2-type decay parameter, T2*, which is due to the irreversible effects of true T2-decay, along with signal loss due to magnetic field non-uniformities and magnetic susceptibility differences across a voxel. The frequency-encoding gradient is exactly reversed so that the effect of the frequency-encoding gradient on T2*-decay is cancelled out (see the fourth line of Figure 5.4). Similarly, the slice-select gradient, which must be turned on while the RF pulse is sent into the patient, is reversed so that the slice-select gradient does not contribute to faster T2*-decay across the voxel (second line of Figure 5.4). Any other causes of magnetic non-uniformities during the time TE, however, will add to true T2 effects and increase the rate of T2* decay. The strength of the peak gradient-echo signal at time TE is given by the equation:

$$M_{xy}(TE) = M_{xy}(0)e^{-TE/T2^*} \tag{5.1}$$

$M_{xy}(0)$ is the amount of magnetization flipped into the transverse plane by the θ-degree pulse. Note that T2* controls the rate of decay of transverse magnetization during the time interval TE after the θ-degree pulse. Because T2* contains additional causes of transverse magnetization dephasing beyond true T2-decay, T2* < T2.

Variants of Gradient-echo Imaging

Before we discuss contrast in gradient-echo imaging, it is important to mention that there are a number of variants of gradient-echo imaging, depending on how the transverse magnetization is treated after signal measurement and before the next θ-degree pulse. If transverse magnetization is eliminated or "spoiled" before starting the next repetition of the pulse sequence, then fast low-angle shot (FLASH) imaging or "spoiled" gradient-recall steady-state gradient (spoiled-GRASS or SPGR) imaging is being performed.[3] This is the type of gradient-echo imaging described above and the type used for most breast imaging, including 3D imaging, as it delivers the strongest T1-weighting of the different variants of gradient-echo imaging. Recall that T1-weighting is needed because the effect of gadolinium-chelate administration is greatest on T1 (rather than T2 or T2*), so enhancing lesions show up best on T1-weighted images.

Transverse magnetization can be "spoiled" by making TR sufficiently long (several times T2*, which in breast tissue would be 100 to 200 ms) so that there is little or no transverse magnetization present on the next repetition of the gradient echo sequence. If shorter TR values are desired, the transverse magnetization can be spoiled by applying a series of gradient pulses or RF pulses after signal measurement but before the start of the next sequence so that the transverse magnetization is intentionally erased.

There are several other variants of gradient-echo imaging that fall under the general category of "coherent" or "steady-state" gradient-echo imaging. In this form of gradient-echo imaging, the transverse magnetization is not spoiled but feeds back into the signal that is measured on the next repetition of the pulse sequence. These variants will be discussed briefly later. We will now discuss spoiled gradient-echo imaging in detail, as it is the type of gradient-echo sequence used for T1-weighted contrast-enhanced breast imaging.

Signal Dependence on TR, TE, and θ in Spoiled Gradient-echo Imaging

The complete signal dependence of spoiled gradient-echo imaging on TR, TE, and θ is:

$$S_{ge}(TR,TE,\theta) = \frac{N[H]\sin(\theta)(1-e^{-TR/T1})e^{-TE/T2^*}}{(1-e^{-TR/T1}\cos(\theta))} \tag{5.2}$$

Just as in spin-echo imaging, measured signal strength is directly proportional to the spin-density of the voxel, N[H]. The T2*-term described above, $e^{-TE/T2^*}$, is also a multiplicative factor in the gradient-echo signal expression, as the T2-term was in spin-echo imaging. The only change is that in gradient-echo imaging, T2* replaces T2.

The biggest change between spin-echo and gradient-echo imaging is that the T1-factor of spin-echo imaging is replaced by a factor that depends both on T1 and θ in gradient-echo imaging:

$$T1\text{-}Factor = \frac{\sin(\theta)\left(1-e^{-TR/T1}\right)}{(1-e^{-TR/T1}\cos(\theta))} \tag{5.3}$$

If θ = 90°, then sin(90°) = 1 and cos(90°) = 0, so the T1-factor just reduces to $(1-e^{-TR/T1})$, the same T1-factor as in spin-echo imaging. Then the signal from gradient-echo imaging is:

$$M_{ge}(TR,TE,90°) = N[H](1-e^{-TR/T1})e^{-TE/T2^*}, \tag{5.4}$$

which is identical to the spin-echo sequence expression (see Eq. 4.3) except that T2* has replaced T2. The signal from gradient-echo imaging with a 90° pulse will be less than that from a spin-echo sequence with the same TR and TE, since T2* < T2. The signal from gradient-echo imaging with less than a 90° pulse will be even smaller because the T1-factor is less than one for θ < 90°. The main advantage of gradient-echo imaging, however, is that its shorter TR values speed image acquisition.

Figure 5.6 shows the dependence of the spoiled gradient-echo T1-factor on TR for several different θ values and on θ for several different TR values. It is apparent from these graphs that in spoiled gradient-echo imaging, the T1-factor is more stongly affected by θ than by TR.

In spoiled gradient-echo imaging, heavily T1-weighted images, as used in contrast-enhanced breast imaging, are achieved by selecting TE to be as short as

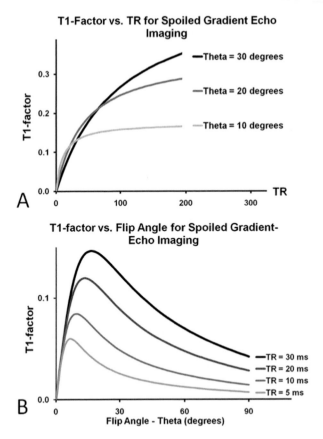

Figure 5.6 The T1-factor in spoiled gradient-echo imaging. (A) Dependence of the T1-factor on TR for several different θ values. (B) Dependence of the T1-factor on θ for several different TR values.

possible to minimize T2* weighting. Signal is maximized in T1-weighted spoiled gradient-echo imaging by setting TR and θ in a coupled manner according to the formula:

$$\theta_{max} = \cos^{-1}(e^{-TR/T1}), \tag{5.5}$$

where θ_{max} is the flip angle that maximizes signal for a given user-selected TR in gradient-echo imaging and T1 is the longitudinal relaxation time of the tissue of interest (see Figure 5.7). This angle that maximizes signal is referred to as the "Ernst angle," after Richard R. Ernst, 1991 Nobel laureate in chemistry for his work on pulsed NMR spectroscopy.

Short TR is desired to speed image acquisition and to maximize signal-to-noise ratios in gradient-echo imaging. For those short TR values, according to Eq. 5.5,

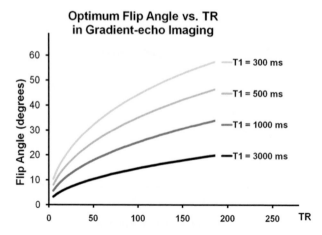

Figure 5.7 The dependence on TR of the Ernst angle, θ_{max}, the flip angle that maximizes signal in spoiled gradient-echo imaging, for various T1 values.

maximum contrast is achieved by making the flip angle relatively small. Consequently, to maximize the signal from a gadolinium-containing enhancing breast lesion (with a T1 of approximately 300 ms), for TR set at 5 ms, θ_{max} is 10°. For longer TR values, the optimum flip angle increases, as shown in Figure 5.7. This figure shows that at the same TR value, the signal from tissues with longer T1 values are maximized by using even smaller flip angles.

Contrast in Spoiled Gradient-echo Pulse Sequences

For contrast-enhanced breast imaging, the goal is to maximize the contrast between enhancing lesions and background breast tissues in subtracted images where pre-contrast images have been subtracted from post-contrast images. Unenhanced background breast tissue will have no signal in properly acquired and subtracted images and will therefore be black. The goal of selecting gradient-echo imaging parameters is to maximize the signal difference between an unenhanced breast cancer in pre-contrast images and an enhanced breast cancer in post-contrast images, so that enhancing lesions will have maximum contrast against the black background. Let us assume that an unenhanced breast cancer has a T1 of 1000 ms and a T2* of 80 ms, and that an enhanced breast cancer has a T1 of 300 ms and a T2* of 40 ms because gadolinium chelates have shortened both T1 and T2*. Because the only difference is the uptake of contrast agent, the spin density will remain the same between unenhanced and enhanced states of the same lesion. We can optimize conspicuity of the enhancing lesion in subtracted images by maximizing the signal difference between an enhanced and an unenhanced breast cancer. This signal difference is plotted as a function of θ for several choices of TR in

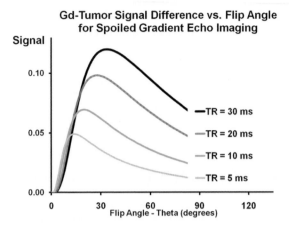

Figure 5.8 Signal difference between enhanced breast cancer and an unenhanced breast cancer in spoiled gradient-echo imaging, assuming TE = 2 ms, the unenhanced breast cancer has a T1 of 1000 ms and a T2* of 80 ms, and the enhanced breast cancer has a T1 of 300 ms and a T2* of 40 ms. Signal difference is plotted versus θ for several different TR values.

Figure 5.8, assuming that TE = 2 ms (the TE value affects the height of the each curve in Figure 5.8, but does not affect the locations at which maxima occur, since that depends only on the T1-factor). Note that the contrast curves in Figure 5.8 are similar in shape to the signal curves in Figure 5.6, but the maximum of each curve has shifted toward a slightly higher flip angle in the contrast curves in Figure 5.8. The slight shift in maxima is because we are plotting the difference in signals between two tissues (an enhanced and an unenhanced cancer) rather than simply maximizing the signal from a single tissue (an enhancing cancer). If our assumptions about T1-values of enhanced and unenhanced cancers are correct, Figure 5.8 indicates that for a TR of 5 ms, the flip angle that would maximize enhancing lesion conspicuity in subtracted images is approximately 15°, while for a TR of 10 ms, the optimum flip angle is approximately 20°.

Steady-state Gradient-echo Imaging

A variant of gradient-echo imaging that differs from spoiled gradient echo imaging is "coherent" or "steady-state" gradient echo imaging. In this form of gradient-echo imaging, the transverse magnetization is not spoiled but is intentionally fed back into the longitudinal magnetization so that it can affect the signal measured on the next repetition of the pulse sequence. The term "coherent" or "steady-state" gradient-echo imaging reflects this feedback of transverse magnetization into the longitudinal magnetization. Gradient-recalled acquisition in the steady-state (GRASS) and fast imaging with steady-state precession (FISP) are manufacturer's names for coherent or steady-state gradient-echo imaging. The signal expression in steady-state gradient echo imaging is slightly different than that in Eq. (5.2). In brief, for small flip angles and short TE values, steady-state gradient-echo imaging is primarily spin-density weighted. For larger flip angles, this sequence is predominately weighted by the T2/T1 ratio, which tends to be higher (so signal is brighter) for fat and for fluids such as CSF and non-bloody cysts. Steady-state gradient-echo sequences with longer TE values are sometimes used to obtain T2/T1-weighted images that closely resemble T2-weighted images. To date, these sequences have not been used much in breast MRI.

Total Acquisition Time in 2D Gradient-echo Imaging

The time it takes to collect a 2D gradient-echo image is given by the same formula as for spin-echo imaging. The pulse sequence must be repeated enough times, each time with a different phase-encoding gradient strength, to collect adequate data for a complete image. Thus, the formula for total imaging time is:

$$T_{total} = (TR)(N_{pe})(N_{ex}), \tag{5.6}$$

where N_{pe} is the number of phase-encoding steps and N_{ex} is the number of repetitions of each phase-encoding step. In gradient-echo imaging, N_{ex} is usually 1, with the caveat that N_{ex} can be set to be between 0.5 and 1 on some MR scanners (eg, GE), indicating that phase-symmetry (half-Fourier or three-quarters-Fourier imaging; see Chapter 3) is being used to further speed image acquisition.

Because there is no need to wait for recovery of the longitudinal magnetization to get adequate signal, the TR values used with gradient-echo pulse sequences can be much shorter than for spin-echo. While the shortest TR values used in spin-echo are typically 200 to 500 ms, in gradient echo imaging TR values as short as 3 to 5 ms can be used. With TR = 5 ms, N_{pe} = 256, and N_{ex} = 1, the time required to collect a single slice gradient-echo image is:

$$T_{total} = (TR)(N_{pe})(N_{ex}) = (0.005s)(256)(1) = 1.28\,s. \tag{5.7}$$

The limit on how short TR can be has to do with gradient rise times and rates of data collection. Very fast systems have been designed to perform gradient-echo imaging in near "real-time" (20 to 30 frames per second, or with total imaging times of 0.05 to 0.033 seconds) with limited spatial resolution. This "MR fluoroscopy" technology has the potential to guide placement of needles for marking, sampling, or guiding treatment of lesions in real-time, but is not widely available on existing commercial systems.

With very short TR values, there is not sufficient time for multi-slice acquisitions. In fast gradient-echo imaging, collection of multiple 2D images is achieved by sequential single-slice acquisitions at different locations in the patient. For example, with a single-slice acquisition time of just 1.28 s, it would be feasible to obtain a series of 30 to 40 gradient-echo slices in just under a minute. By reducing in-plane spatial resolution and using half-Fourier techniques (where only slightly more than half of the phase-space samples are obtained), 30 to 40 slices could be obtained in a single breath-hold (10 to 20 s).

For longer TR values in gradient-echo imaging, the same multi-slice approach used in spin-echo imaging can be applied. As with SE, the limit on the number of slices depends on TR, TE, and the time constant that reflects the time required to complete data acquisition, turn off the slice-select gradient, and re-initiate the pulse sequence. If the time constant for those operations is T_c, then the maximum number of slices that can be acquired is:

$$N_{Slices}(max) = TR/(TE+T_c), \qquad (5.8)$$

For example, with TR = 200 ms, TE = 3 ms, and T_c = 2 ms, the maximum number of slices would be:

$$N_{Slices}(max) = TR/(TE+T_c) = (200 \, ms)/(3 \, ms + 2 \, ms) = 40 \, slices. \qquad (5.9)$$

This means that for longer TR values, gradient-echo image acquisitions could by multi-slice acquisitions where a large number of T1-weighted images could be acquired in the same time needed for a single slice. According to Equation 5.6, the time to obtain these 40 slices with multislice gradient-echo imaging with 256 phase-encoding steps and N_{ex} = 1 would be:

$$T_{total} = (TR)(N_{pe})(N_{ex}) = (0.20s)(256)(1) = 51.2 \, s.$$

This multislice approach with longer TR has a signal advantage over the sequential single-slice gradient-echo approach with shorter TR. To obtain 40 slices with each approach takes exactly the same amount of time: 51.2 s for the multislice approach with TR = 200 ms and, by coincidence, 51.2 s for the sequential single-slice method with TR = 5 ms (see Eq 5.7): 1.28 s × 40 slices = 51.2 s with the same spatial resolution of 256 phase-encoding steps. In multislice imaging with TR = 200 ms, however, the signal is 12.4 times higher than in sequential single-slice imaging with a TR = 5 ms, assuming T1 = 300 ms and that flip angles are optimized for each TR value: for TR = 5 ms, θ_{max} = 10°; for TR = 200 ms, θ_{max} = 59°. Thus, if 2D gradient-echo imaging was being performed, it would make sense to use longer TR values (and larger flip angles) in a multi-slice acquisition than to acquire multiple single-slice acquisitions with short TR (and small flip angles).

3D Gradient-echo Imaging

One of the biggest advantages of the gradient-echo pulse sequence is that it can be performed quickly enough to enable 3DFT (volume) data acquisitions. In 3DFT imaging, a volume or slab of tissue is excited, rather than merely a thin slice of tissue. This is done by using a broader-band RF pulse or a weaker slice-select gradient and

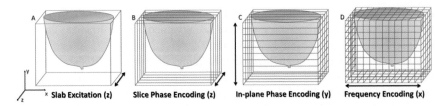

Slab Excitation (z)   Slice Phase Encoding (z)   In-plane Phase Encoding (y)   Frequency Encoding (x)

Figure 5.9 Schematic of 3DFT image acquisition. (A) The slice-select gradient is used to select a slab or volume of tissue. (B) Phase-encoding gradients are used to resolve tissue in both the slice-select direction and (C) in-plane phase encoding direction. (D) Frequency-encoding is used to resolve tissue in the other in-plane direction.

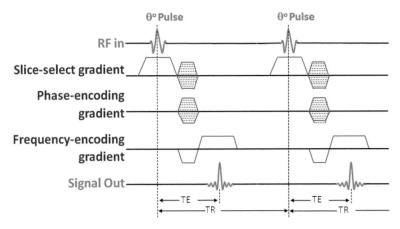

Figure 5.10 The 3D (volume) gradient-echo pulse sequence diagram. A different amount of phase-encoding is used in both the slice-select and in-plane phase-encoding direction on each repetition of the pulse sequence.

thereby selecting a wider slab of tissue each time a transmitted RF pulse is sent into the patient (Figure 5.9A). Two separate phase-encoding gradients are used, one in the slice-select direction (Figure 5.9B) and the other in one of the two in-plane directions (Figure 5.9C) to resolve the volume into individual voxels. Frequency-encoding is still used to distinguish tissue in the other in-plane direction (Figure 5.9D).

The pulse sequence diagram for 3D gradient-echo imaging is shown in Figure 5.10. As with 2D imaging, the slice-select gradient is turned on during each RF transmission. In 3D imaging, however, an entire volume (or slab) of tissue is excited with each RF pulse. Following slab excitation, the slice-select gradient and in-plane phase-encoding gradient are turned on multiple times, each time with a different gradient strength, to resolve the excited volume into slices within the slab and pixels within each slice. The frequency-encoding gradient, as in 2D imaging, is turned on during signal measurement from the entire volume, to resolve each slice into strips the frequency-encoding direction.

The time required for performing 3D gradient-echo imaging is:

$$T_{total} = (TR)(N_{slices})(N_{pe})(N_{ex}), \tag{5.10}$$

where the new term N_{slices} is the number of slices in the excited volume. This additional multiplicative time factor is due to the need to use phase-encoding in a second direction, the slice-select direction, to distinguish slices in the excited slab, as shown in Figure 5.9B. Enough phase-encoding steps must be used to distinguish one slice from another in the slice direction for each phase-encoding step performed in-plane (to distinguish each slice into pixels in the phase-encoding direction) (Figure 5.9C), so the two phase resolution factors, N_{slices} and N_{pe}, are multiplicative.

For example, in transaxial breast imaging, a 3D volume can be selected to cover both breasts. This can be done by selecting 64 3 mm slices (N_{slices} = 64), which would cover 3×64 mm = 192 mm = 19.2 cm in the head-to-foot direction. With TR = 5 ms, N_{pe} = 256, and N_{ex} = 1,

$$T_{total} = (TR)(N_{slices})(N_{pe})(N_{ex}) = (5\,\text{ms})(64)(256)(1) = 82\,\text{s}. \tag{5.11}$$

If the axial 3D gradient-echo pulse sequence described above is repeated without a time gap between successive repetitions, it provides 82 s (1.4 minute) temporal resolution. It is easy to see that with TR values typical of spin-echo imaging, for example TR = 200 ms, performing a 3D imaging sequence with the same spatial parameters as above would take 40 times longer (200 ms/5 ms = 40), and the total imaging time would be 3277 seconds (54.6 minutes), which would be impractical. Gradient-echo imaging with short TR values makes 3D imaging feasible and is used almost exclusively for contrast-enhanced breast MRI.

The 3D approach has several other advantages. Unlike 2D excitations, the slice profiles of 3D slices separated by phase-encoding are rectangular (meaning that an equal contribution to signal comes from every hydrogen nucleus in the slice) rather than Gaussian (where most of the signal comes from the center of the slice and little signal from the edges). Figure 5.11 illustrates this difference. As a result, more of each slice's hydrogen nuclei contribute to the image in 3D acquisitions. Second, in 3D imaging, slices are contiguous rather than having gaps between them. Most importantly, 3D imaging is more efficient than 2D imaging because signal is being collected from an entire volume of tissue, rather than from just a single slice, on each signal measurement. This improves the SNR of 3D imaging compared to 2D imaging, at least for the same TR value. For example, if 3D imaging is compared to sequential 2D single-slice acquisition with the same TR value, each planar image acquired in 3D would have a factor of $(N_{slices})^{1/2}$ higher SNR than each 2D image, not accounting for slice profile differences. In the case cited above where N_{slices} = 64, this would be a factor of 8 difference in SNR. Slice profile differences would contribute another factor of 1.5 to 2.0 advantage in SNR to 3D acquisitions, for an overall SNR factor of 12–16 for 3D compared to 2D acquisitions. As we saw in the previous section, using a multislice 2D approach with TR = 200 ms enabled the acquisition of 40 slices in the same time as 40 slices could be obtained in a sequential single-slice mode with a TR = 5 ms, but with 12.4 times the signal with the

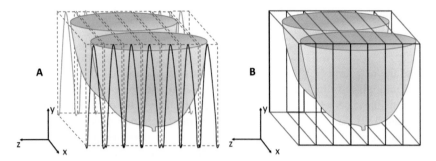

Figure 5.11 Schematic of slice profiles in (A) 2D versus (B) 3D image acquisitions. In A, 2D (planar) acquisition slice profiles are Gaussian (solid black curves), meaning that more signal comes from tissue at the center of each slice than near the edges. Here, the 2D acquisition is shown to have slight gaps between selected slices (dotted blue lines), which is used commonly to reduce cross-talk between slices. In B, 3D (volume) acquisition slice profiles are always rectangular and slices are always contiguous, as shown by the solid black lines. This means that signal derives uniformly from all tissue in each slice, without cross-talk.

multi-slice approach. Our estimate above is that the 3D approach would generate 12 to 16 times the SNR as in a single slice approach with a TR of 5 ms, so the signal or SNR in a 3D approach (taking 82 s) would be comparable to or slightly higher than that in a 2D multi-slice approach taking 51 s.

The main disadvantage of 3D imaging is that it requires longer acquisition times, since phase encoding must be used to distinguish tissue into voxels in both the slice-select and in-plane phase encoding directions. A secondary disadvantage of 3D imaging is that the gradient-echo sequence is more susceptible to signal loss due to magnetic field inhomogeneities (through T2* decay) and artifacts (primarily magnetic susceptibility artifacts) than is the SE sequence. Still, the efficiency of collecting a volume of data on each signal acquisition, rather than single slices of data, overcome these disadvantages and make 3D gradient-echo imaging the sequence of choice for contrast-enhanced breast MRI.

Chapter Take-home Points

- Gradient-echo pulse sequences speed image acquisitions by using partial flip angles (less than 90°) and gradient-reversal to form a signal echo, leaving longitudinal magnetization undisturbed after the initial RF pulse.
- The gradient-echo pulse sequence has three user-selectable parameters: TR, TE, and flip angle θ.
- The T1-weighting of gradient echo imaging is determined primarily by θ and to a lesser extent by TR.
- The T2*-weighting of gradient-echo imaging is determined by TE.

- For contrast-enhanced breast MRI, T1-weighted gradient-echo imaging is performed by choosing a short TR, small flip angle (based on TR), and very short TE.
- The very short TR values enabled by gradient-echo imaging make 3D (volume) acquisitions feasible with scan times of a few minutes or less.
- Total scan time in 3D gradient-echo imaging is determined by the product of TR, the number of slices (N_{slice}), the number of in-plane phase-encoding steps (N_{pe}), and the number of excitations per phase-encoding step (N_{ex}).

References

1. Haase A, Frahm J, Matthaei D, et al. Regional physiological functions depicted by sequences of rapid magnetic resonance images. Lancet 1985; 2: 893.
2. Haase A, Frahm J, Matthaei D, et al. FLASH imaging. Rapid NMR imaging using low flip-angle pulses. J Magn Reson 1986; 67: 258–266.
3. Frahm J, Haase A, Matthaei D. Rapid NMR imaging of dynamic processes using the FLASH technique. Magn. Reson. Med 1986; 3: 321–327.
4. Haase A, Matthaei D, Hanicke W, et al. Dynamic digital subtraction MR imaging using the FLASH method. Radiology 1986; 160: 537–541.
5. Frahm J, Haase A, Matthaei D, et al. Rapid three dimensional MR imaging using the FLASH technique. J Comput. Assist. Tomogr. 1986; 10: 363–368.
6. Haacke EM, Tkach JA. Fast MR imaging: techniques and clinical applications. American Journal of Roentgenology 1990; 155: 951–964.
7. Hendrick RE. Image contrast and noise. In Stark DD, Bradley WG, eds. Magnetic Resonance Imaging, 3rd Edition. St. Louis: Mosby Publishing Co., 1999, Vol 1, Ch. 4, p. 43–68.

Suggested Reading

Frahm J, Haenicke W. Rapid scan techniques. In: Stark DD, Bradley WG, eds. Magnetic Resonance Imaging, 3rd edition. New York: C.V. Mosby Publishing, 1999:87–124.

Haacke EM, Brown RW, Thompson MR, et al. Magnetic Resonance Imaging: Physical Principles and Sequence Design. Ch 18. New York: John Wiley & Sons, 1999: 451–512.

Harms SE, Flamig DP, Hensley KL, et al. MR imaging of the breast with rotating delivery of excitation off-resonance: clinical experience with pathologic correlation. Radiology 1993; 187:493–501.

Heywang SH, Wolf A, Pruss E, et al. MR imaging of the breast with Gd-DTPA: use and limitations. Radiology 1989; 171:95–103.

Chapter 6
Fast-spin Echo, Echo Planar, Inversion Recovery, and Short-T1 Inversion Recovery Imaging

This chapter covers other pulse sequences used for breast MRI. Most sites use fast spin-echo (FSE), also sometimes called turbo spin-echo (TSE), in place of normal spin-echo (SE) sequences for both T1- and T2-weighted imaging, as FSE speeds image acquisition compared to SE.[1,2] Echo-planar imaging is an extremely fast imaging technique that has been used for cardiac imaging and in breast imaging research applications requiring very high temporal resolution at the cost of lower spatial resolution.[2,3] Echo-planar imaging has not found clinical application in breast imaging but may in the future as echo-planar techniques become more refined. Inversion-recovery has been used since the earliest days of clinical MRI to provide heavily T1-weighted images.[4,5] Short-TI inversion recovery (STIR) imaging is used by some breast MRI sites in place of T2-weighted SE or FSE, as STIR can provide more resilient fat-suppression than the chemical-shift techniques used in SE and FSE.[5-7] STIR has the added benefit of being the only pulse sequence in which T1, T2, and spin-density effects of diseased tissues add constructively to enhance image contrast. Each of these techniques will be described in this chapter.

Fast Spin-echo Imaging

Spin-echo imaging with multiple echoes has been used since the early days of clinical MRI. In multi-echo SE, additional echoes are collected after a 90° and 180° pair by applying additional 180° pulses to form additional echoes, as shown in Figure 6.1. In multi-echo SE imaging, different echo signals are compiled separately to form different images, each image having a different degree of T2-weighting due to different TE values. With long TR values, echoes with short TE are more spin-density weighted, while echoes at long TE are more T2-weighted. Unevenly spaced dual-echo SE imaging is sometimes used to collect both a long TR, short TE spin-density weighted first-echo image and the same long TR, long TE T2-weighted second echo image. In multi-echo SE, the same phase-encoding gradient is applied prior to all echoes following a 90° pulse.

R.E. Hendrick (ed.), *Breast MRI: Fundamentals and Technical Aspects.*
© Springer 2008

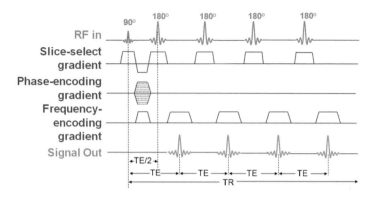

Figure 6.1 Basic pulse sequence for multi-echo spin-echo imaging, with 4 echoes per excitation pulse. In multi-echo SE, the phase-encoding gradient is applied prior to the first echo, but not between echoes. Each echo at a different TE value is compiled to a different image, so four images with four different degrees of T2W would result. For 256 × 256 spatial resolution, the basic pulse sequence would be repeated 256 times, each time with a different amount of phase-encoding.

Fast spin-echo was developed by Hennig in 1986 as RARE (rapid acquisition with relaxation enhancement).[1] It is now called FSE by some manufacturers (GE, Toshiba, Hitachi) and turbo spin-echo (TSE) by others (Siemens and Philips)[2]; here we will use the acronym FSE. In FSE, additional echoes are formed after each 90° RF pulse by applying additional 180° pulses, just as in multi-echo SE. In FSE, however, each echo collected after the 90° pulse is collected as a different phase-encoding view of a single image. The number of echoes collected after each 90° pulse is referred to as an echo-train length (ETL). For example, if four evenly spaced 180° pulses are applied after the 90° pulse to form four evenly spaced echoes, then the ETL=4. The total image acquisition time is reduced by a factor equal to the ETL. Acquiring more than one phase-encoding view per excitation means that more than one line in k-space is acquired after a single excitation pulse; this data collection method is referred to as "segmented k-space."

For 2D (planar) FSE imaging, the formula for total imaging time is:

$$T_{total} = (TR)(N_{pe})(N_{ex})/ETL. \tag{6.1}$$

Thus, with an ETL of 4, the total image acquisition time can be reduced by a factor of 4 compared to SE imaging with the same TR setting and the same number of phase-encoding steps. It makes no sense to use a N_{ex} greater than 1 with FSE, since the goal is to speed image acquisition. It is more likely that partial-Fourier techniques might be combined with FSE, so N_{ex} might be set between 0.5 and 1.0 to further speed image acquisition.

Figure 6.2 illustrates the FSE pulse sequence with ETL=4, with the phase-encoding gradient applied just after each 180° pulse to make each echo a different phase-encoding view; just after each signal measurement, the phase-encoding gradient is reversed to help rephrase signal. In FSE, different echoes at different TE

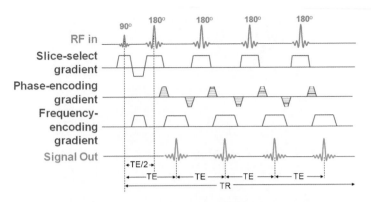

Figure 6.2 Basic pulse sequence for FSE, with ETL=4. For FSE, phase-encoding gradients are applied before each echo to permit collection of a different phase-encoding view with each echo. These different views are compiled to the same image, thus reducing the scan time by a factor equal to the ETL. For example, to achieve 256 × 256 spatial resolution, this basic pulse sequence would be repeated 64 times. Each repetition of the basic pulse sequence would collect four horizontal lines in k-space.

values provide different degrees of T2-weighting to different phase-encoding views. This gives FSE images a different overall weighting than the TE$_{eff}$ might indicate (based on SE imaging) and can result in slight image blurring compared to SE images.

Typical ETL factors range from 2 to 32. Higher ETL factors usually are used for T2-weighted FSE than for T1-weighted FSE because the use of larger ETLs extends the effective TE, adding greater T2-weighting. This is desirable in T2-weighted FSE, but not in T1-weighted FSE, since T2-weighting counteracts T1-weighting. Larger ETL values also can cause greater image blurring. Figure 6.3 compares SE to FSE on a normal volunteer for T1-weighted imaging, demonstrating little difference in image quality or contrast. Figure 6.4 compares FSE with a low ETL to FSE with a high ETL for T2-weighted imaging, again with only slight changes in image appearance. In general, it is not practical to perform SE imaging with the long TRs used in FSE (> 3 seconds), so typically FSE rather than SE is used for T2W imaging. For example, if SE had been used with the TR value and spatial parameters specified in Figure 6.4, image acquisition would have taken over 17 minutes. With FSE and ETL=4, image acquisition time was less than 5 minutes.

Attention to details within the FSE sequence can offset some of the variable T2-weighting effects caused by collecting different echoes at different TE values for the same image. Recall from Chapter 3 that most of the contrast in an image comes from image data collected near the center of k-space (that is, for low spatial frequency k_x and k_y). This feature of MR imaging is used to advantage in FSE by making sure that the views collected near the center of k-space (with the weakest phase-encoding gradients applied) are biased toward the desired weighting of the FSE sequence. For example, if T1-weighted FSE is prescribed, then in addition to

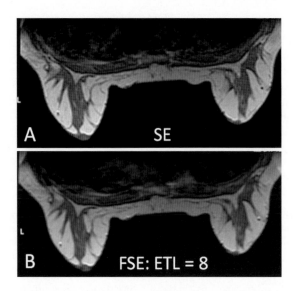

Figure 6.3 Comparison of T1-weighted SE and FSE in the same volunteer. (A) SE image with TR = 650 ms, TE = 8 ms. (B) FSE with ETL = 8, TR = 650 ms, TE_{eff} = 14 ms.

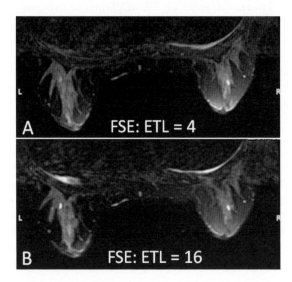

Figure 6.4 Comparison of T2-weighted FSE in the same volunteer. (A) FSE with ETL = 4, TR = 5.1 s, TE_{eff} = 56 ms. (B) FSE with ETL = 16, TR = 5.4 s, TE_{eff} = 84 ms.

using relatively short TR values and collecting echoes with short echo-to-echo time gaps (small TE values), the phase-encoding views with the smallest k_y values (assuming that the phase-encoding gradient is in the y-direction) are those with the shortest TE values. This shortens the effective TE and gives the image a more T1-weighted appearance.

Similarly, if a T2W FSE is prescribed, in addition to using longer TR and longer echo-to-echo gaps (longer TE values), the phase-encoding views with the smallest k_y values are collected at the longest possible TE values. This lengthens the effective TE and gives the FSE images a more T2-weighted appearance.

Since higher ETLs are used with T2-weighted images, which have longer TR values, the total time required for a T2-weighted FSE sequence is not that much greater than that required for a T1-weighted FSE. For example, for T1-weighted 2D FSE, TR might be set to 600 ms and ETL=4. For $N_{pe}=512$ and $N_{ex}=1$, the total imaging time would be:

$$T_{total} = (TR)(N_{pe})(N_{ex})/ETL = (600\,ms)(512)(1)/4 = 77\,s = 1.3\,min \qquad (6.2)$$

For a T2-weighted 2D FSE, TR might be set to 3000 ms and ETL=12. For the same N_{pe} and N_{ex} as above,

$$T_{total} = (TR)(N_{pe})(N_{ex})/ETL. = (3000\,ms)(512)(1)/16 = 128\,s = 2.1\,min \qquad (6.3)$$

One limitation of multislice FSE is that the number of slices that can be acquired with a given effective TE is smaller than that in multislice SE, since the echo train in FSE takes longer to collect then a single echo. In FSE, the number of slices that can be collected for a given TR is

$$N_{Slices}(max) = TR/(ETL*TE + T_c), \qquad (6.4)$$

where TE is the time spacing between successive echoes (not the effective TE) of the pulse sequence. For T1-weighted FSE, TE might be 5 ms, so for the example above (TR=600 ms, ETL=4) and with $T_c=4$ ms,

$$N_{Slices}(max) = TR/((ETL)(TE)+T_c) = (600\,ms)/(4*5\,ms+4\,ms)$$
$$= (600\,ms)/(24\,ms) = 25\,slices$$

In the case of T2-weighted FSE, with TE=15 ms, TR=3000 ms, ETL=12, and $T_c=4$ ms, the maximum number of slices would be:

$$N_{Slices}(max) = TR/((ETL)(TE)+T_c) = (3000\,ms)/(12*15\,ms+4\,ms)$$
$$= (3000\,ms)/(184\,ms) = 16\,slices.$$

This might require doubling the total imaging time to 4.2 minutes if between 17 and 32 slices were prescribed, or tripling the total imaging time to 6.3 minutes if between 33 and 48 slices were prescribed. The number of slices required in a study is determined by the required range of anatomic coverage in the slice-select direction, the slice thickness, and the slice gap factor, which is the ratio of the gap between slices to the slice thickness. Typical gap factors are 10% to 25% (0.1 – 0.25) of the slice thickness.

$$\text{Number of Slices} = (\text{Range of Coverage})/((t_{slice})(1+\text{Gap Factor})) \qquad (6.5)$$

For transaxial breast imaging, the typical range of coverage in the slice-select direction is 12–18 cm, depending on breast size. For 15 cm of required coverage in the head-to-foot direction, 3 mm slices, and a 20% gap,

$$\text{Number of Slices} = (\text{Range of Coverage})/((t_{slice})(1+\text{Gap Factor}))$$
$$= (15\,\text{cm})/((3\,\text{mm})(1.2)) = (150\,\text{mm})/(3.6\,\text{mm}) = 42 \text{ slices}$$

The MR technologist setting up the scanning protocol should adjust TR and ETL to minimize imaging time while achieving the desired slice thickness and number of slices needed for full breast coverage in FSE imaging. For example, with exactly the timing and spatial parameters prescribed above, three measures of the 2D T2-weighted FSE sequence would be required to cover 15 cm in the slice-select direction by collecting 42 slices, which would take 6.3 minutes (3*2.1 minutes) (see Equation 6.3). By increasing TR to 3870 ms with all other parameters remaining the same, 21 slices could be obtained per measure. Then collecting 42 slices would require only 2 measures of the T2-weighted FSE sequence and would take a total time of 5.5 minutes (2*3.87 s*512/(12*60 s/min), which would be slightly more efficient (and also slightly more T2-weighted) than the 3 measures required if TR were kept at exactly 3000 ms.

Another option would be to increase slice thickness and gap spacing between slices, but increasing either of these to obtain more efficient imaging times can have adverse effects on image quality. For example, with T2-weighted FSE keeping TR = 3000 ms, slice thickness would need to be increased to 4.0 mm with a 20% gap (which would increase the gap from 0.6 mm to 0.8 mm) so that only 32 slices would be needed to cover 15 cm. This would then require only 2 measures of the T2-weighted FSE sequence, reducing the total acquisition time to 4.2 minutes but at the cost of greater partial volume effects (due to thicker slices) and larger gaps between slices.

Echo-planar Imaging

Echo planar imaging (EPI) is the ultimate extension of fast imaging, where the echo-train length equals the number of phase encoding views desired to form the image ($\text{ETL} = N_{pe}$). In true EPI, the entire image is collected after a single 90° RF pulse (or set of excitation pulses). In EPI, repeated echoes are formed by gradient reversal rather than by 180° pulses. The use of a 90° RF pulse means that the maximum possible magnetization, M_0, is flipped into the transverse plane prior to the collection of multiple echoes. This also means that there is no TR, since there is only one excitation pulse per slice, and, as a result, no T1-weighting to the conventional echo-planar sequence. EPI acquired in this fashion can be either spin-density or T2*-weighted.

Historically, EPI predates FSE and even SE sequences. EPI was developed in the earliest days of MRI research by Dr. Peter Mansfield, who made many contributions to the development of clinical MRI and improved pulse sequences for clinical imaging.[3] Dr. Mansfield shared the 2003 Nobel Prize in Physiology or Medicine with Dr. Paul Lauterbur for his contributions to the development of MRI techniques.[8]

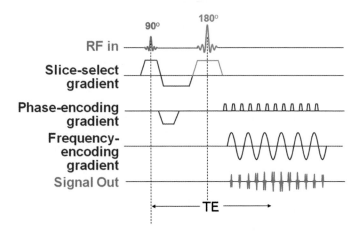

Figure 6.5 The pulse sequence diagram for echo-planar imaging. In traditional EPI, the 180° pulse and gradient lobe below it (both shaded lighter) are not present; in spin-echo EPI, they are all phase-encoding views are collected after a single excitation pulse. The frequency-encoding gradient is shown to oscillate during signal collection, forming a series of echoes. Peak echo signal occurs at time TE after the 90° pulse (and TE/2 after the 180° pulse). The phase-encoding gradient is blipped prior to each echo, so that each echo collects a different phase-encoding view.

The pulse sequence diagram for traditional EPI is shown in Figure 6.5. The repeated echoes are formed by read gradient reversal, as in gradient-echo imaging, but done rapidly and repeatedly after the initial 90° pulse. The phase-encoding gradient is turned on negatively prior to the collection of all echoes to start data collection with the most negative phase. Prior to each echo (after the first), the phase-encoding gradient is turned on very briefly or "blipped" so that each echo collects a different, slightly more positive phase-encoding view. This steps the data collection upward along the k_y-axis in k-space for each succeeding echo, as shown in Figure 6.6.

Because gradient-echoes are used, the decay parameter governing the strength of the signal at each repeated echo is T2*. If TE is the time between repeated echoes, then the transverse magnetization measured on the nth echo at time n(TE) will be:

$$M_n = M_0 e^{-n(TE)/T2*} \tag{6.6}$$

EPI can be biased toward spin-density weighting by making TE very short and limiting the number of echoes collected, which also limits spatial resolution in the phase-encoding direction. EPI is biased toward T2*-weighted imaging by making TE longer, which makes the effective TE longer. As in other pulse sequences, most of the contrast-weighting of the pulse sequence comes from the data collected near the center of k-space, where k_y is near zero. This means that the "effective TE" of the EPI sequence (thinking of TE as the degree of T2*-weighting, as in a gradient-echo pulse sequence) is near the middle of data acquisition, at n(TE)/2 (where the TE in this formula is the time gap between successive echoes). A limitation of EPI is that all n echoes, each of which represents a different phase-encoding view, must

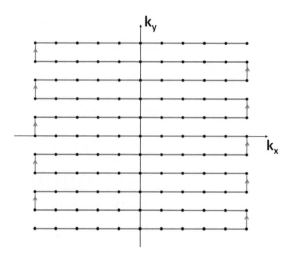

Figure 6.6 The k-space diagram for echo-planar imaging. Each echo in Figure 6.5 corresponds to collection of a horizontal line of k-space data. The negative phase-encoding gradient applied before data collection shifts data acquisition of the first echo to the bottom horizontal line of k-space. The gradient blip before each subsequent echo steps the horizontal line of acquired data upward, as shown by the arrows. Only 11 x- and y- points are shown in this diagram (instead of 64, 128, or more) to simplify the diagram.

be collected before the transverse magnetization disappears. Thus, n(TE) should not be greater than 2 or 3 times T2*.

Since an entire slice can be collected in 40 to 100 ms, EPI is typically implemented in a 2D format with sequential slice acquisition. With $T_{total} = 40$ ms, 40 slices can be acquired in 1.6 s. With sequential acquisition, each slice would have its full magnetization M_0 prior to excitation by the 90° pulse.

EPI can also be implemented in 3D format, with phase-encoding used to separate both slices and in-plane phase-encoding views.[2] In 3D implementation, there would be repeated excitations of the same volume so that different phase-encoding views could be used to separate tissue in the slice-select direction, so a TR value would be introduced as the time between successive volume excitations. If TR were comparable to or shorter than T1, then EPI would have some degree of T1-weighting. To minimize T2*-weighting, n(TE)/2 should be short compared to T2*.

Figure 6.7 illustrates 2D EPI in a breast volunteer. EPI is more typically used for body applications and it sometimes has limitations on the field-of-view (FOV), requiring larger FOV, and on matrix size, limiting the number of phase-encoding steps to 128. This means that rather large pixels are acquired, which limits its applicability to breast MRI. In this example, the sagittal EPI was acquired on a 20 cm FOV with 128 phase-encoding steps (vertically) and 256 frequency-encoding steps (left-to-right).

EPI can also be implemented in a spin-echo version, where initially a 90° and 180° pulse are applied, with subsequent echoes formed by gradient reversal of the frequency-encoding gradient while the phase-encoding gradient is blipped

Figure 6.7 Example of 2D EPI with a 256 (FE) × 128 (PE) matrix. Total acquisition time was 8 s for 11 slices.

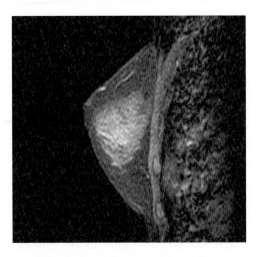

(Figure 6.5). In SE-EPI, the center of the gradient echoes should occur at the time of the spin-echo formed by the 180° pulse. SE-EPI is more resistant than EPI to magnetic field non-uniformities and magnetic susceptibility artifacts.

There are many different variations on ways to sample k-space in EPI, including applying a weak, constant phase-encoding gradient to acquire diagonal lines in k-space, multiple repetitions of EPI or SE-EPI to segment the collection of data in k-space, and use of oscillating gradients to further speed data acquisition. Typically, clinical breast MRI does not require the speed of EPI (Chapter 8) and seeks better spatial resolution and image quality than is often achievable with EPI (Chapter 9), so the sequence has not been used for clinical breast MRI.

Inversion Recovery and Short-T1 Inversion Recovery Imaging

Inversion recovery (IR) is one of the earliest imaging methods developed for clinical MRI.[5,6] It employs an initial 180° pulse, followed by either a single 90° pulse (IR) or by the 90° and 180° pair used in SE imaging (for IR spin-echo imaging, referred to as IRSE). IRSE is preferred over IR for clinical imaging and is shown in Figure 6.8. The time between the initial 180° pulse and the 90° pulse is TI, the inversion time. The signal echo is formed at time TE after the 90° pulse, just as in SE imaging. The time TR is the time between successive repetitions of the basic 180° - 90° - 180° pulse train.

The purpose of the initial 180° pulse is to invert the longitudinal magnetization opposite to its original direction, as shown in Figure 6.9A-J. Prior to the 180° inverting pulse, the magnetization from a voxel of tissue is positive, as shown in **A**. Just after the 180° pulse, whatever positive magnetization existed in the voxel just before the 180° pulse is inverted, as shown in **B**. During the interval TI that follows,

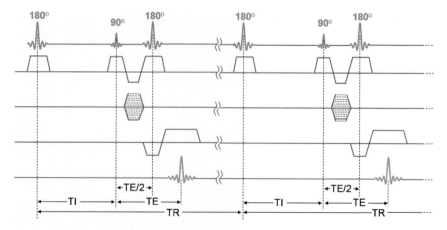

Figure 6.8 Sequence diagram for the inversion-recovery spin-echo (IRSE) pulse sequence. (From Hendrick RE. (6) Adapted with permission from Elsevier).

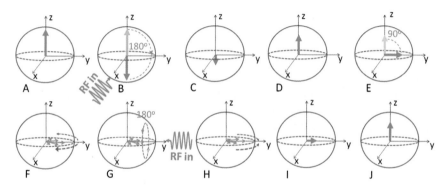

Figure 6.9 Schematic illustration of the longitudinal and transverse magnetization in the IRSE pulse sequence. (From Hendrick RE. (7) Adapted with permission from Elsevier).

the longitudinal magnetization recovers from a negative value back towards $+M_0$, as shown in **C and D**. How much recovery occurs and whether the magnetization is negative, zero, or positive at the time of the 90° pulse depends on the length of TI and on the tissue parameter T1; recovery is exponential and is governed by the rate $(1-e^{-TI/T1})$. The 90° pulse flips whatever longitudinal magnetization exists into the transverse plane (**E**), where it dephases during the interval TE/2 after the 90° pulse (**F**). The second 180° pulse (around the axis perpendicular to that of the first 180° and 90° pulses) (**G**) is performed to rephase the transverse magnetization during the subsequent period TE/2 (**H**) to form the measured signal echo (**I**). During the subsequent interval (TR-TI-TE), the longitudinal magnetization grows to the value it attains before the next repetition of the entire pulse sequence (**J**). The length of this interval has a mild effect on the T1-weighting of the IRSE sequence. If this interval TR-TI-TE is very long compared to T1, then most of the longitudinal magnetization will recover and the longitudinal magnetization prior to the next repetition of the pulse sequence will be near M_0.

As with SE and gradient-echo imaging, the IRSE pulse sequence can be broken down into its T1, T2, and spin density components.[7] For TR >> TE (which is true in most clinical applications), the expression for the IRSE signal strength as a function of user-selectable parameters TR, TI, and TE is:

$$M_{IR}(TR, TI, TE) = N[H](1 - 2e^{-TI/T1} + e^{-TR/T1})e^{-TE/T2}. \qquad (6.7)$$

The spin-density factor, N[H], is identical to that in SE and gradient-echo imaging. The T2 factor, $e^{-TE/T2}$, is identical to that in SE imaging, since a spin-echo is formed to measure the transverse magnetization. The T1-factor for IRSE is $(1 - 2e^{-TI/T1} + e^{-TR/T1})$, which depends on two user-selectable parameters, TR and TI, along with the tissue parameter T1. Figure 6.10 illustrates the T1-factor as a function of TI for fixed TR (3 s) for three tissues: fat (T1 = 260 ms at 1.5 T; see Table 6.1), normal breast fibroglandular tissue (T1 = 700 ms) and cyst (T1 = 3 s).

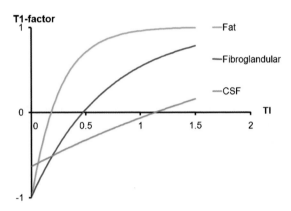

Figure 6.10 The T1-factor in real-reconstructed IRSE as a function of TI for fixed TR (3 s) for three tissues: fat (T1 = 260 ms at 1.5 T), normal breast fibroglandular tissue (T1 = 700 ms) and cyst (T1 = 3 s).

Table 6.1 T1 Values for Fat and TI Null Points as a Function of Magnetic Field Strength, 0.15 to 3.0 Tesla

Magnetic Field Strength (Tesla)	T1 of Fat (ms)	TI_{null} (ms)
0.15	174	121
0.25	190	132
0.5	214	148
1.0	242	168
1.5	260	180
3.0	310	215

T1 values for fat at 0.15 to 1.5 T from Reference 5. Each was measured to stated value ± 28 ms.

Note that all tissue signals are negative for short TI and become positive for longer TI: the larger the T1 of the tissue, the higher the TI value at which the signal crosses zero, called the "null point". As we will see later, short TI inversion recovery (STIR) imaging takes advantage of this null point to cancel the signal from fat, which is done by choosing TI appropriately.

Real and Magnitude Reconstructions of IR Spin-echo Signal

In MR imaging, both a real part and an imaginary part of the signal are measured.[7,8] This reflects the fact that two quantities, both real and imaginary parts, or both magnitude and phase, are present in any vector quantity. The magnetization in a voxel of tissue is such a vector quantity and is the quantity on which MR signal is based. In most cases, the grayscale image that is presented is a "magnitude image", a composite of real and imaginary parts added in quadrature; that is, the square-root of the sum or their squares:

$$S_{magnitude} = (S_{real}^{2} + S_{imaginary}^{2})^{1/2}. \tag{6.8}$$

In addition to the magnitude image, a phase image can be constructed, which describes the phase relation between real and imaginary parts of the measured signal. The phase image is rarely presented, as it seldom contains diagnostic information and, when it does, is more difficult to interpret. The magnitude image is always positive (or zero), so any sign information contained in the MR signal is lost. Hence, while IRSE with phase-corrected or phase-preserving reconstruction has the signal value shown in Equation 6.7 and Figure 6.11, magnitude reconstructed IRSE has the signal value:

$$S_{IRSE}(TR, TI, TE) = N[H] \, | \, (1 - 2e^{-TI/T1} + e^{-TR/T1}) \, | \, e^{-TE/T2}. \tag{6.9}$$

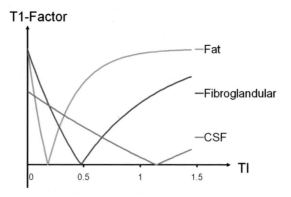

Figure 6.11 The T1-factor in magnitude-reconstructed IRSE as a function of TI for fixed TR (3 s) for three same three tissues illustrated in Figure 6.10.

where absolute value signs surround the T1-factor. This means that signals that were negative in Equation 6.7 will always be positive in magnitude-reconstructed images, as shown in Equation 6.9 and Figure 6.11. Magnitude reconstruction has the effect of reducing the dynamic range of the T1-factor to be between 0 and 1, therefore reducing the dynamic range of the signal measured in IRSE to be between 0 and N[H].

Short T1 Inversion Recovery Imaging

As mentioned above, an important feature of IR or IRSE sequences is the ability to null the signal from a single tissue. As Figure 6.11 illustrates, the proper choice of TI could null the signal from fat (180 ms at 1.5 T), fibroglandular tissue (475 ms at 1.5 T), or cystic fluid (1140 ms at 1.5 T). The general formula for the TI value that can null signal from a single tissue is:

$$TI_{null} = T1 * \ln(2/(1 + e^{-TR/T1})), \tag{6.10}$$

where T1 is the longitudinal relaxation time of the tissue of interest and ln( ) is the natural logarithm of the argument within parentheses. Where T1 << TR, as is the case for fat with a TR = 3 s, the null point can be approximated by $TI_{null} = T1*\ln(2)$. This feature of IRSE is used to advantage in short TI inversion recovery (STIR) pulse sequences, where the TI is set as close as possible to the null point of fat. IRSE with properly set TI is particularly effective as a fat suppression technique for lower magnetic field strength systems where magnetic field homogeneity is far worse than 1 part per million and chemical shift fat suppression techniques are ineffective (see Chapters **9** and **11**). Since STIR does not depend on magnetic field homogeneity to achieve fat suppression, it is far more effective in suppressing the signal from fat over a large volume of tissue where field homogeneity is compromised. Table 6.1 lists T1 values of fat as a function of magnetic field strength from 0.15 to 3.0 T and the corresponding TI values that null the signal from fat. Figure 6.12 illustrates fat suppression for various TI values in STIR imaging at 1.5 T.

Signal Strength as a Function of TR, TI, and TE in IR Spin-echo

We have illustrated the T1-factor for both real- and magnitude-reconstructed STIR as a function of TI. We go on to illustrate the signal strength in magnitude-reconstructed IRSE as a function of user-selectable parameters TR, TI, and TE for the same three tissues at 1.5 T: fat (T1 = 260 ms, T2 = 84 ms, N[H] = 0.9) normal breast glandular tissue (T1 = 700 ms, T2 = 70 ms, and N[H] = 1.0), and cyst (T1 = 3 s, T2 = 300 ms, and N[H] = 1.1). Because magnitude-reconstruction is used, the T1-factor is always positive, between 0 and 1, as shown in Figure 6.11 for an assumed TR value of 3 s. The dashed lines in Figure 6.13 show the T1-factor multiplied by N[H]

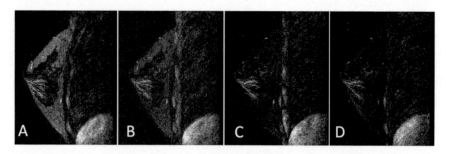

Figure 6.12 STIR imaging at 1.5 T for various TI values around the null point of fat. (A) TI = 135 ms. (B) TI = 150 ms. (C) TI = 165 ms. (D) TI = 180 ms. The null point of fat occurs for a TI of 165 to 180 ms.

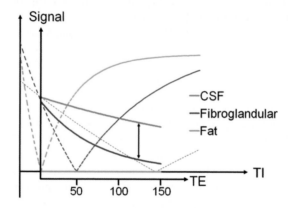

Figure 6.13 Signal factors for three different tissues at 1.5 T: fat (T1 = 260 ms, T2 = 84 ms, N[H] = 0.9) normal breast glandular tissue (T1 = 700 ms, T2 = 70 ms, and N[H] = 1.0), and cyst (T1 = 3 s, T2 = 300 ms, and N[H] = 1.1). Magnitude-reconstructed T1-factors multiplied my N[H] for the three tissues are shown as dashed lines. Signal values consisting of N[H], T1, and T2 factors multiplied together are shown as solid lines as a function of TE (inset) for an assumed TI value of 180 ms, which nulls the signal from fat and makes this IRSE sequence a STIR sequence. Note that in STIR, N[H], T1, and T2 factors all work in concert to make cyst (or any tissue with longer T1, longer T2, and higher N[H]) brighter than fibroglandular tissue (or any tissue with shorter T1, shorter T2, and lower N[H]). Maximum contrast between cyst and fibroglandular tissue occurs for a TE value of 125 ms (vertical black arrow).

for each of the three tissues. Setting an assumed TI value of 180 ms to null the signal from fat, the T2-factor as a function of TE can be added, resulting in the signals from fibroglandular tissue and cyst as shown by the thicker solid lines in Figure 6.13.

T1, T2, and N[H] for these tissues are correlated in that each tissue parameter is higher for cyst than for normal fibroglandular tissue and higher for fibroglandular tissue than for fat. Comparison of Figures 6.11 and 6.13 demonstrates that all three tissue parameters add constructively to make cysts brighter than fibroglandular tissue in STIR. Adding the spin-density factor to the T1-factor elevates cyst signal relative to fibroglandular tissue signal. Adding the T2-factor to T1 and N[H] factors

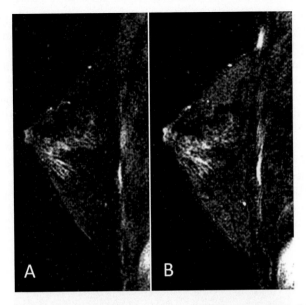

Figure 6.14 Comparison of fat suppression techniques at 1.5 T: (A) STIR IRSE with TI set to null fat signal (TI = 180 ms), (B) T2-weighted FSE with chemical fat suppression in the same subject. Both images have been cropped LR. Artifacts along the chest wall are due to image wrap along the phase-encoding direction, which is head-to-foot or vertical in these images (see Chapter 11).

(Figure 6.13) further increases the difference between cyst signal and fibroglandular tissue signal for any TE value, with maximum signal difference at a TE of 125 ms. Magnitude-reconstructed IRSE is the only pulse sequence in which all three tissue parameters add constructively to increase signal for tissues with larger T1, T2, and N[H] values.

In the early implementation of IRSE sequences, like SE, typically only one phase encoding view was collected after each 180° - 90° - 180° pulse series. Now, just as in FSE, "fast IRSE" or "fast STIR" acquisitions can be made by collecting multiple echoes in the shadow of the 180° - 90° - 180° pulse train. This increases the efficiency of IRSE acquisitions by the ETL factor, which is usually a factor of 2 to 16, and makes fast STIR IRSE a practical alternative to T2-weighted FSE. Figure 6.14 compares STIR IRSE with TI set to null fat signal to T2-weighted FSE with chemical fat suppression in the same subject at 1.5 T, showing little difference. Figure 6.15 shows a similar comparison in a different subject at 3 T.

Chapter Take-home Points

- Fast spin-echo (FSE) sequences provide similar contrast weighting to SE sequences, but with reduced scan times.

- The echo train length (ETL) in FSE describes the number of echoes acquired after each excitation; each echo corresponds to a different phase-encoding view (or line in k-space).
- Echo planar imaging (EPI) acquires extremely fast images but at limited spatial resolution and contrast weighting; EPI typically is not used in breast imaging.
- Short TI inversion recovery (STIR) sequences provide fat suppression by selection of a TI value that nulls the signal from fat; STIR is a useful substitute for fat-suppressed T2W SE or FSE sequences.
- STIR imaging is the only pulse sequence in which T1, T2, and spin-density effects all add constructively; tissues with higher T1, T2, and spin-density values are brighter than other tissues.
- "Fast STIR" imaging collects multiple phase-encoding views (or lines in k-space) for each 180° - 90° - 180° pulse train, making it a practical alternative to FSE for obtaining fat-suppressed T2-weighted breast images.

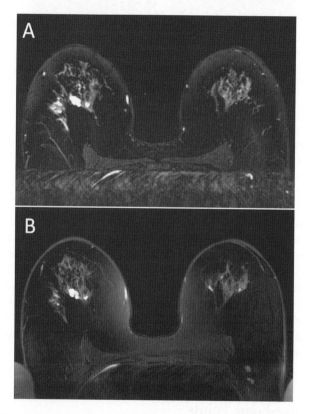

Figure 6.15 Comparison of fat suppression techniques at 3 T: (A) STIR IRSE with TI set to null fat signal (TI = 230 ms), (B) T2-weighted FSE with chemical fat suppression in the same subject. Both images have been cropped in the AP direction. Note that fat suppression is not completely uniform in either image. In general, fat-suppression is more challenging at 3 T than at 1.5 T.

References

1. Hennig J, Nauerth A, Friedburg H. RARE imaging: a fast imaging method for clinical MR. Mag. Reson. Med. 1986; 3: 823–833.
2. Bradley WG, Chen D-Y, Atkinson DJ, Edelman RE. Fast spin-echo and echo-planar imaging. In Stark DD, Bradley WG. Magnetic Resonance Imaging, 3rd Edition. St. Louis: Mosby Publishing Co., Vol 1, Ch 7, 1999; 125–157.
3. Mansfield P. Multi-planar image formation using NMR spin echoes. J. Phys. Chem. 1977; 10: L55–L58.
4. Smith FW, JR Mallard, Reid A, et.al. Nuclear magnetic resonance tomographic imaging in liver disease. Lancet 1981; 1: 963–966.
5. Bydder GM, Hajnal JV, Young IR. Use of the inversion recovery pulse sequence. In Stark DD, Bradley WG. Magnetic Resonance Imaging, 3rd Edition. St. Louis: C.V. Mosby Publishing Co. 1999, Vol 1, Ch 5, 69–86.
6. Hendrick RE. Image contrast and noise. In Stark DD, Bradley WG. Magnetic Resonance Imaging, 3rd Edition. St. Louis: Mosby Publishing Co., 1999, Vol 1, Ch 4, p. 43–68.
7. Haacke EM, Brown RW, Thompson MR, et.al. Magnetic Resonance Imaging: Physical Principles and Sequence Design. New York: John Wiley & Sons, 1999, especially Ch. 19,; 513–568.
8. *Les Prix Nobel. The Nobel Prizes 2003*, Editor: Tore Frängsmyr, [Nobel Foundation], Stockholm, 2004. Found on the Internet at: http://nobelprize.org/nobel_prizes/medicine/laureates/2003/mansfield-autobio.html (last accessed September 25, 2006).

Chapter 7
Signal, Noise, Signal-to-Noise, and Contrast-to-Noise Ratios

In previous chapters we have discussed signal values for various pulse sequences as a function of user-selectable parameters. Formal definitions of signal, noise, signal-to-noise ratios (SNR), and contrast-to-noise ratios (CNR) appear below. This chapter then presents general SNR and CNR considerations, including the effect of user-selectable imaging parameters on SNR and CNR. SNR is important, as it is a good measure of image quality. In detecting lesions in the body, however, high SNR alone will not guarantee that sufficient contrast exists to make the lesion detectable. CNR between lesion and background is important, as it serves as a quantitative metric for low-contrast lesion detection: the higher the CNR between lesion and background, the more likely the lesion's detection.[1]

Magnetic Resonance Signal

Signal is a representation of the measured MR magnetization from a voxel or collection of voxels.[2,3] When measured in a collection of voxels, as in a region-of-interest (ROI) encompassing a lesion, organ, or region prescribed on a uniform background, the signal is averaged over each of the N pixels in the ROI:

$$S_{mean} = \frac{1}{N} \sum_{i=1}^{N} S_i \qquad (7.1)$$

where S_i is the signal in the ith pixel, and the summation Σ adds up the signal from all N pixels, i = 1 to N. Dividing by N takes the mean of those N signal measurements.

When image data are being acquired, RF receiver gain values are adjusted to ensure that measured signals are in the correct dynamic range for collection and storage. Since MRI signals are stored in digital format, the typical dynamic range of a voxel's signal is a power of two: 12-bit digitization results in 2^{12} or 4,096 possible signal values, 14-bit digitization results in 2^{14} or 16,384 possible signal values, just as in digital mammography. Since zero typically is included, magnitude signals measured on an MR scanner range from 0 to 4095 for 12-bit digitization, or

R.E. Hendrick (ed.), *Breast MRI: Fundamentals and Technical Aspects.*
© Springer 2008

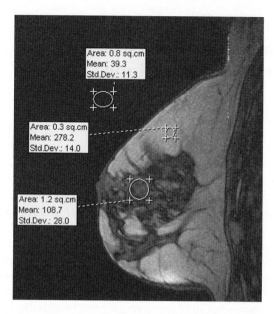

Figure 7.1 Signal (and standard deviation) measurements from a T1W pre-contrast sagittal gradient-echo image without fat-saturation. Imaging parameters were TR = 6.6 ms, TE = 2.8 ms, 25° flip angle. The mean signal in the background region outside the breast is 39.3, in fat is 278.2, and in a heterogeneous area of fibroglandular tissue is 108.7. These values show that in standard image presentation, tissues with higher signal are assigned brighter grayscale values.

0 to 16,383 for 14-bit digitization. Figure 7.1 illustrates signal measurement from several ROIs in a clinical image, showing that higher signals are represented by brighter pixels.

Noise in a Magnetic Resonance Image

Noise is a general term describing pixel-to-pixel variations in signal.[1-3] The noise in a local region-of-interest (ROI) can be described by the standard deviation of the pixel signal values in that region:

$$\sigma = \frac{1}{(N-1)}\sqrt{\left(\sum_{i=1}^{N}(S_i - S_{mean})^2\right)} \tag{7.2}$$

where σ is the standard deviation of signal value, N is the number of pixels contained in the ROI, the symbol Σ indicates summation over all N pixels in the ROI, and the sum taken is of the square of the difference between each individual pixel's signal (S_i) and the mean of the signals averaged over all N pixels, S_{mean}, defined in Eq. 7.1. The square root is taken of the entire sum before dividing by the number of degrees of freedom, N-1. The larger the deviations from the mean for each individual pixel, the larger the measured standard deviation or noise. Figure 7.1 displays standard deviation values for the three regions of interest. In the background region outside the breast, the standard deviation is 11.3 units of signal. In the fairly uniform fat region, the standard deviation is 14.0. In the fibroglandular region, the standard deviation is twice that in fat (28.0) due to greater tissue heterogeneity.

There are two primary types of noise. The first is Gaussian noise, also described as random noise or "quantum mottle", which is unstructured signal variation from pixel to pixel. This is the type of noise appearing in the background region of Figure 7.1. Gaussian noise is responsible for the "salt and pepper" appearance of an image of a uniform phantom. It is due to random fluctuations in the measured signal from data point to data point or view to view, even in a uniform object. It can be due to fluctuations in electronics or signal fluctuations in the sample. The second type of noise is structured noise, which appears as lines, streaks, or blotches that are lighter or darker than normal tissue. The tissue heterogeneities in and around the lower ROI in Figure 7.1 are an example of structured noise. Structured noise is the type of noise occurring in image artifacts (eg, motion ghosting, truncation artifacts, wrap artifacts). Both quantum mottle and structured noise can confound image interpretation by masking the conspicuity of low-contrast lesions. Figure 7.2 illustrates the effect of noise on low-contrast lesion detection using the ACR phantom. As noise is decreased by increasing the number of excitations per phase-encoding step (N_{ex}), more low-contrast objects become visible in the phantom. We will discuss minimizing structured noise in the form of image artifacts in Chapter 11.

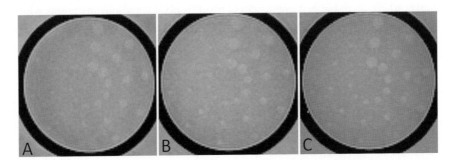

Figure 7.2 A low-contrast detection section of the ACR MRI Accreditation phantom consists of 10 radial rows of low-contrast objects, 3 objects per row, with object diameter decreasing for holes further in the clockwise direction. The phantom was imaged with the same T1W pulse sequence, delay times, and spatial parameters, but with different numbers of excitations per phase-encoding step (N_{ex}). (A) N_{ex} = ½ (half-Fourier imaging), (B) N_{ex} = 1, (C) N_{ex} = 2. Using a scoring method that requires all 3 objects to be visible above background noise levels to count the row as detected, 5 rows are visible in A, 8–9 rows are visible in B, and 9–10 rows are visible in C. Theoretically, SNR increases as the $\sqrt{N_{ex}}$, so SNR in B should be 1.41 times that in A and SNR in C should be twice that in A. SNR measurements in A-C indicate that SNR in B is 1.37 times that in A, while SNR in C is 1.60 times that in A.

This chapter is concerned primarily with the first type of noise, random or Gaussian-distributed image noise. Even in a perfectly uniform object, variations in signal from pixel-to-pixel occur because the imaging system is not perfect in measuring the signal from each pixel. In random or Gaussian-distributed noise that is responsible for quantum mottle, a histogram of signal values measured in a ROI will have a peak at the mean signal, with the number of pixels having signal values differing from the mean falling off on either side of the peak, as shown in Figure 7.3. This is a characteristic Gaussian or "normal" distribution. The part of the peak ranging from $S_{mean} - \sigma$ to $S_{mean} + \sigma$ (+ or − one standard deviation) contains 68.3% of the pixels. The range about the mean from -2σ to $+2\sigma$ (two standard deviations) contains 95.4% of the pixels, and the range from -3σ to $+3\sigma$ (three standard deviations) contains 99.7% of the pixels.

Noise is best measured from the background of a clinical image (Figure 7.1) or on a uniform phantom, as shown by the central regions (where no low-contrast objects exist) in the phantom images displayed in Figure 7.2. This ensures that pixel-to-pixel variations represent signal variations from a uniform source rather than signal variations due to tissue non-uniformities, as occur in the breast tissues in Figure 7.1, especially in the lowest ROI that is placed in fibroglandular tissue. The goal in quantifying noise is to measure the pixel-to-pixel variations due to the choice of pulse sequences, user-selectable parameters, and the system itself, not due to inherent tissue variations. Hence, basing noise measurements on a uniform phantom is desirable.

Recall from Chapter 3 that in 2D or 3D MR imaging, data are collected to fill out k-space in 2 or 3 dimensions and 2D or 3D Fourier transforms are taken to reconstruct planar images or a volume of image data. A general property of 2DFT- and 3DFT-reconstructed MRI is that Gaussian noise is propagated uniformly across the image. Thus, the pixel-to-pixel variations occurring in the background of an image, where no tissue is present, reflect pixel-to-pixel variations in regions where

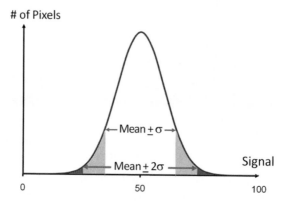

Figure 7.3 A Gaussian or normal distribution of signal values within an image ROI. The peak signal is at the mean. The range from $S_{mean} - \sigma$ to $S_{mean} + \sigma$ includes 68.3% of pixels within the ROI, shown by the white area under the curve. The range from $S_{mean} - 2\sigma$ to $S_{mean} + 2\sigma$ includes 95.4% of pixels within the ROI, shown by the white plus light blue areas under the curve.

tissues exist. As a result, a simple way to measure noise in the form of quantum mottle and avoiding tissue heterogeneity effects is to place a ROI in the background, where no signal-producing tissues exist, and to measure the standard deviation in that region, as shown in Figure 7.1 (upper ROI).

There is one caveat to this method of measuring image noise. In MR images that are magnitude-reconstructed images, as most clinical images are, the standard deviation in the background does not capture the full range of pixel variations because negative image signals have been made positive.[4] Magnitude reconstruction does not affect signal values in bright tissues, where all signals are positive, but affects signal values in the background, where signal values are near zero. This means that a standard deviation measured in the background of a magnitude-reconstructed image underestimates noise compared to either a brighter region where no signals are negative or a background region where negative signals are allowed. The noise measured in the background of a magnitude-reconstructed image will yield a result that is 0.665 of the Gaussian noise in a signal-producing tissue, σ_{image}, where signals are not close to zero or in a background region where negative signal values are allowed. This provides a simple way to correct noise measurements taken in the background:

$$\sigma_{image} = \sigma_{bkgd}/0.665 = 1.50\,\sigma_{bkgd}. \qquad (7.3)$$

If no artifacts are present, we can also get a good estimate of image noise from the signal measured in the background, S_{bkgd}:

$$S_{bkgd} = 1.253\sigma_{image} \text{ so } \sigma_{image} = 0.80\,S_{bkgd}. \qquad (7.4)$$

For example, in Figure 7.4, the ROI placed in the background gave signal mean and standard deviation values of 10.4 ± 5.7. Using Eq. 7.3 and the standard deviation measured in the background gives an estimate of image noise as:

$$\sigma_{image} = 1.50\,\sigma_{bkgd} = (1.50)(5.7) = 8.6.$$

Using Eq. 7.4 and the mean signal measured in the background gives an estimate of image noise as:

$$\sigma_{image} = 0.80\,S_{bkgd} = (0.80)(10.4) = 8.3.$$

As shown in Figure 7.4, the standard deviations measured in relatively uniform signal-producing tissues in the image itself (cyst and muscle) gave standard deviations of 9.1 and 8.7, respectively, in good agreement with image noise estimated from background measurements (8.6 and 8.3). Figure 7.5 shows three measurements of signal mean and standard deviation in the same image, but from fat. The upper ROI includes a relatively uniform region of fat where tissue heterogeneities do not dominate the standard deviation measurement. In that upper ROI, the standard deviation is comparable to the image noise determined in (A) (10.0 in uniform fat vs. 8.3–9.1). The two lower ROIs in Figure 7.5 illustrate improper ROI selection

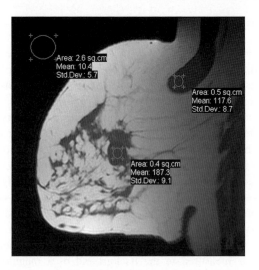

Figure 7.4 Non-fat suppressed T1-weighted sagittal image of a breast with a large cyst. (A) Signal mean and standard deviation measurements are shown for three ROI: upper left ROI in the background of the image, $S_{mean} = 10.4$, $\sigma = 5.7$; pectoral muscle, $S_{mean} = 117.6$, $\sigma = 8.7$; cyst, $S_{mean} = 187.3$, $\sigma = 9.1$. Based on the background standard deviation and Eq 7.3, image noise is estimated to be $\sigma_{image} = 8.6$. Based on the background signal and Eq 7.4, image noise is estimated to be $\sigma_{image} = 8.3$. Both are in good agreement with ROI measurements of standard deviation within relatively homogeneous regions of muscle and cyst fluid.

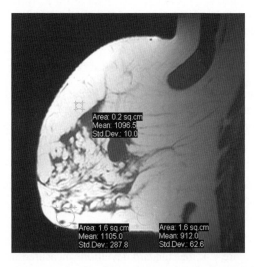

Figure 7.5 ROI measurements taken in various regions of fat in the same image as Figure 7.4. The upper ROI, a relatively homogeneous area of fat, has mean signal of 1096.5 and standard deviation of 10.2, approximately the same standard deviation as other image noise estimates in Figure 7.4, even though fat signal is much higher than that of cyst or muscle in this image. The standard deviations measured in the two lower ROIs are much higher because they are taken in heterogeneous tissues where tissue signal differences dominate over image noise. Reliable noise measurements are best made using ROIs in the background and estimating image noise as shown in Eq 7.3 or 7.4. Signal measurements, on the other hand, should be made by taking the mean signal in a relatively uniform area of the tissue of interest, as in the upper ROI in this image.

to estimate image noise, as tissue heterogeneities dominate standard deviations measurements (of 287.8 and 62.6) in those two regions.

System Parameters Affecting Noise

Some parameters inherent to the MRI system, such as magnetic field strength and system electronics, affect both signal and noise in an image.[1-3] Others, such as RF receiver coil volume and bandwidth, affect only image noise. These two parameters and their effects on image noise are discussed below.

Volume of the Radiofrequency Receiver Coil

A general feature of noise in an MR image is that it is influenced by the sensitive volume of the RF receiver coil. Larger receiver coils capture more noise, due to the larger volume of tissue contributing noise to the image. Use of a larger coil does not typically affect signal (other than different sized coils possibly having different signal sensitivities), as the same limited volume of tissue (a voxel, plane, or volume) will yield the same measured signal, assuming the same pulse sequence and spatial parameters are used.

The effect of the sensitive volume of the receiver coil on noise is the primary reason that in clinical applications, the RF receiver coil should be no larger than needed to cover the anatomic region of interest. It explains why dedicated breast RF receiver coils are used rather than the body coil, which has a much larger sensitive volume and consequently, more noise, as illustrated in Figure 7.6. It also explains why the contralateral breast coil should be turned off when doing unilateral imaging. The contralateral coil, if left on, will add noise to the image, without contributing additional signal to the unilateral image. It may also introduce wrap artifacts into the breast of interest that could be reduced or eliminated by turning off the contralateral coil (see Chapter 11, Figure 11.4).

Receiver Bandwidth

The bandwidth of the RF receiver coil is the range of frequencies over which signal is recorded. The bandwidth needs to be broad enough to record the range of frequencies emitted by the entire slice or volume during frequency encoding, but should not be broader than necessary, as image noise is directly proportional to the square root of RF receiver bandwidth:

$$\sigma_{image} \propto \sqrt{BW} \qquad\qquad (7.5)$$

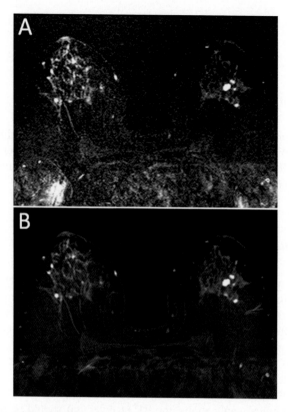

Figure 7.6 Comparison of SNR in a transaxial bilateral breast image acquired at 3 Tesla using (A) the body coil as the receiver coil versus (B) a dedicated bilateral breast coil as the receiver coil. The same pulse sequence (STIR, TR = 4.25 s, TE = 63 ms, TI = 205 ms), imaging parameters, subject, and slice were used in A and B. SNR in B is 7.0 times higher than in A due to the more restricted volume of the dedicated breast coil.

That's because the broader the range of received frequencies, the more noise that's collected on each signal measurement and the more noise that will occur in the reconstructed image. Bandwidth is also related to the sampling time (T_s) and number of pixels recorded in the frequency-encoding direction (N_x), which is equal to the number of separate signal measurements taken during the signal measurement interval T_s:

$$BW = N_x/T_s. \tag{7.6}$$

Signal-to-Noise Ratios

Signal-to-noise ratios (SNR) describe the signal in a single tissue relative to the pixel-to-pixel variations in that tissue or the pixel-to-pixel variations in a background tissue. Signal-to-noise ratios better represent image quality than signal or noise alone, as both signal and noise affect the ability to detect low-contrast structures or lesions.

For an image region with signal S and noise σ, SNR is defined as the ratio of the two:

$$SNR = S/\sigma. \qquad (7.7)$$

SNR is a good metric for overall image quality, as it quantitatively describes how much the signal rises above pixel-to-pixel variations. In general, the higher the SNR in an image, the smoother and more appealing the image is to the reader.

For example, when using a RF receiver coil with a larger sensitive volume, the signal is unaffected (assuming the same coil signal sensitivity), while the noise is increased in proportion to the square root of the volume of tissue from which signal is received. Thus, SNR is decreased by using a larger receiver coil, as illustrated in Figure 7.6.

Effect of Magnetic Field Strength on Signal-to-Noise Ratios

Increasing the strength of the primary magnetic field, B_0, affects SNR by increasing the magnetization from each voxel of tissue. For magnetic field strengths above 0.5 T, SNR goes up approximately linearly with magnetic field strength.[2] This means that doubling the magnetic field strength will approximately double the measured SNR. This is the primary motivation behind higher magnetic field strengths for patient imaging. One cannot, however, merely turn up the field strength on an MR system. Clinical imaging systems are designed to have a fixed magnetic field strength; their associated RF systems are tuned accordingly to match the Larmor frequency of the fixed magnetic field. Thus, going from 1.0 T to 1.5 T or from 1.5 T to 3.0 T requires a forklift upgrade, replacing the entire MR system. A comparison of image quality and image SNR on the same volunteer at 1.5 T and 3.0 T is given in Chapter 13 (Figure 13.3).

Higher field strength poses some additional technical challenges. As magnetic field strength increases, RF penetration into tissue decreases. For a long time, there was a controversy about whether MRI could be done at magnetic field strengths above 0.5 T due to the problems of RF penetration. Those questions have been put to rest with the development of 3 T, 4 T, and even 7–10 T whole-body MR systems and software that can correct for signal non-uniformities. There are still problems with achieving high magnetic field homogeneities and coil uniformities at higher magnetic field strengths. Another minor issue is that T1 values are longer at higher magnetic field strength, so that less T1 recovery occurs for the same TR value and total imaging time. T1 values do not go up linearly with magnetic field strength, but as the cube root or square root of the magnetic field strength. This increase in T1 with B_0 slightly lessens the measured signal, and thus, slightly reduces the SNR from increasing linearly with higher magnetic field strength.

Effect of User-selectable Image Acquisition Parameters on Signal-to-Noise Ratios

It is instructive to consider the effects of user-selectable spatial parameters on signal, noise, and SNR. Table 7.1 summarizes these effects. A simple parameter affecting SNR is N_{ex}, the number of excitations per phase encoding step. For any pulse sequence, doubling N_{ex} (from 1 to 2 or from 2 to 4) doubles the total image acquisition time. Doubling N_{ex} doubles the total signal attributed to each pixel, as the additional collected signals are added together. This additive process increases the noise, as well, but noise adds in quadrature (that is, as the square root of the sum of the squares), which has the effect of increasing image noise by a factor of $\sqrt{2} = 1.41$, a 41% increase in noise, as a result of doubling N_{ex}. Thus, doubling N_{ex} causes signal to double and noise to goes up by $\sqrt{2}$, so SNR goes up by a factor of $2/\sqrt{2} = \sqrt{2} = 1.41$, so SNR increases by 41%. An example of the effect of increasing N_{ex} is shown in Figure 7.7.

Effects of TR, TE, and Flip Angle on Signal-to-Noise Ratios

The effects on signal of altering TR, TE, and, where relevant, TI or flip angle, have already been given in Chapters 4–6. These parameters have little or no effect on noise. Hence, their effect of SNR is identical to their effect on signal.

Effect of Spatial Parameters on Signal-to-Noise Ratios

Spatial parameters include slice thickness (Δz) and in-plane pixel sizes (Δx and Δy), which are in turn determined by the in-plane fields-of-view, L_x and L_y, and

Table 7.1 Effect of doubling each user-selectable MR parameters on signal, noise, and SNR or CNR

User-Selectable Parameter	Effect of Doubling on Signal	Noise	Effect of Doubling on SNR or CNR
Magnetic Field Strength (B_0)	$\times 4$	$\times 2$	$\times 2$
Bandwidth	–	$\times \sqrt{2}$	$\times 1/\sqrt{2}$ or $\times 0.71$
Number of Ex-citations per Phase-encoding Step (N_{ex})	$\times 2$	$\times \sqrt{2}$	$\times \sqrt{2}$ or 1.41
Slice Thickness (Δz)	$\times 2$	–	$\times 2$
Pixel Size in Frequency-encoding Direction (Δx)	$\times 2$	–	$\times 2$
Pixel Size in Phase-encoding Direction (Δy)	$\times 2$	$\times \sqrt{2}$	$\times \sqrt{2}$ or 1.41

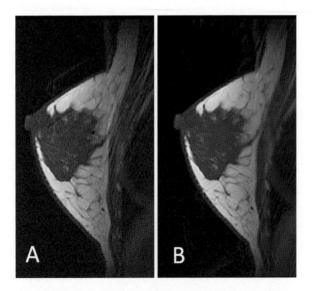

Figure 7.7 A volunteer imaged with the same pulse sequence delay times and spatial parameters, but with different SNR values by using different N_{ex} values. (A) $N_{ex} = 1$, (B) $N_{ex} = 4$. SNR in B is approximately twice that in A and motion ghosting is reduced by signal averaging.

the number of pixels, N_x and N_y, in the frequency- and phase-encoding in-plane directions, respectively:

$$\Delta x = L_x / N_x \text{ and } \Delta y = L_y / N_y \tag{7.8}$$

For example, with a 20 cm FOV and 256 pixels in each in-plane direction,

$$\Delta x = \Delta y = 20 \text{ cm}/256 = 0.078 \text{ cm} = 0.78 \text{ mm}.$$

Effect of Slice Thickness on Signal-to-Noise Ratios

When doubling the slice thickness (Δz) in 2DFT imaging, the volume of tissue contributing signal from each voxel doubles and, consequently, the measured signal doubles. Doubling the slice thickness has no effect on noise, since the noise level is set by the volume of tissue in the sensitive volume of the receiver coil, not just the selected slice. Hence, doubling slice thickness doubles SNR, which improves low-contrast lesion detection at the expense of increasing partial volume effects. In general, this will mean that low-contrast lesions are better detected, as long as the lesion is not so small in the slice-select direction that it is "partial-volumed" away; that is, that the lesion occupies less than the full

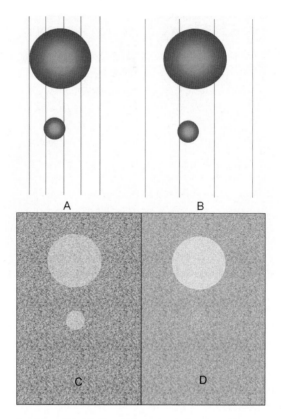

Figure 7.8 Schematic of the effect of slice thickness on lesion detection. (A) and (B) illustrate the relation of slice thickness to lesion size; (C) and (D) illustrate the appearance of the two lesions in an MR image in the case of thinner and thicker slices, respectively. Slice thickness in (A) is smaller than both lesions. When slice thickness is doubled (B), SNR is higher and the larger lesion is more visible, as shown in (D), but the smaller lesion is less visible due to partial volume effects.

width of the slice, so that the slice contains part lesion, part other tissues (see Figure 7.8).

Effect of the Number of Frequency-encoding Steps

Doubling the voxel dimension in the frequency-encoding direction (Δx) doubles the signal measured from that voxel, again without any change in noise, so SNR is doubled. The trade-off for this increased SNR is poorer spatial resolution in the frequency-encoding (x) direction, resulting in images looking more blurred (see Figure 7.9). Altering the voxel size in the frequency-encoding direction has no effect on total imaging time.

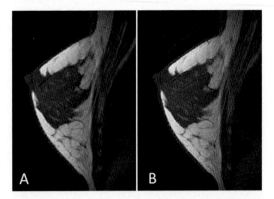

Figure 7.9 Illustration of the effect of the number of frequency-encoding steps on image quality in T1W gradient-echo imaging. (A) 256 frequency-encoding steps. (B) 512 frequency-encoding steps. Frequency-encoding is in the LR (horizontal) direction in both images. TR = 300 ms, TE = 9 ms, flip angle = 25°, FOV = 20 cm × 20 cm, and the number of phase-encoding steps was 256 in each image. Scan time was identical (77 seconds) to collect 13 3-mm slices in both image acquisitions. Both images have been cropped to a rectangular FOV for display. Motion artifacts are visible as light-dark line pairs just posterior to the nipple in both images.

Effect of the Number of Phase-encoding Steps

Doubling voxel size in the phase-encoding direction (Δy) is slightly more complicated. Doubling Δy doubles the signal measured from the voxel on each phase-encoding view due to twice as much hydrogen contributing to each voxel's signal. Doubling Δy halves the number of phase-encoding views collected to form the image, assuming the FOV in the phase-encoding direction, L_y, is unchanged; this reduces the SNR by the square root of two due to only half as many phase-encoding views contributing to the image. Thus, the net effect of doubling Δy is to increase SNR by a factor of $2/\sqrt{2} = \sqrt{2}$ (a factor of 1.41), so overall SNR would be increased by 41%. More generally, increasing Δy by a factor of N increases SNR by a factor of $\sqrt{N}$. Cutting the number of phase-encoding views in half (or 1/N, where in this case N = 2) reduces the total imaging time by a factor of 2 (N), but spatial resolution is made poorer in the phase-encoding direction by a factor of 2 (N), which increases image blur. Figure 7.10 illustrates the effect of changing the number of phase-encoding steps on image quality.

Putting Together All Factors Affecting Signal-to-Noise Ratios

When considering the dependence of SNR on all user-selectable parameters, it is best to separate the cases of 2D (planar) and 3D (volume) imaging.

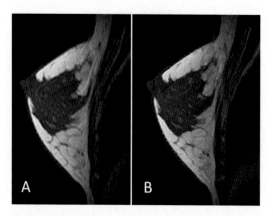

Figure 7.10 Demonstration of the effect of the number of phase-encoding steps on image quality. (A) 128 phase-encoding steps. (B) 256 phase-encoding steps. Phase-encoding is in the HF (vertical) direction in both images. The same imaging parameters as in Figure 7.9 were used, with 256 frequency-encoding steps in each image. Imaging time for 13 slices was 38 seconds for A, 77 seconds for B. Both images have been cropped to a rectangular FOV for display. Motion artifacts are visible just posterior to the nipple in both images, primarily as bright lines in A and dark lines in B.

Signal-to-Noise Ratios in 2D (Planar) Imaging

Combining all of the user-selectable factors affecting signal or noise in 2D imaging into a single formula helps summarize the discussion above:

$$SNR = S/\sigma \; \alpha \; (\Delta x)(\Delta y)(\Delta z) \sqrt{N_{pe}} \sqrt{N_{ex}} \sqrt{T_s} \, S(TR,TE,TI,\theta), \qquad (7.8)$$

where α is a proportionality sign, T_s is the total sampling time for signal measurement, $S(TR,TE,TI,\theta)$ is the generic signal from any 2D pulse sequence, given specifically for SE, FSE, IR, EPI, and gradient-echo imaging in Chapters 3-6.

The total sampling time, T_s, depends on the number of frequency-encoding samples taken, N_x, and the time taken to measure each sample (Δt):

$$T_s = N_x (\Delta t). \qquad (7.9)$$

Since bandwidth (BW) is inversely proportional to Δt, Eq. (7.9) can be rewritten in terms of BW as:

$$T_s = N_x /(BW) \qquad (7.10)$$

and Eq. (7.8) can be rewritten in terms of BW as:

$$SNR = S/\sigma \; \alpha \; (\Delta x)(\Delta y)(\Delta z) \sqrt{(N_{pe} N_{ex} N_x /BW)} S(TR,TE,TI,\theta), \qquad (7.11)$$

For the more mathematically inclined reader, this formula can be used to predict the effect of changing any of the user-selectable parameters in 2D MRI. Similar formulas are built into some scanner's software, so that the technologist or other user at the MRI console can see the effects of changing user-selectable parameters on image SNR.

Signal-to-Noise Ratios in 3D (Volume) Imaging

Combining all of the user-selectable factors affecting image quality in 3D imaging gives a single formula comparable to Eq (7.8):

$$SNR = S/\sigma \; \alpha \; (\Delta x)(\Delta y)(\Delta z) \sqrt{N_z} \sqrt{N_{pe}} \sqrt{N_{ex}} \sqrt{T_s} \, S(TR, TE, TI, \theta). \qquad (7.12)$$

where N_z is the number of slices separated by phase-encoding in the slice-select (z) direction. The only difference between Eq (7.8) and Eq. (7.12) is the extra term $\sqrt{N_z}$ in Eq. (7.12), due to a factor of N_z additional phase-encoding views acquired in 3D imaging compared to 2D imaging to divide the volume into individual slices.

Contrast and Contrast-to-Noise Ratios

Contrast refers to the signal difference between a lesion and its background. Contrast-to-noise is defined as the ratio of signal difference (contrast) to the noise level in the image:

$$CNR = \frac{(S_{lesion} - S_{background})}{\sigma} \qquad (7.13)$$

CNR is an excellent quantitative metric for low-contrast lesion detection, as it describes how much the difference between lesion signal and background signal rises above pixel-to-pixel variations, either in the background or in both tissues (see Figure 7.11). It is common practice to measure the standard deviation (noise) in the background tissue alone, as that is the background on which the lesion must be detected. Moreover, the noise in the background is usually representative of the noise in the lesion itself, since noise propagates uniformly across an MR image. If the noise levels in the lesion and background are dissimilar due to tissue heterogeneity differences, then σ in Eq (7.4) can be better estimated by combining the noise from each tissue in quadrature:

$$\sigma = (1/2) \sqrt{(\sigma^2_{lesion} + \sigma^2_{bkgd})}. \qquad (7.14)$$

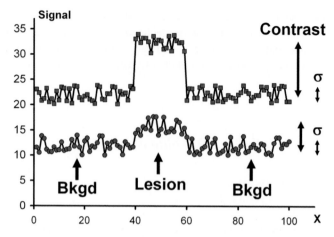

Figure 7.11 Two-dimensional schematic illustrating two different contrast-to-noise ratios. Each curve represents the pixel values along a line parallel to the x-axis through a 2-dimensional image. In both the upper and lower curves, the "lesion" is the set of elevated signal values in the center portion of the x-axis (points 40–59). In the upper curve, the contrast between lesion and background is approximately 5 times the noise level (σ) in each tissue (CNR = 5), making the lesion easily detectable. In the lower curve, the contrast between lesion and background is approximately 2 times σ in each tissue (CNR = 2), making the lesion more difficult to detect. The human eye averages over similar signal values to attempt to detect a difference between lesion and background, as described by the Rose model.

Tissue heterogeneities can add to image noise to make it more difficult to detect low-contrast lesions on a subtly different background.

The Rose Model[5]

Along with contrast and noise, the area of the lesion in a planar image affects lesion detection. In general, the larger the area, the lower the contrast necessary between lesion and background for a given noise level to detect a lesion. The Rose model describes the relationship between lesion area, contrast, and noise for lesion detection.[5] The Rose model is based on detailed experiments of low-contrast lesion detection carried out with dozens of observers and accounts for lesion size by modifying the CNR expression. In the case of a pixilated image, as occurs in MRI, lesion size is determined by the number of image pixels comprising the lesion, N_{pixels}. The effective CNR is defined by:

$$CNR_{eff} = \sqrt{N_{pixels}} (S_{lesion} - S_{bkgd}) / \sigma = \sqrt{N_{pixels}} \, CNR, \qquad (7.15)$$

assuming that the noise is the same in lesion and background.

Table 7.2 Rose model estimation of the CNR needed between lesion and background to ensure lesion detection as a function of the number of pixels comprising the lesion. Area refers to the area (in mm²) of a lesion in a noise-limited 256 × 256 image with a 20 cm FOV

N_{pixels}	Area (mm²)	Minimum CNR
1	0.61	4.00
2	1.22	2.83
3	1.83	2.31
4	2.44	2.00
5	3.05	1.79
10	6.10	1.26
15	9.16	1.03
20	12.2	0.89
25	15.3	0.80
30	18.3	0.73
40	24.4	0.63
50	30.5	0.57
100	61.0	0.40

The Rose criterion for lesion detection is that the effective CNR in Eq (7.15) should be 3–5. Table 7.2 details the Rose model's estimation of the minimum CNR required to ensure lesion detection as a function of the number of pixels comprising the lesion, assuming that an effective CNR of 4 is adequate for lesion detection. Of course, the higher the effective CNR, the more confident the reader is that a lesion is present in a noisy image.

Effect of Image Addition on Signal, Noise, Signal-to-Noise Ratios and Contrast-to-Noise Ratios

Acquiring two or more identically-acquired images and adding them pixel by pixel adds the signal in each pixel, so that the combined signal is approximately double (or N times) the signal from either image (or N images). While signal adds linearly, noise adds in quadrature. This means that combining two images adds the noise from each image as the square root of the sum of the squares (that is, the noise variance is additive):

$$\sigma_{combined} = \sqrt{(\sigma_A^2 + \sigma_B^2)}. \qquad (7.16)$$

For two identically-acquired images with identical noise, $\sigma_A = \sigma_B$, then

$$\sigma_{combined} = \sqrt{2}\,\sigma_A.$$

When N identically-acquired images are combined,

$$\sigma_{combined} = \sqrt{N}\,\sigma_A, \tag{7.17}$$

where σ_A is the noise from a single image. Therefore, when adding N images,

$$SNR_{combined} = \sqrt{N}\,SNR_A, \tag{7.18}$$

where SNR_A is the signal-to-noise ratio from a single image. Similarly, when adding N identically-acquired images, the CNR between lesion and background in the combined image is:

$$CNR_{combined} = \sqrt{N}\,CNR_A, \tag{7.19}$$

where CNR_A is the contrast-to-noise ratio between lesion and background from a single image. This is exactly what happens when multiple repetitions of each phase-encoding view (N_{ex}) are collected, with $N = N_{ex}$ in Eqs (7.17) – (7.19).

Effect of Image Subtraction on Signal, Noise, Signal-to-Noise Ratios and Contrast-to-Noise Ratios

In contrast-enhanced MRI, pre-contrast images are subtracted from post-contrast images with the goal of improving the detection of enhancing lesions relative to unenhanced background tissue. Image subtraction subtracts signal from the two images pixel-by-pixel. Image noise, however, adds in quadrature between the two images, just as in image addition. When subtracting image A from image B,

$$S_{subtracted} = S_B - S_A, \tag{7.20}$$

while

$$\sigma_{subtracted} = \sqrt{(\sigma_B^{\,2} + \sigma_A^{\,2})}. \tag{7.21}$$

If noise is approximately the same in the two images, as is usually the case in subtracted breast MRI, then the noise in the subtracted image is a factor of $\sqrt{2}$ greater in the subtracted image than in the post-contrast image. Thus, to make the lesion more conspicuous in the subtracted image than in the post-contrast image alone, lesion enhancement must more than compensate for the 41% greater noise in all tissues in the subtracted image. This is usually the case for focal lesions, where contrast enhancement increases lesion signal by greater than 50%, often increasing lesion signal by several hundred percent, above the background lesion signal. The amount of lesion signal increase can be read from the time-enhancement curve (see Chapter 10). The exception to this can occur in diffuse lesions (such as some cases of ductal carcinoma in-situ, DCIS) where enhancing lesion is mixed with non-enhancing normal tissue. Especially when thicker slices are used, partial volume effects can make DCIS difficult to detect in subtracted images because net signal increase per voxel does not exceed 50%. The thicker the slice, the lower the net signal increase per voxel when partial volume averaging occurs.

Chapter Take-home Points

- Signal is best measured by a small ROI in tissue or a uniform phantom.
- Noise is best measured as the standard deviation in the background of an MRI.
- Both quantum mottle and structured noise occur in MRI.
- Quantum mottle is uniformly distributed across an MR image by the 2DFT or 3DFT reconstruction process.
- Quantum mottle increases as the square root of the receiver bandwidth.
- Image SNR increases approximately linearly with static magnetic field strength above 0.5 Tesla.
- Image SNR increases linearly with slice thickness and with pixel size in the frequency-encoding direction.
- Image SNR increases as the square root of the pixel size in the phase-encoding direction.
- When two similarly acquired images are added or subtracted, the resulting image has a noise level that is $\sqrt{2}$ higher than that in either image.
- The Rose model describes the relationship between lesion area, contrast, and noise for lesion detection; the larger the lesion area or contrast, and the lower the noise, the easier the lesion is to detect.

References

1. Hendrick RE. Image contrast and noise. In Stark DD, Bradley WG, eds. Magnetic Resonance Imaging, 3rd Edition, St. Louis: Mosby Publishing Co., 1999, Vol 1, Ch. 4, p. 43–68.
2. Edelstein WA, Glover GH, Hardy CJ, Redington RW. The intrinsic signal-to-noise ratio in NMR imaging. Magn. Reson. Med. 1986; 3: 604–618.
3. Haacke EM, Brown RW, Thompson MR, et.al. Magnetic Resonance Imaging: Physical Principles and Sequence Design. New York: John Wiley & Sons, 1999, especially Ch 15, 331–380.
4. Henkelman RM. Measurement of signal intensities in the presence of noise in MR images. Med. Phys.1985; 12: 232–233.
5. Rose A. Vision: human and electronic. New York: Plenum Press, 1973.

Chapter 8
Contrast Agents in Breast Magnetic Resonance Imaging

This chapter begins the breast-specific section of this book. The discussion of contrast agents is placed at the beginning of the breast section, as the imaging requirements for breast MRI are dictated by the spatial and temporal requirements of detecting and evaluating breast lesions enhanced by contrast media.

A Brief History of Contrast Media in the Breast

After the introduction of clinical MRI in the early 1980s, the hope was that breast cancers could be distinguished from fibroglandular tissues and benign breast lesions based on their T1 and T2 values or based on their signal intensities in T1- or T2-weighted images. This early hope was dispelled by detailed evaluations of breast tissue relaxation times and signal values in T1- and T2-weighted imaging. Breast cancers, on average, were found to have T1 and T2 values higher than those of normal fibroglandular tissues, but lower than those of many benign breast lesions, as shown in Table 8.1.[1–5] This would tend to make breast cancers appear slightly darker than normal fibroglandular tissues on unenhanced T1-weighted images and somewhat brighter than normal fibroglandular tissues on unenhanced T2-weighted images (Figure 8.1). In addition, due to the heterogeneity of both benign and malignant breast lesions, significant overlap was found between the T1 and T2 values of breast cancers and benign breast lesions such as fibroadenomas.

By the mid-1980s, contrast agents based on the rare-earth element gadolinium (Gd) were being developed to enhance cancers in the brain and spinal cord. The first Gd-based contrast agent was approved by the U.S. Food and Drug Administration (FDA) for central nervous system (CNS) indications in 1988.

Gadolinium-based Contrast Agents

Gadolinium is a paramagnetic ion due to the presence of three unpaired electrons in its outer shell. When placed in a strong magnetic field, these unpaired electrons align with the field and their electron magnetic dipole moments add together, creating

R.E. Hendrick (ed.), *Breast MRI: Fundamentals and Technical Aspects.*
© Springer 2008

Table 8.1 T1 and T2 values of tissues in the breast, including breast cancers

Tissue Type	$N_{samples}$	T1	T2
Fat	28	265 ± 2	58 ± 1
Normal fibroglandular	23	796 ± 21	63 ± 4
Benign lesions	17	1049 ± 40	89 ± 8
Malignant lesions	11	876 ± 29	75 ± 4

Source: Data from Merchant TE, et al., (5).

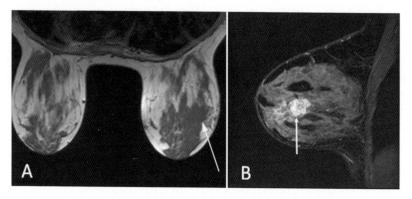

Figure 8.1 (A) Unenhanced T1-weighted bilateral transaxial SE image without fat-suppression. Breast on right contains a recently biopsied 2-cm invasive breast cancer (arrow), which is slightly darker than normal fibroglandular tissues due to its longer T1 value. (B) Unenhanced T2-weighted fat-suppressed sagittal STIR image of the right breast demonstrating the same invasive breast cancer (arrow), which is brighter than normal fibroglandular tissues due to its longer T2 value. Post biopsy changes may also increase lesion signal on T2-weighted images.

a strong, local magnetic field in the vicinity of the Gd ion. The property of having a strong local magnetic field caused by an externally applied magnetic field is the property of paramagnetism. It is the strong local magnetic field of the Gd ion that decreases the T1, T2, and T2* values of hydrogen nuclei in the vicinity of the Gd ion (see Chapter 2).

Elemental gadolinium is toxic. It can be formed into chloride, sulfate, or acetate compounds, but these are easily dissociated in the body and are not well-tolerated. To make gadolinium safe for human injection, it is chelated by a molecule that renders the Gd-compound non-toxic. A *chelate,* from the Latin word *chelae* or "claws," is defined as "a heterocyclic chemical compound whose molecules consist of a metal ion attached to at least two nonmetal ions".[6]

The first group to demonstrate the use of Gd-chelates to aid breast cancer detection was Sylvia Heywang-Kobrunner and collaborators in 1985.[6] Since then, many studies have confirmed that administration of Gd-chelates at the same concentrations as recommended for CNS lesions, 0.1 millimoles per kilogram of body mass (mmol/kg), increases the sensitivity of breast MRI to invasive breast cancer. Current estimates of sensitivity to invasive breast cancer using Gd-chelates are discussed later in this chapter.

Invasive breast cancers tend to exhibit more rapid and more focal uptake of contrast agent than normal fibroglandular tissues or benign breast lesions. After uptake, invasive breast cancers tend to exhibit irregular margins and some exhibit washout of contrast agent, which is not typical of benign lesions. The time after injection during which invasive breast cancers demonstrate greater enhancement than surrounding fibroglandular tissues is usually 5 to 10 minutes, with increasing contrast between lesion and normal fibroglandular tissues for the first 1 to 3 minutes after injection and slowly decreasing contrast after that. By 6 to 10 minutes after injection, normal fibroglandular tissues have increased in signal intensities to the point that invasive breast cancers are far less distinct relative to background fibroglandular tissues, as shown in Figure 8.2.

The first FDA-approved chelated paramagnetic gadolinium-based contrast agent was gadopentetate dimeglumine (Gd-DTPA, sold under the brand name Magnevist™, Berlex Inc., Wayne, NJ, a subsidiary of Bayer Schering Pharma AG, Berlin Germany), approved for adult CNS applications in the U.S. in 1988. Four other Gd-chelates have been approved by the FDA since that time: gadoteridol (Gd-HP-DO3A, sold under the brand name Prohance™, Bracco Diagnostics, Inc., Princeton, NJ, a subsidiary of Bracco Group, Milan, Italy), gadodiamide (Gd-DTPA-BMA, sold under the brand name Omniscan™, by Nycomed Amersham, now part of GE Healthcare, Milwaukee, WI), gadoversetamide (Gd-DTPA-BMEA, sold under the brand name Optimark™, Mallinckrodt, Inc., St. Louis, MO), and gadobenate dimeglumine (Gd-BOPTA, sold under the brand name Multihance™, Bracco Diagnostics, Inc.).[7]

Table 8.2 summarizes some of the physical properties of these FDA-approved MRI contrast agents. These gadolinium chelates have molecular weights ranging

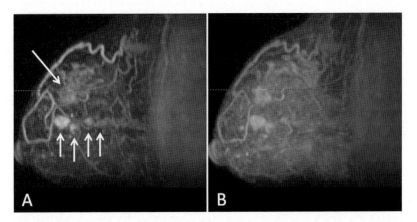

Figure 8.2 Sagittal 3D maximum-intensity projections of subtracted images of a breast containing both invasive breast cancer (long arrow) and DCIS (short arrows). Each image set was acquired transaxially with 1-minute temporal resolution. (A) First post-contrast subtracted series (first post-contrast series minus pre-contrast series). (B) Last post-contrast subtracted series acquired 6 to 7 minutes after injection. Progressive enhancement of normal parenchyma masks enhancing cancers in (B).

Table 8.2 Properties of Gd-chelated contrast agents

Agent	Chemical Formula	Common Name	Molecular Weight	Density (g/mL)	Viscosity (cP) 37°C	Relaxivities α_1	α_2
Magnevist (Gd-DTPA)	$C_{28}H_{54}GdN_5O_{20}$	gadopentetate dimeglumine	938	1.195	2.9	4.9	6.3
Prohance (Gd-HP-DO3A)	$C_{17}H_{29}N_4O_7Gd$	gadoteridol	559	1.137	1.3	4.6	5.3
Omniscan (Gd-DTPA-BMA)	$C_{16}H_{28}GdN_5O_9 \cdot xH_2O$	gadodiamide	574	1.14	1.4	4.8	5.1
Optimark (Gd-DTPA-BMEA)	$C_{20}H_{34}N_5O_{10}Gd$	gadoverset-amide	662	1.16	2.0	*	*
Multihance (Gd-BOPTA)	$C_{22}H_{28}GdN_3O_{11} \cdot 2C_7H_{17}NO_5$	gadobenate dimeg-lumine	1058	1.22	5.3	9.7	12.5

Notes: Densities measured at 20°C or 25°C
Viscosities are measured in centiPoise at 37°C
(Viscosity of water is 1.002 cP)
* = Not given in labeling information
Relaxivities α_1 and α_2 are given in units of $(mmole/L)^{-1}s^{-1}$

from 559 to 1058, meaning that the weight of the entire chelated molecule is between 559 and 1058 times the weight of a single hydrogen atom. All have densities slightly greater than water, ranging from 1.14 to 1.22 grams/milliliter (g/mL) at 20°C to 25°C (water has a density of 1.00 g/mL, so these chelated compounds have densities 14% to 22% higher than the density of water). All are considerably more viscous than water, with viscosities ranging from 1.4 to 5.3 centiPoise (cP) at a human body temperature of 37°C (water has a viscosity of 1.002 cP). Contrast agents with higher viscosities are more resistant to injection, making use of a power injector more important for achieving consistent injection rates.

A contrast agent's most important property is its effect on MR relaxation times. Relaxation rates r1 and r2 are defined as the inverse of relaxation times T1 and T2, respectively:

$$r_1 = 1/T1 \text{ and } r_2 = 1/T2. \tag{8.1}$$

Since relaxation times are given in units of time (in seconds or milliseconds), relaxation rates are given in units of inverse time (usually s^{-1}).

Relaxivity, which is different from relaxation rates, describes a contrast agent's effect on relaxation rates per unit concentration. Relaxivity (α_1 or α_2) is expressed in units of inverse seconds per millimolar concentration ($s^{-1}mM^{-1}$), where M stands for molar concentration in moles/liter (mol/L); equivalently, relaxivity can be expressed in units of inverse seconds per millimole per liter ($s^{-1}(mmol/L)^{-1}$). Relaxivity can be determined by measuring the relaxation rate (r_1 or r_2) at several different concentrations of the contrast agent and fitting the measured relaxation rates as a function of concentration of the contrast agent assuming a linear relationship. For example, the relaxivity α_1 is determined by measuring the relaxation rate r_1 as a function of concentration C, where C is in units of mmol/L:

$$r_1 = 1/T1 = r_{10} + \alpha_1 \cdot C \tag{8.2}$$

The intercept constant $r_{10} = 1/T1_0$ is the inverse of T1 in tissue at zero concentration of contrast agent. The relaxation rate r_1 can then be measured at several different concentrations of contrast agent. The relaxivity α_1 is the slope parameter determined by a best fit of measured relaxation rates r_1 to the known concentrations, C. The larger the relaxivity α_1, the greater the effect of the contrast agent on relaxation rate for a given molar concentration of the agent.

α_1 is the relaxivity for longitudinal magnetization (T1) and α_2 is the relaxivity for transverse magnetization (T2). The relaxivities α_1 and α_2 of most of the FDA-approved contrast agents are given in Table 8.2. As stated in Chapter 2, the fractional change in T1 is greater than the fractional change in T2 for a given dose of Gd-chelated contrast agent, so it is an agent's effect on T1 that is of primary interest. This is the main reason that T1-weighted pulse sequences are used, rather than T2- or $T2^*$-weighted sequences, to monitor the uptake of contrast: because heavily T1-weighted sequences are more sensitive to the effects of paramagnetic contrast agents.[8]

As Table 8.2 indicates, gadobenate dimeglumine (Gd-BOPTA, sold as Multihance™) has relaxivities that are approximately twice those of the other four FDA-approved contrast agents. These increased α_1 and α_2 values are attributed to weak, transient binding of the Gd-BOPTA molecule to serum proteins, in particular to serum albumin.[9] The mechanism of uptake and washout of Gd-BOPTA has been confirmed to be similar to that of Gd-DTPA and the other Gd-chelates listed in Table 8.2.[9–11]

These properties suggest that Gd-BOPTA should improve the conspicuity of enhancing breast lesions by increasing the signal in those lesions when used at the same concentration as other Gd-chelates. Percent signal increase in enhancing breast lesions is defined as the difference between enhanced signal (S_{post}) and unenhanced signal (S_{pre}) relative to the amount of unenhanced signal:

$$\text{Percent Signal Increase} = \frac{(S_{post} - S_{pre})}{S_{pre}} \times 100\% \tag{8.3}$$

in an ROI that is fully contained within the enhancing lesion, using the same ROI placement for pre- and post-contrast images.

For example, Equation 8.2 can be used to estimate that 0.1 mmol/kg of Gd-DTPA to a 70 kg woman (a total dose of 7 mmol of Gd-DTPA) would reduce the T1 of an enhancing breast lesion from 1000 ms (pre) to 356 ms (post), a 64% reduction in T1. If a TR of 10 ms and a 10° flip angle were used in spoiled 3D gradient-echo imaging, Equations 5.3 and 8.3 can be used to determine that a signal increase of 64% would occur from the T1-factor alone due to the lowered T1 value of the enhanced lesion. Similarly, a 0.1 mmol/kg dose of Gd-BOPTA to the same 70-kg woman (again 7 mmol) would reduce the T1 of the same breast lesion from 1000 ms (pre) to 219 ms (post), a 78% decrease in T1, resulting in a 90% increase in signal between the unenhanced and enhanced lesion from the T1-factor for the same TR and flip angle values. The $T2^*$-factors from the two different contrast agents would affect the overall signal only slightly, assuming that a very short TE value was used in gradient-echo imaging. For example, with TE = 2 ms, the $T2^*$-factor would alter the total signal increase with 0.1 mmol/kg of Gd-DTPA from 64% to 62%, while with Gd-BOPTA the $T2^*$-factor would alter the signal increase from 90% to 87%. Using a heavily T1-weighted pulse sequence with TE very short, T1 brightening of an enhancing lesion far outstrips $T2^*$ darkening of that lesion. Moreover, the higher α_2 value for Gd-BOPTA compared to Gd-DTPA does not come close to offsetting the signal increase from the higher α_1 value of Gd-BOPTA.

Preliminary clinical breast MRI studies indicate that Gd-BOPTA at a dose of 0.1 mmol/kg produces more conspicuous enhancement of lesions than 0.1 mmol/kg of Gd-DTPA.[12,13] Signal changes, sensitivities, and positive and negative predictive values appear to be significantly improved with this new agent. A CNS study found that Gd-BOPTA exhibited the same safety and efficacy as Gd-DTPA-BMA (Omniscan) for imaging of CNS lesions, even at higher dose levels for each agent.[14]

The gadolinium-based contrast agents listed in Table 8.2 were all originally approved by the FDA as CNS agents. Most have now been approved for body applications as well. To date, these agents are not FDA-approved or labeled specifically for use in breast cancer detection,[7] but they are used routinely for this purpose.

The Physiologic Basis of Contrast Enhancement

The mechanism for enhancement of invasive breast cancers compared to normal fibroglandular breast tissues relies on the extracellular nature of Gd-chelates. These contrast agents consist of relatively small molecules that can diffuse from the intravascular space to the interstitium or extravascular space. Studies of the vascular beds of breast cancers, like many other cancers in the body, show that invasive breast cancers greater than a few millimeters in size have higher densities of microvessels to support tumor growth (Figure 8.3). The density of microvessels alone, however, is not sufficient to explain the remarkable degree of enhancement that Gd-chelates cause in invasive breast cancers. These newly formed blood vessels are also leakier than more established microvessels. This is because newly formed vessels have permeable intercellular connections that permit proteins to pass through to extracellular spaces. These permeable connections also permit Gd-chelates to pass more freely between the intravascular bed and extracellular space in the vicinity of newly formed breast cancers. Vascular endothelial growth factor (VEGF) is known to affect vascular permeability, and VEGF has been shown to be higher in invasive breast cancers than in normal fibroglandular tissues and most benign breast lesions.[15]

The increased density and increased permeability of newly formed microvessels explain the preferential uptake of Gd-chelates in invasive breast cancers. These two

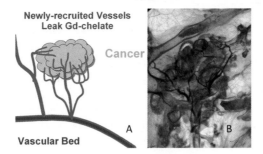

Figure 8.3 Tumor angiogenesis. (A) Schematic of a small invasive breast cancer recruiting vessels to support its growth. VEGF supports tumor growth and makes vessels more permeable. (B) Subgross, thick section (1.5 mm) 3D histologic image of ducts distended by high grade cancer (corresponding to the thickened wall and darker stained tissue) within the ducts. The spider's web-like net around the cancer-filled terminal ductal lobular unit is neoangiogenesis, supporting tumor growth. (Image provided by Dr. Laszlo Tabar, Professor of Radiology, University of Uppsala School of Medicine, Uppsala, Sweden, and Medical Director, Department of Mammography, Falun Central Hospital, Falun, Sweden).

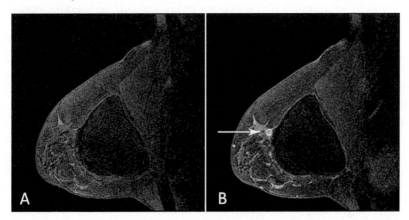

Figure 8.4 (A) Pre-contrast and (B) first post-contrast images of a breast containing a 4-mm invasive ductal carcinoma demonstrating rim enhancement (arrow) just distal to a silicone implant. Acquisition parameters for sagittal images were 18 × 18 cm FOV and 256×256 matrix, resulting in 0.7 × 0.7 mm in-plane pixels, with 1 mm slice thickness. Small in-plane pixel sizes and thin slices enable identification of important lesion characteristics that correlate with suspicion of cancer, such as margin characteristics and presence of rim enhancement.

factors also explain why breast cancers often exhibit a heterogeneous, ring pattern of enhancement, as shown in Figure 8.4. The newly formed microvasculature supporting tumor growth is near the surface of the lesion; those newly formed vessels are the most permeable, permitting Gd-chelates to leak into extracellular spaces. This feature also explains a distinguishing difference between invasive breast cancers and fibroadenomas. While fibroadenomas have microvascular densities that are similar to those of invasive breast cancers in terms of numbers,[16] the distribution of microvessels is more uniform in fibroadenomas than in invasive breast cancers. Invasive breast cancers have fewer microvessels in their central regions than in their peripheral regions, while fibroadenomas have more uniform vascular densities. Fibroadenomas also tend to have smoother margins than invasive breast cancers and, with adequate spatial resolution, internal septations within fibroandenomas are often visible.

These differences make it clear why high spatial resolution in breast MRI is imperative. To distinguish features that help identify cancers on a background of fat and normal fibroglandular tissue and help distinguish cancers from benign lesions, high spatial resolution is essential. These requirements are met by having smaller in-plane pixel sizes to avoid averaging over distinguishing features and by having thinner slices to avoid partial volume effects that can average away distinguishing morphology after uptake of contrast media.

Dosage of Gadolinium-chelated Contrast Agents

The labeled dosage of Gd-chelated contrast agents for adult central nervous system (CNS) studies is 0.1 millimoles/kilogram (mmol/kg). For a-110-lb (50-kg) woman, the recommended administration is (0.1 mmol/kg) * (50 kg) = 5 mmol. Since the concentration of each of the Gd-chelate contrast agents in standard dosage is 0.5 mmol per milliliter (ml), a 2 ml (or 2 cubic centimeter (cc)) volume contains 1 mmol of contrast agent. Thus, the labeled dosage in terms of volume is 0.2 ml/kg of body mass (or 0.2 cc/kg body mass), which is equivalent to a dose of 0.1 mmol/kg body mass. A simple rule to achieve the recommended dosage of 0.1 mmol/kg is to administer 1 ml of Gd-chelated contrast agent for each 11 lbs of body weight. Again, for a 110-lb woman, this rule would specify administering 10 ml of 0.5 mmol/ml contrast agent, or 5 mmol of Gd-chelated agent.

A flush of at least 5 ml of 0.9% saline solution should follow contrast agent injection to flush contrast agent from the tubing; 20 ml of saline solution typically follows contrast agent injection to flush the agent from both tubing and arm vein. A dual-headed MR-compatible power injector is recommended to deliver both contrast and saline at consistent injection volumes and rates. The labeled rate of injection of Gd-DTPA is at a rate not to exceed 10 ml per 15 seconds. Most other approved Gd-chelate agents have labeled injection rates of 1 to 2 ml per second, which is equal to 1 to 2 cubic centimeters per second (cc/s). A number of research studies have used injection rates of 2 to 4 cc/s without adverse effects.

Safety of Gadolinium-chelated Contrast Agents

Properties of the five FDA-approved Gd-chelated contrast agents related to their safety are summarized in Table 8.3.[7,17] All of these contrast agents are rendered non-toxic by their chelating compounds. These light-weight molecules are small enough to leak through newly formed vessel walls and occupy extravascular spaces.

One measure of the relative safety of a MRI contrast agent is its osmolality. The "osmole" defines the number of moles of a chemical compound contributing to the osmotic pressure of a solution. *Osmolality* describes the number of osmoles per kg

Table 8.3 Properties of Gd-chelated contrast agents

Agent	Injection pH	Osmolality (mOsmol/kg)	Recommended Injection Rate	LD_{50} (mmol/kg)
Magnevist	6.5–8.0	1960	≤ 0.67 mL/s	6–7
Prohance	6.5–8.0	630	> 1 mL/s	12
Omniscan	5.5–7.0	789	*	>30
Optimark	5.5–7.5	1110	1–2 mL/s	*
Multihance	6.5–7.5	1970	*	*

Notes: Osmolality of blood plasma = 285 mOsmol/kg.
LD_{50} = dose of agent at which 50% of laboratory animals (usually mice) die.
* = Not specified or reported in labeling information.
Data taken from manufacturers' product labeling.[7]

of solution; the *osmolarity* describes the number of osmoles per liter of solution. Osmolality is stated in units of Osmol or milliOsmol (mOsmol) per kg of solution (see Table 8.3). The osmolality of Gd-chelated contrast agents ranges from 630 to 1970 mOsmol/kg. Assuming an administered dose of 0.1 mmol/kg for these MRI contrast agents, a 70-kg patient would receive a total osmotic load ranging from 8.8 to 27.5 mOsmol. This can be compared to a total osmotic load of between 100 and 300 mOsmol from standard doses of iodine-based X-ray contrast agents.[17]

Gd-chelates have been used as a substitute for iodinated contrast agents in CT exams of patients with allergic reactions to iodine.[18] The high atomic number of gadolinium (64, compared to an atomic number of 53 for iodine) provides good X-ray attenuation per atom. The total attenuation of Gd-DTPA per molar concentration, however, is not as good as that of iodinated contrast agents due to fewer Gd ions per Gd-chelate molecule (one) than iodine atoms per iodinated contrast agent molecule (three). Thus, the density of Gd ions in Gd-DTPA is lower than the density of iodine atoms in standard X-ray contrast agents (16.8% vs 46.4%). As a result, in the CT study replacing iodinated contrast agents with Gd-chelates, Gd-DTPA was used at 3 to 4 times the label-recommended dose (of 0.1 mmol/kg) to provide X-ray attenuation comparable to a normal dose of iodinated contrast agent (30–60 g of iodine).[18]

One way of measuring the toxicity of any drug is by assessing the median lethal dose (LD_{50}) to laboratory animals (usually mice). The reported LD_{50} values of Gd-chelates in mice ranges from 6 to 30 mmol/kg, approximately 60 to 300 times the recommended doses per unit body mass in humans.

Possible Adverse Events Resulting from Gadolinium-chelates

Another way of assessing drug toxicity is by reporting the incidence of adverse events resulting from human administration. Adverse events based on recommended administration levels and at higher doses are reported in each product's FDA-required label. The most common reported adverse side effects of gadolinium-chelates at a standard dose of 0.1 mmol/kg are headache, dizziness, nausea, and emesis. Any single adverse event is reported in less than 1% of patients, and any adverse event at all is reported in less than 5% of patients.[17] Other types of adverse events are injection site pain, warmth or burning sensation, and localized edema. Delayed-onset adverse events include erythema, swelling, and pain at, and proximal to, the injection site. These delayed-onset events usually occur 1 to 4 days after intravenous injection, peak, and then resolve within a few days.[7,17] Other adverse events that have been reported include chest pain or tightness, fever, fatigue, arthralgias, rigors, asthenia, hot flashes, flushed feeling, malaise, weakness, facial edema, neck rigidity, abdominal cramps, itching, watery eyes, a tingling sensation in the throat, and generalized coldness.[7,17]

An assortment of other adverse events have been reported including gastrointestinal reactions, cardiovascular symptoms, respiratory events, anaphylactoid reactions, and other events, but the incidence of such events is quite low. For example, the true incidence of anaphylactoid reactions appears to be less than 1 in 100,000. Nonetheless, MR sites should be equipped to manage any adverse event as a result of a possible reaction to Gd-based contrast agents. The labeling of the specific contrast agent used should be consulted to get a more accurate estimate of the likelihood of adverse events.

Gadolinium-based contrast agents are cleared from the body by glomerular filtration and eliminated primarily through the urine, with approximately 95% of the agent eliminated within 24 hours. Patients with renal insufficiency or renal failure are of particular concern, as the agent may take longer to clear. This gives more time for dissociation of the Gd ion from its chelating ligand and may lead to the accumulation of free gadolinium within the body. Concerns have been raised about the use of off-label higher doses of Gd-chelates due to their potential for nephrotoxicity.[19] Careful attention should be given to the labeling of the specific agent administered.

Nephrogenic Systemic Fibrosis: A New Adverse Event of Gadolinium-chelates

As of December 21, 2006, the FDA has reported the occurrence of a new disease in approximately 90 patients in the U.S. with moderate to end-stage kidney disease who received Gd-based contrast agents.[20–22] Approximately 215 cases had been reported worldwide. The new disease, called nephrogenic systemic fibrosis (NSF) or nephrogenic fibrosing dermopathy (NFD), is characterized by extensive skin thickening, often occurring with hyperpigmentation and, in some cases, papules and subcutaneous nodules. The FDA is advising the public with the following warning: "Patients who develop NSF/NFD have areas of tight, rigid skin and may have scarring of their body organs. The signs of NSF/NFD also include: burning, itching, swelling, hardening and tightening of the skin; red or dark patches on the skin; yellow spots on the whites of the eyes; stiffness in joints with trouble moving or straightening the arms, hands, legs, or feet; pain deep in the hip bones or ribs; and muscle weakness."[21] Some patients have died from the disease.

This new disease has occurred anywhere from 2 days to 18 months after administration of Gd-based contrast agents. It has been noted that the great majority of patients suffering this new disease had severe renal disease or end-stage renal disease at the time of receiving Gd-chelated contrast agents. Many were on kidney dialysis when they received gadolinium-based contrast agent. No cases of NSF have been reported in patients with normal kidney function or in those with mild to moderate kidney insufficiency.

About 90% of the NSF cases reported to the FDA followed the administration of Omniscan™. Six cases have been reported following administration of Magnevist™, and two following administration of Optimark™.[20] To date, there have been no NSF cases reported following administration of MultiHance™ or ProHance™ alone. To get current information on the connection between NSF and Gd-chelate administration, consult the FDA website at: www.fda.gov/cder/drug/infopage/gcca/default.htm. As of May 23, 2007, the FDA was requiring all five approved Gd-chelate manufacturers to revise product labeling to include a warning about the potential for causing NSF. Additional information about NSF can be found at: www.icnfdr.org.

Currently, the FDA and other organizations advise MRI facilities that any patient scheduled to receive a Gd-chelated contrast agent in conjunction with their MRI exam be screened for the presence of moderate to end-stage kidney disease (defined by the FDA as a glomerular filtration rate of less than $30\,ml/min/1.73\,m^2$). Also considered at risk are patients with acute renal insufficiency of any severity due to hepato-renal syndrome or patients in the peri-operative liver transplantation period. If such conditions exist, every effort should be made to find an alternative exam that does not involve the administration of Gd-based contrast agents. If the exam must be performed, kidney dialysis is recommended following the MRI exam.[21]

Sensitivity and Specificity of Contrast-enhanced Breast Magnetic Resonance Imaging

Following the pioneering work of Heywang-Kobrunner and colleagues,[6] numerous studies have shown that contrast-enhanced breast MRI is highly sensitive to breast cancer. Results depend on study groups, imaging techniques, and other factors, but the sensitivity of contrast-enhanced breast MRI is consistently reported to be between 71% and 100%, with most studies reporting sensitivities in excess of 90%. In studies involving screening of high-risk women with breast MRI, mammography, ultrasound, and physical breast examination, breast MRI has had consistently higher sensitivities than other screening methods (see Table 8.4).

An early study compared the accuracy of standard dosage Gd-DTPA to higher doses in the breast.[29] They found that a dose of 0.16 mmol/kg had higher accuracy than the standard dose of 0.1 mmol/kg. Specifically, based on lesions larger than the

Table 8.4 Summary of the sensitivities reported in screening studies of women at high risk for breast cancer

Site	Investigators	$N_{subjects}$	Modality Sensitivities		
			Mammo	US	MRI
Dutch Multicenter	Kriege, et al[23]	1909	33%	–	80%
Bonn	Kuhl et al[24]	462	43%	47%	96%
Rotterdam	Tilanus-Linthorst, et al[25]	109	0%	–	100%
Nijmegen	Stoutjesdijk, et al[26]	179	46%	–	100%
Toronto	Warner, et al[27]	293	44%	41%	72%
Memorial-Sloan Kettering	Morris et al[28]	367	–	–	100%

slice thickness of their 3D images (4 mm), using a diagnostic criterion of 20% signal increase with injection of 0.1 mmol/kg gave a sensitivity of 94% and a specificity of 52%; using a diagnostic criterion of 60% signal increase with injection of 0.16 mmol/kg gave a sensitivity of 100% and a specificity of 73%. These results suggest that higher doses of contrast agent might increase sensitivity and specificity, but this needs further confirmation with current MR imaging techniques.

A more recent clinical study comparing three different doses of Gd-BOPTA (Multihance™), 0.05, 0.1, and 0.2 mmol/kg, found that sensitivity to breast cancer was highest with a 0.1 mmol/kg dose.[12] This study found that a higher dose of 0.2 mmol/kg, in addition to not increasing sensitivity, led to a higher false-positive rate than either of the other two doses. Finally, this study showed that evaluation of unenhanced, enhanced, and subtracted images, including a MIP image of the first post-contrast subtraction, was superior to the evaluation of enhanced images alone.[12]

An unpublished survey of 21 MR sites involved with the American College of Radiology Imaging Network (ACRIN) MR study of the contralateral breast in women with a known breast cancer found that contrast injection techniques varied considerably from site to site: 12 sites injected 0.1 mmol/kg of Gd-chelate, 6 sites injected 0.2 mmol/kg, and 3 sites injected fixed amounts of contrast agent regardless of body mass. Of those three sites injecting a fixed amount of contrast agent, one site injected 15 cc (7.5 mmol), one injected 20 cc (10 mmol), and one site injected 40 cc (20 mmol) for all patients. The label-recommended limit on injection of Gd-DTPA is 0.3 mmol/kg, which could easily be exceeded by a fixed dose independent of body mass to a small woman. For example, a fixed dose of 40 cc would exceed the FDA maximum dose of 0.3 mmol/kg to a woman who weights less than 66.7 kg (147 lbs). The other problem with using a fixed dose of contrast agent regardless of body mass is that the diagnostic criterion for degree of enhancement deemed suspicious would then vary with patient body mass.

Just as important as total <u>amount</u> of Gd-DTPA injected are the <u>rate</u> and <u>method</u> of injection. A recent abstract demonstrated that enhancement rates and time to peak enhancement are strongly affected by injection rate.[30] The authors compared injection rates of 0.5 ml/second and 2 ml/second for administration of fixed 20 ml doses of Gd-DTPA by injecting 27 women with two doses administered on different days. They found that breast cancers demonstrated a more rapid enhancement rate and earlier time to peak enhancement with the higher injection rate. Mean enhancement rates were 6.2 signal units per second for the 0.5 ml/s injection rate and 12.9 signal units per second for the 2.0 ml/s injection rate. Mean times to peak enhancement were approximately 3.5 minutes (209 s) for the 0.5 ml/s injection rate and 1.9 minutes (113 s) for the 2.0 ml/s injection rate. Surprisingly, peak enhancement factors of cancers, the ratio of peak post-contrast lesion signal to pre-contrast signal, did not differ significantly for the two injection rates: enhancement factors were 2.4 (240%) for 0.5 ml/s and 1.71 (171%) for 2.0 ml/s (p = 0.08).

Timing of Pulse Sequences After Contrast Injection

The timing of pulse sequences after contrast agent injection is determined by the rate of uptake and washout of the fastest enhancing lesions, which are invasive breast cancers. Typical invasive breast cancers reach maximum enhancement (and therefore maximum signal difference between cancer and background fibroglandular tissues) between 1 and 3 minutes after the end of contrast injection, assuming injection of 0.1 mmol/kg at a steady injection rate of 1 to 3 cc/s. Some focal cancers wash out after peaking 1 to 3 minutes after injection, while other cancers maintain near peak enhancement for the next few minutes. A small fraction of invasive breast cancers do not peak early but continue to enhance for more than 3 minutes after injection.

Kuhl et al. showed the importance of measuring enhancement curve shape as a way to add specificity to contrast-enhanced breast MRI.[31] Their study group consisted of 266 enhancing lesions in 230 patients, with 101 breast cancers. A standard dose of 0.1 mmol/kg of Gd-DTPA was administered, and imaging was performed every 42 seconds. Curve shapes were divided into 3 groups as illustrated in Figure 8.5. Type 1 curves with continuous uptake were shown to correspond to cancers in only 6% of cases. Type 2 curves with a rapid uptake and plateau corresponded to cancer in 64% of lesions, and Type 3 curves with rapid uptake followed by washout were cancer in 87% of lesions. Combining lesion morphology with curve shape information (Type 1 negative, Types 2 and 3 positive where morphology was equivocal) gave an overall specificity of 83%, with 91% sensitivity. When degree of enhancement alone was considered, using an 80% increase in lesion signal as the criterion for cancer, specificity was only 37%, again with 91% sensitivity. This study indicates the importance of capturing curve shape information, not just degree of enhancement, to increase the specificity of contrast-enhanced breast MRI.

The results of Kuhl and colleagues demonstrate that both Type 2 and Type 3 curves are highly suggestive of cancer.[31] Some radiologists refer to Type 2 curves as "indeterminate," which is a misnomer based on their study's results. A 64% probability of cancer is hardly indeterminate, especially when compared to the positive predictive values of other imaging tests, such as mammography. Other users have not necessarily duplicated the Kuhl, et al. data on the positive predictive value of morphology plus curve shape, but in some cases those studies lacked adequate temporal resolution to test the hypothesis that curve shape adds to the specificity of breast MRI. Kuhl et al. have demonstrated the importance of accurately

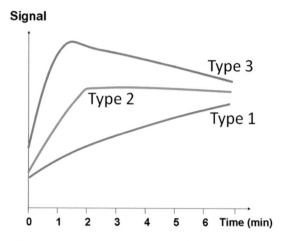

Figure 8.5 Three time-enhancement curve shapes correlate with suspicion of cancer. Type 1 curve (blue) with continuous uptake is indicative of a low probability of cancer. Type 2 curve (green) with rapid uptake and plateau is indicative of a higher probability of cancer. Type 3 curve (red) with rapid uptake and washout is most suspicious for breast lesions.

measuring time-enhancement curve shape, not as a replacement for morphology, but to be evaluated in conjunction with morphology.

Temporal Resolution in Contrast-enhanced Breast Magnetic Resonance Imaging

The time needed to acquire a complete set of 2D slice or 3D volume acquisitions through the breast can be considered the temporal resolution of a repeated series of pulse sequences, assuming those series are acquired in a repeated manner without time gaps. A pulse sequence that collects signal from both breasts and requires one minute of scan time provides 1-minute temporal resolution, as new measurements of signal from each pixel would be collected every minute. The particular time point within each series at which the measurement is most heavily weighted in terms of contrast is the point at the center of k-space in the phase-encoding direction, where $k_y = 0$. For most 3D gradient-echo pulse sequences, this point occurs about one-third of the way through the total acquisition. So for a repeated series with 1-minute temporal resolution, the specific time point at which that series can be considered to be most heavily weighted in terms of contrast is about 20 seconds after the start of acquisition. Some MR systems explicitly report the time point at which the center of k-space (in the phase-encoding direction), is collected. This is the most heavily contrast-weighted point in the pulse sequence.

Figure 8.6 illustrates the "sampling problem" in contrast-enhanced breast MRI. The green curve in each figure represents the most rapidly changing pattern of any

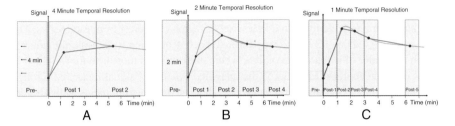

Figure 8.6 The most rapidly changing tissues in the breasts are invasive breast cancers with Type 3 curves, as illustrated by the green curve in each of these three diagrams. (A) Pre- and post-contrast series with 4-minute temporal resolution record a curve shape shown by the red curve, failing to capture the true curve shape and thereby underestimating the level of suspicion of some breast cancers. (B) Pre- and post-contrast series with 2-minute temporal resolution fails to correctly capture peak signal location but correctly replicates the true curve shape, giving a good estimate of lesion suspicion. (C) Pre- and post-contrast series with 1-minute temporal resolution capture both peak location and true curve shape accurately.

tissue in the breast, and the one that you would most like to measure because it represents the signature of lesions most suspicious for breast cancer. To correctly measure the curve shape, the temporal resolution of the contrast-enhanced series should be short enough to capture a pattern of rapid uptake and washout. A prerequisite to extracting quantitative time-enhancement data is running precisely the same pulse sequence once before administration of contrast agent (pre-contrast) and multiple times after contrast injection to sample the time-enhancement curve at multiple points (post-contrast). It is also essential that the same pulse sequence be repeated without resetting transmit or receiver gain so that each measurement of signal is recorded on the same scale. Re-tuning the scanner or allowing the scanner to auto-tune between successive acquisitions may change the scale of signal from measurement to measurement, rendering the time-enhancement curve shape inaccurate. On most modern scanners, it is possible to set up the entire series of pre-contrast and post-contrast scans as multiple measurements at different "phases" with a single pre-tuning prior to the *pre-contrast scan*. This practice is highly recommended to avoid errors in measuring the time-enhancement curve. Some sites set up separate series for the single pre-contrast and multiple post-contrast acquisitions, inadvertently re-tuning between the pre-contrast and post-contrast series. This captures the correct curve shape but may render measurement of *degree of enhancement* inaccurate. The correct procedure is to avoid re-tuning the scanner between the pre-contrast and any of the post-contrast scans. On some manufacturers' scanners with older software, multiple repetitions of the same pulse sequence require manual initiation of each series. In such cases, it is important to manually initiate each post-contrast series without re-tuning the scanner, both to minimize time gaps between series and to avoid the re-setting of gain factors within the multi-phase acquisition.

Figure 8.6A illustrates a contrast series with 4-minute temporal resolution. A single series identical to each post-contrast scan is collected before contrast administration to measure the pre-contrast point shown at t = 0. The solid blue dots represents the weighted average signal measured in a voxel or region of interest from each series. The dots are placed about 1/3 of the way through each acquisition to indicate the point at which the center of k-space is acquired, where each series is most heavily weighted in terms of tissue contrast. Each dot is the weighted average of signal measured through the entire 1-minute acquisition. Connecting those signal measurements with straight (red) lines depicts the *measured* time-enhancement curve. Ideally, the measured curve shape would match the actual curve shape. With 4-minute temporal resolution, however, the measured (red) curve fails to correctly demonstrate a signal peak or washout. Temporal resolution in excess of approximately 2 minutes is too slow to measure the correct curve shape for rapidly enhancing lesions. As a result, the true curve shape is "aliased away" by inadequate sampling; the result is that the level of suspicion of the enhancing lesion is underestimated. The measured curve in Figure 8.6A appears to have continuous uptake (a Type 1 curve) rather than a peak with washout (a Type 3 curve) due to inadequate temporal resolution in the contrast series.

Figure 8.6B shows a contrast series with 2-minute temporal resolution. As above, the solid blue dots represent the signal measured by each series and the red curve constructed by connecting the dots with straight lines shows the curve shape actually measured by the 2-minute temporal resolution series. While sampling every 2 minutes does not perfectly capture the location of the true enhancement curve's peak, it does a reasonable job of capturing the general curve-shape, showing both a peak and washout.

Figure 8.6C shows a post-contrast series with 1-minute temporal resolution. The measured time-enhancement curve accurately determines both the time of peak enhancement and the curve shape. The measured red curve shows rapid enhancement followed by washout, the signature of the Type 3 curve most suspicious for breast cancer. Taking more closely spaced time points with less than 1-minute temporal resolution would provide essentially the same curve shape information but with less SNR per pixel or poorer spatial resolution due to shorter acquisition time.

In addition to imaging with adequate temporal resolution, the techniques used to extract time-enhancement curves are important. Basing curve shape or degree of enhancement on an ROI encompassing an entire lesion can be misleading, due to the presence of necrotic areas and components with lower neovascularity. Hence, it is important to base enhancement curve analysis on the most rapidly enhancing areas of a tumor, with the exclusion of visible enhancing blood vessels. Smaller ROIs, encompassing 3 to 10 pixels, placed on the brightest areas of the enhancing lesion while looking at the first or second post-contrast image (whichever shows the lesion as being brighter) will result in the most accurate measurement of curve shape.[32] It is important to analyze unsubtracted images, not subtracted images, to measure degree of enhancement, basing enhancement on the signal strength of the unenhanced lesion within the specified ROI. It is also essential that identically acquired pre- and post-contrast images are used for curve shape extraction. Thus, the exact same pulse sequence should be run from one series to the next, the images in the same slice location should be analyzed, and exactly the same ROI size and location should be used for analysis. In addition, re-tuning the scanner's center frequency, transmit gain, or receiver gain between pre- and any post-contrast series is counterproductive to obtaining accurate time-enhancement curves.

Automated methods of generating time-enhancement intensity curves pixel-by-pixel exist on some MR systems and on most third party computer-aided diagnosis (CAD) systems. These methods will be discussed in Chapter 10.

Trade-offs Between Adequate Temporal Resolution and Adequate Spatial Resolution

In the past, imaging techniques forced a compromise between having adequate temporal resolution (1 to 2 minutes) and adequate spatial resolution (in-plane pixels less than 1 mm in both directions), thin slices (< 3 mm), and full coverage of both breasts. Techniques that opted for high spatial resolution, such as the traditional RODEO technique introduced in the early 1990s, often sacrificed breast coverage (RODEO as originally implemented imaged only one breast) and temporal resolution (RODEO had 4 to 5 minute temporal resolution) in order to gain sub-millimeter in-plane pixels with relatively thin (1.4 mm) slices.[33] Users that opted for higher temporal resolution (1 minutes or less) often sacrificed breast coverage or used larger pixels and thicker slices to gain detailed dynamic information.[31]

A recent paper by Kuhl et al, tested the relative tradeoffs of higher temporal resolution and higher spatial resolution.[34] Specifically, a series of 30 subjects with 54 enhancing lesions were given two separate contrast-enhanced imaging studies, one with approximately 1-minute temporal resolution (1 minute, 9 seconds) and larger pixels (1.25 mm in each in-plane direction), the other with 2-minute temporal resolution (1 minute, 56 seconds) and smaller pixels (0.8 × 0.6 mm in-plane). In both cases, other factors remained the same: 3 mm slice thickness, with 0.1 mmol/kg of Gd-DTPA injected at a rate of 3 mL/s by power injection, followed by a 20 mL saline flush.

Receiver-operating curve (ROC) analysis showed that the higher spatial resolution protocol had a significantly higher ROC curve area than the higher temporal resolution protocol, with ROC curve areas of 0.945 and 0.877, respectively ($p < 0.05$, indicating a statistically significant difference in favor of the higher spatial resolution protocol). With the higher spatial resolution protocol, the BIRADS ratings of 10 of 28 benign lesions were correctly downgraded, primarily because of the ability to better visualize lesion margins and internal septations in fibroadenomas. The higher spatial resolution protocol also correctly upgraded the BIRADS rating of 13 of 26 cancers, four from BIRADS 3 to BIRADS 4 or 5, nine from BIRADS 4 to BIRADS 5. Relaxing temporal resolution from just over 1 minute to just under 2 minutes had only minor effects on curve shape classification.

Some readers have interpreted the outcome of this study to mean that dynamic information is less important that spatial information or that dynamic information is useless in separating benign from malignant lesions. Neither conclusion is correct. A more accurate interpretation of the results of this important study is that little is lost by dropping temporal resolution from 1 minute to 2 minutes, while a great deal of morphologic detail is sacrificed by going from sub-millimeter in-plane pixels to pixels greater 1 mm in size.

This paper, along with the graphic illustration of temporal resolution give above, supports the concept that temporal resolution of 1 to 2 minutes is adequate, while in-plane spatial resolution should be sub-millimeter. We know that imaging with faster than 1-minute temporal resolution does not add additional clinical information by better measuring curve shape but causes a loss in SNR or spatial resolution. Can more information be gained by going to even higher spatial resolution? Probably, as long as the higher spatial resolution is not at the cost of SNR falling too low or slice thickness being made too large (or both), such that small contrast-enhanced lesions and vessels in the breast are missed. Use of gadolinium contrast agents takes enhancing breast lesions, as well as vessels, from being low-contrast structures to being high-contrast structures relative to their background, especially in subtracted images. In this situation, as long as low SNR and excessive partial voluming are avoided, the smaller the in-plane pixel size, the better.

Obtaining High Temporal Resolution and High Spatial Resolution Contrast-enhanced Studies

Earlier in this chapter we stated that in the past, MR users had to choose between high temporal resolution (1 to 2 minutes) and high spatial resolution (sub-millimeter in-plane pixels and thin slices). Modern MR imaging techniques have made that trade-off unnecessary. In particular, high-field scanners with stronger gradients and shorter rise-times have made it possible to acquire 3D gradient-echo images with very short TR and TE values. This has made it possible to achieve 1 to 2 minute temporal resolution while imaging both breasts with sub-millimeter pixels and thin slices (down to 1 millimeter). The techniques to achieve both high temporal resolution and high spatial resolution, requirements driven by the dynamics and spatial requirements for imaging contrast-agents in the breast, are described in detail in the Chapter 9.

Enhancement of Normal Fibroglandular Tissues in Pre-menopausal Women

One exception to the general rule that normal fibroglandular tissues enhance more slowly than breast cancers is the case of fibroglandular enhancement in pre-menopausal women. The fibroglandular tissues in pre-menopausal women are estrogen-responsive, changing their vasodilation and capillary permeability through a histamine-like response to estrogen.[35] Hence, pre-menopausal women can show a cyclic response to varying estrogen levels during their menstrual cycle. This cyclic response alters both tissue relaxation times and uptake of contrast agent during the menstrual cycle.

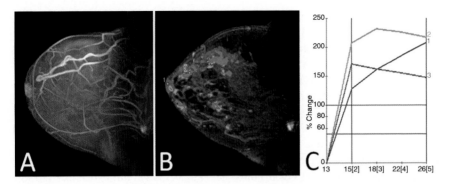

Figure 8.7 (A) Maximum intensity projection (MIP) of subtracted sagittally acquired images of an otherwise normal lactating breast. (B) Color map overlaying a single sagittal slice of the same lactating breast. (C) The inset graph displays three time-enhancement curves of three representative pixels (labeled 1, 2, and 3 in B and C) placed in normal lactating parenchymal tissue and illustrating the presence of all three curve types in a normal lactating breast. See Chapter 10 for a more detailed explanation of MIPs, color maps, and time-intensity curves.

Several studies performing repeated contrast agent administration to normal pre-menopausal women have shown a cyclic uptake of Gd-chelated contrast agents in normal fibroglandular tissue, with highest uptake in weeks 1 and 4 after menses.[36,37] During these times, spurious uptake of contrast agent occurred in enhancing foci, either focally or diffusely, with greater than 50% to 80% increase in signal during the first 1 to 2 minutes after contrast agent administration. More than 90% of this spurious enhancement in pre-menopausal women exhibited Type 1 curves, with continuous uptake. Spurious enhancement in less than 10% exhibited Type 2 curves (rapid uptake followed by a plateau; none exhibited Type 3 curves, with rapid uptake followed by washout). Most spurious enhancement was bilateral. A general rule resulting from these studies is that it is best to perform contrast-enhanced breast MRI on pre-menopausal women during the second or third week following menses to minimize the chance of spurious, hormonally induced parenchymal enhancement.[36,37]

Another subgroup in which spurious enhancement of fibroglandular tissues can occur is women who are lactating. Proliferation of milk-producing lobules and ducts often causes enhancement characterized by type 2 or type 3 curves, as shown in Figure 8.7.

Chapter Take-home Points

- Gd-chelate administration is essential for high sensitivity to breast cancer.
- Gd-chelates' primary effect is marked shortening of T1; thus heavily T1-weighted sequences are essential for high sensitivity to breast cancer.

- The recommended dose of all current Gd-chelates is 0.1 mmol/kg of body mass, which is equal to 0.2 mL/kg, a dose of 1 mL per 11 pounds of body weight.
- Gd-chelate contrast agents have the potential to cause a new, potentially serious disease (nephrogenic systemic fibrosis or NSF) in patients who have moderate to end-stage kidney disease at the time of administration of contrast agent
- Gd-chelate time-intensity curve shapes can add specificity to breast cancer detection.
- To measure time-intensity curves of cancers accurately, a temporal resolution of about 2 minutes or less is required.
- To capture morphologic information of enhancing lesions accurately, in-plane pixel sizes should be less than 1 mm.
- To be sensitive to small focal lesions of 5 mm or less and diffuse enhancement, slice thickness should be less than 3 mm.
- As will be shown in the next chapter, modern MR scanners should be able to capture both high spatial resolution and adequate temporal resolution of both breasts simultaneously with good SNR.

References

1. Ross RJ, Thompson JS, Kim K, et al. Nuclear magnetic resonance imaging and evaluation of human breast tissue: preliminary clinical trials. Radiology 1982; 143: 195–205.
2. El Yousef SJ, Alfidi RJ, Duchesnau RH, et al. Initial experience with nuclear magnetic resonance (NMR) imaging of the human breast, J Comput Assist Tomogr. 1983; 7: 215.
3. McSweeney MB, Small WC, Cerny V, et al. Magnetic resonance imaging in the diagnosis of breast disease: use of transverse relaxation times. Radiology 1984; 153: 741–744.
4. Wiener JI, Chako AC, Merten CW, et al. Breast and axillary tissue MR imaging: correlations of signal intensities and relaxation times with pathologic findings, Radiology 1986; 160: 299–305.
5. Merchant TE, Thelissen GRP, de Graaf PW, et al. Application of a mixed imaging sequence for MR imaging characterization of human breast disease. Acta Radiol 1993; 34: 356–361.
6. Heywang SH, Hahn D, Schmid H, et al. MR imaging of the breast using gadolinium-DTPA. J. Comput. Assist. Tomogr. 1986; 10: 199–204.
7. The labeling information of each FDA-approved Gd-based contrast agent was consulted for the data in this section: Magnevist, Document NDA 19-596/S-033, available at: http://www.fda.gov/cder/foi/label/2005/19596s033lbl.pdf, last accessed: 5-17-07, Berlex Imaging, 2004; Prohance, Document F1/3.5281.96, Bracco Diagnostics, Revised April 2006, available at: http://dailymed.nlm.nih.gov/dailymed/fda/fdaDrugXsl.cfm?id=1069&type=display, last accessed 6-17-07. Multihance, Document F1/3.5410.37, Bracco Diagnostics, revised January 2005, available at: http://www.bracco.com/NR/rdonlyres/B78D4E76-2E3D-4C88-81A7-C8C5B875DD28/0/MULTIHANCEPIJan2005.pdf, last accessed on 6-17-07; Optimark, Document NDA 20-937/20-975/20-976/S-009 Mallinckrodt Inc, Revised January 2003, available at: http://www.fda.gov/cder/foi/label/2006/020937,020975,020976s009lbl.pdf, last accessed on 6-17-07; Omniscan, ONC-2P-OSLO, GE Healthcare, October 2005, revised March 2007, available at: http://dailymed.nlm.nih.gov/dailymed/drugInfo.cfm?id=3425, last accessed on 6-17-07.
8. Hendrick RE, Haacke EM. Basic physics of MR contrast agents and maximization of image contrast. J. Magn. Reson. Imaging 1993; 3: 137–148.
9. Cavagna FM, Maggioni F, Castelli PM, et al. Gadolinium chelates with weak binding to serum proteins: a new class of high-efficiency general purpose contrast agents for magnetic resonance imaging. Invest. Radiol. 1997; 32: 780–796.

10. Kirchin MA, Pirovano G, Spinazzi A. Gadobenate dimeglumine (Gd-BOPTA): an overview. Invest. Radiol. 1998; 33: 798–809.

11. Spinazzi A, Lorusso V, Pirovano G, et al. Safety, tolerance, biodistribution and MR imaging enhancement of the liver with gadobenate dimeglumine. Acad. Radiol. 1999; 6: 282–291.

12. Knopp MV, Bourne MW, Sardanelli F, et al. Gadobenate dimeglumine – enhanced MRI of the breast: analysis of dose response and comparison with gadopentetate dimeglumine. AJR 2003; 181: 663–676.

13. Pediconi F, Catalano C, Occhiato R, et al. Breast lesion detection and characterization at contrast-enhanced MR mammography: Gadobenate dimeglumine versus gadopentetate digeglumine. Radiology 2005; 237: 45–56.

14. Runge VM, Armstrong MR, Barr RG, et al. A clinical comparison of the safety and efficacy of MultiHance (gadobenate dimeglumine) and Omniscan (gadodiamide) in magnetic resonance imaging in patients with central nervous system pathology. Invest Radiol 2001;36:65–71.

15. Knopp MV, Weiss E, Sinn HP, et al. Pathophysiologic basis of contrast enhancement in breast tumours. J. Magn. Reson. Imaging 1999; 10: 260–266.

16. Weind KL, Maier CF, Rutt BK, et al. Invasive carcinomas and fibroadenomas of the breast: comparison of microvessel distributions – implications for imaging modalities. Radiology 1998; 208: 477–483.

17. Shellock FG, Kanal E. Safety of magnetic resonance imaging contrast agents. J Magn Reson Imaging 1999; 19: 477–484.

18. Remy-Jardin M, Dequiedt P, Ertzbischoff O, et al. Safety and effectiveness of gadolinium-enhanced multi-detector row spiral CT angiography of the chest: preliminary results in 37 patients with contraindications to iodinated contrast agents. Radiology 2005; 235: 819–826.

19. Becker J, Thompson H. Renal safety of gadolinium-based contrast agent for ionizing radiation imaging (Letter to the editor). Radiology 2006; 240: 301–302.

20. Kuo PH, Kanal E, Abu-Alfa AK, Cowper SE. Gadolinium-based MR contrast agents and nephrogenic systemic fibrosis. Radiology 2007; 242: 647–649.

21. U.S. FDA Public Health Advisory: Information for Healthcare Professionals: Gadolinium-based Contrast Agents for Magnetic Resonance Imaging. Published on-line May 23, 2007 at: http://www.fda.gov/cder/drug/infopage/gcca/default.htm or http://www.fda.gov/cder/drug/InfoSheets/HCP/gcca_200705HCP.pdf. Last accessed on June 17, 2007.

22. Broome DR, Girguis MS, Baron PW, et al. Gadodiamide-associated Nephrogenic Systemic Fibrosis: why radiologists should be concerned. Am. J. Roentgenol., 2007; 188: 586 – 592.

23. Kriege M, Brekelmans CT, Boetes C, et al. Efficacy of MRI and mammography for breast-cancer screening in women with a familial or genetic predisposition. N Engl J Med. 2004; 351: 427–437.

24. Kuhl CK, Schrading S, Leutner CC, et al. Mammography, breast ultrasound, and magnetic resonance imaging for surveillance of women at high familial risk for breast cancer. J Clin Oncol 2005; 23: 8469–8476.

25. Tilanus-Linthorst MM, Obdeijn IM, Bartels KC. MARIBS study. Lancet. 2005; 366: 291–292.

26. Stoutjesdijk MJ, Boetes C, Jager GJ, et al. Magnetic resonance imaging and mammography in women with a hereditary risk of breast cancer. J Natl Cancer Inst. 2001; 93: 1095–102.

27. Warner E, Plewes DB, Hill KA, et al. Surveillance of BRCA1 and BRCA2 mutation carriers with magnetic resonance imaging, ultrasound, mammography, and clinical breast examination. JAMA. 2004; 292: 1317–1325.

28. Morris EA, Liberman L, Ballon DJ, et al. MRI of occult breast carcinoma in a high-risk population. AJR 2003; 181: 619–626.

29. Heywang-Kobrunner SH, Haustein J, Pohl C. Contrast-enhanced MR imaging of the breast: comparison of two different doses of gadopentetate dimeglumine. Radiology 1994; 191, 639–646.

30. Joe BN, Bae KT, Chen VY, et.al. Dynamic MR contrast enhancement characteristics of breast cancer: effect of contrast injection rate (Abstract). Radiology 2003; RSNA Annual Meeting Abstracts, p. 289.

31. Kuhl CK, Peter Mielcareck P, Klaschik S, et. al. Dynamic breast MR imaging: are signal intensity time course data useful for differential diagnosis of enhancing lesions? Radiology 1999; 211: 101–110.

32. Liney GP, Gibbs P, Hayes C, et al. Dynamic contrast-enhanced MRI in the differentiation of breast tumors: user-defined versus semi-automated region-of-interest analysis. J Magn Reson Imaging 1999; 10: 945–949.

33. Harms SE, Flamig DP, Hensley KL, et al. MR imaging of the breast with rotating delivery of excitation off-resonance: clinical experience with pathologic correlation. Radiology 1993; 187: 493–501.

34. Kuhl CK, Schild HH, Morakkabati N. Dynamic bilateral contrast-enhanced MR imaging of the breast: trade-off between spatial and temporal resolution. Radiology 2005; 236: 789–800.

35. Zeppa R. Vascular response of the breast to estrogen. J. Clin. Endocrinol. Metab. 1969; 29: 695–700.

36. Kuhl CK, Bieling HB, Gieseke J, et. al. Healthy premenopausal breast parenchyma in dynamic contrast-enhanced MR imaging of the breast: normal contrast medium enhancement and cyclical phase dependency. Radiology 1997; 203: 137–144.

37. Muller-Schimpfle M, Ohmenhauser MD, Stoll P, et al. Menstrual cycle and age: influence on parenchymal contrast medium enhancement in MR imaging of the breast. Radiology 1997; 203: 145–149.

Suggested Reading

Padhani AR. (2002) Contrast agent dynamics in breast MRI. In Warren R, Coulthard A, eds. Breast MRI in practice London: Martin Dunitz, pp. 43–52.

Brinck U. (2004) Tumor angiogenesis. In Fischer U. (2004) Practical MR Mammography. Stuttgart: Thieme Publishing Co., p 22.

Brinck U. (2004) Tumor angiogenesis and MR mammography. In Fischer U. (2004) Practical MR Mammography. Stuttgart: Thieme Publishing Co., p 23.

Gore JC, Kennan RP. (1999) Physical and physiological basis of magnetic relaxation. In Stark DD, Bradley WG, eds. (1999) Magnetic Resonance Imaging, 3rd Edition. New York: C.V. Mosby Publishing Co, Vol 1, pp 33–42.

Runge VM, Nelson KL. (1999) Contrast agents. In Stark DD, Bradley WG, eds. (1999) Magnetic Resonance Imaging, 3rd Edition. New York: C.V. Mosby Publishing Co, Vol 1, Ch 12, pp 257–276.

Heywang-Kobrunner SH, Viehwg P. (1999) Breasts. In Stark DD, Bradley WG, eds. (1999) Magnetic Resonance Imaging, 3rd Edition. New York: C.V. Mosby Publishing Co, Vol 1, Ch 15, pp 307–320.

Chapter 9
Breast Magnetic Resonance Imaging Acquisition Protocols

Breast MRI protocols can be divided into image acquisition protocols and image post-processing protocols. Image acquisition protocols should be designed to collect all necessary diagnostic data while minimizing patient scan time. This chapter is devoted to a detailed discussion of image acquisition protocols. Image post-processing protocols are described in Chapter 10.

Essential Elements of an Image Acquisition Protocol

An effective breast MRI protocol for detection or diagnosis of breast cancer has several essential elements:

1. A pre-contrast non-fat-saturated T1-weighted pulse sequence to delineate fat.
2. A pre-contrast fat-saturated T2-weighted pulse sequence to separate cysts from solid masses.
3. A set of contrast-enhanced pulse sequences at different phases to obtain identically acquired pre-contrast and multiple post-contrast views to separate enhancing lesions from other breast tissues. These sequences should meet the temporal and spatial resolution requirements given in Chapter 8. That is, they should have 1- to 2-minute temporal resolution, 1- to 3-mm thick slices, and sub-millimeter in-plane spatial resolution. In addition, they should have adequate signal-to-noise ratios (SNR) to display enhancing lesions and vessels in subtracted or MIP images.

Each of these three requirements and the pulse sequences that meet those requirements, are discussed in detail below. Other pulse sequences are often added to breast MRI protocols for at least two reasons: (1) to obtain the same type of pulse sequences listed above in additional planes to help orient the radiologist to the location of normal breast anatomy, cysts, and enhancing lesions in the breast, and (2) to increase the specificity of breast MRI (that is, to help distinguish benign from malignant lesions). Additional pulse sequences that offer promise of adding specificity to contrast-enhanced breast MRI are discussed further in Chapter 13.

Running additional pulse sequences to help orient the radiologist in the breast is to be discouraged, since additional sequences add additional scan time to breast

R.E. Hendrick (ed.), *Breast MRI: Fundamentals and Technical Aspects.*
© Springer 2008

MRI acquisitions, usually without adding additional diagnostic information. Moreover, with properly acquired T1W, T2W, and pre- and post-contrast-enhanced scans, especially those acquired with nearly isotropic resolution, post-acquisition image reformatting obviates the need for additional primary acquisitions. Eliminating additional pulse sequences speeds image acquisition and minimizes patient time on the scanner. Minimizing patient scan time makes the procedure more tolerable for the patient and can increase patient throughput.

Pre-contrast T1-weighted Non-fat-saturated Pulse Sequence

A pre-contrast T1-weighted non-fat-saturated (T1W-NFS) pulse sequence to delineate fat versus other breast tissues has historically been acquired using SE or FSE sequences with short TR and short TE to maximize T1-weighting. The short T1 of fat relative to other breast tissues makes fat brighter than other tissues, as long as reasonably short TR (under 1 s) is used. The longer T2 value of fat means that TE does not have to be made extremely short to keep fat brighter than other tissues, but short TE values are typically used to permit acquisition of as many slices as possible in 2D multi-slice SE or FSE. The heterogeneity of T1 values in cancers, benign breast lesions, and fibroglandular tissues means that breast lesions are often isointense with, or slightly darker than, normal fibroglandular tissues, making suspicious lesions difficult to detect in T1W sequences without the addition of paramagnetic contrast agent. Exceptions to this rule include cysts containing blood products such as methemoglobin, which can be bright on T1W-NFS sequences.

Most sites acquire pre-contrast T1W-NFS images using multislice 2D (planar) acquisitions rather than 3D acquisitions. With isotropic, or nearly isotropic, fat-saturated T1W 3D gradient-echo pulse sequences that can be obtained bilaterally in 2 minutes or less as the backbone of the contrast-enhanced series, however, the need for a T1W-NFS pulse sequence can be satisfied by simply running a single measure of the same 3D gradient-echo pulse sequence without fat-saturation. This provides a 3D dataset covering both breasts with identical coverage and resolution to the contrast-enhanced series. The isotropic or nearly isotropic dataset can then be reformatted in any planar orientation through post-processing, but in this case with fat brighter rather than dark, as it would be in fat suppressed gradient-echo imaging. Acquisition time for this 3D dataset will not exceed the temporal resolution of the 3D contrast-enhanced series, which should be 2 minutes or less. Since fat has high signal on T1W-NFS sequences, low SNR is seldom a problem, even though voxel size is small. Consequently, spatial resolution is excellent using this approach.

Figure 9.1 illustrates several ways of obtaining T1W-NFS images and illustrates how acquisition times and spatial resolution vary with the choice of pulse sequences. The acquisition of a properly performed bilateral T1W-NFS image set should not add more than 2 to 3 minutes to the breast MRI protocol.

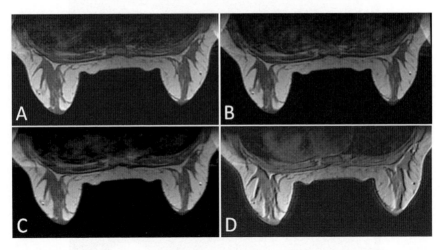

Figure 9.1 T1-weighted non-fat saturated images acquired with different pulse sequences on the same volunteer. In each acquisition, 50, 3-mm thick slices were acquired in the transaxial plane with a 256×256 matrix and a 26 cm square FOV. Images have been cropped vertically (A) 2D multislice SE image, TR = 650 ms, TE = 8 ms, total imaging time = 4:27 min:s. (B) 2D multislice FSE image of the same plane with TR = 450 ms, effective TE = 14 ms, ETL = 4, total imaging time = 3:56 min:s. (C) 2D multislice FSE images, TR = 700 ms, effective TE = 14 ms, ETL = 8, total imaging time = 3:04 min:s. Use of higher ETL values of 12 and 16 resulted in similar total imaging times (3:02 and 3:05) when TR was adjusted to minimize total scan time. (D) 2D multislice gradient-echo NFS images, TR = 525 ms, TE = 3.6 ms, 15° flip angle, total imaging time = 2:01 min:s. Note the dark line chemical shift artifacts at interfaces between fat and water due to use of a gradient-echo (rather than SE or FSE). Chemical shift artifacts are discussed in Chapter 11.

Pre-contrast T2-weighted Sequences

Breast cysts not containing blood have extremely long T1 and T2 values relative to other breast tissues, similar to those of cerebrospinal fluid (CSF), due to their high water content. Cysts typically have few macromolecules to shorten T1 and lack cellular structure to shorten T2 in hydrogen. Thus, cysts appear slightly darker than other breast tissues on heavily T1-weighted sequences due to their longer T1 values, although the higher hydrogen density of cysts partially counteracts the T1-weighted contrast between cysts and other breast tissues in T1-weighted sequences (Figure 9.2A).

Cysts appear much brighter than all other breast tissues on T2-weighted sequences due to their longer T2 values and higher hydrogen spin densities, both of which act in concert to make cysts bright (Figure 9.2B). Cysts are therefore more easily identified as bright areas on fat-suppressed T2-weighted sequences such as spin-echo or fast-spin-echo with long TR (> 2 s) and long TE (≥ 80 ms). Fat suppression in T2W SE or FSE sequences is done by applying one or more fat-saturation pulses prior to each set of 90° and 180° pulses in the SE or FSE sequence. The fat-saturation pulses are done without gradients turned on and act over the entire area of magnetic field

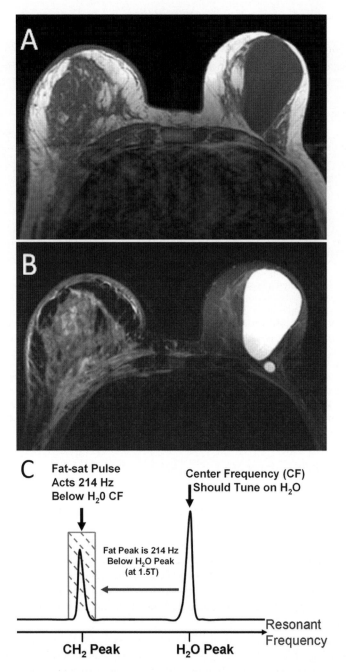

Figure 9.2 (A) Single slice of a T1W non fat-saturated multislice spin-echo sequence demonstrating a very large cyst and a smaller cyst posterolateral to the larger cyst in the breast on the right. Non-bloody cysts are dark on T1W images due to their long T1 values. (B) The same section of the same patient as in (A) acquired using a T2W fat-saturated FSE pulse sequence, showing both cysts to be bright. (C) Schematic of the chemically-selective fat-saturation method used in (B). Chemically selective fat saturation depends on the scanner's center frequency (CF) tuning on the resonant frequency of water and suppressing the signal from fat by applying one

homogeneity in the scanner; however, they act only on the fat peak, not the water peak, because they are applied over a very narrow frequency range (Figure 9.2C). This narrowband fat saturation requires good chemical shift separation of fat and water peaks, which in turn requires high static magnetic field homogeneity across both breasts in bilateral scanning. Magnetic field strengths of 1.0 T or greater are needed to achieve the degree of magnetic field homogeneity needed for good fat suppression across both breasts. Good chemically selective fat suppression during breast imaging can be a challenge on many MRI systems below 1.5 T due to incomplete separation of fat and water peaks at lower magnetic field strengths.

Short TI inversion recovery (STIR) sequences provide an alternative to T2W SE or FSE for achieving good fat suppression without the need for high magnetic field homogeneity. As described in Chapter 6, fat suppression in STIR imaging is performed by selecting a TI value that nulls the signal from fat (a TI value of 150–180 ms at 1.5 T). STIR images have the unique property that correlated T1, T2, and spin density values support one another in producing image contrast. This means that tissues with longer T1 values, longer T2 values, and higher spin densities all contribute coherently to making those tissues bright on STIR images. As a result, cysts are easily identified as being the brightest tissues on a STIR sequence. In addition to choosing TI to null the signal from fat (see Table 6.1), STIR imaging requires long TR values (≥ 3 s) and intermediate to longer TE values (≥ 50 ms).

Most SE, FSE, and STIR pulse sequences are acquired in multi-slice 2D format rather than 3D format because the long TR values needed for these pulse sequences would yield excessively long 3D acquisitions. Frequently, very long TR values (> 4 s) are used in SE, FSE, and STIR pulse sequences to accommodate acquisition of a large number of 2D slices. Use of longer TR values also minimizes T1 effects in SE and FSE, which is beneficial since T1 contrast counteracts T2 and spin-density contrast in these sequences, as shown in Chapter 4.

Contrast-enhanced Sequences

Previous Approaches to Contrast-enhanced Breast Magnetic Resonance Imaging

In the early 1990s, two competing approaches to contrast-enhanced breast MRI (CE-BMRI) emerged. One approach was to emphasize high spatial resolution image acquisitions, imaging once before and once after contrast injection, to be as sensitive as possible to lesions showing uptake of contrast agent. This approach

◄——

Figure 9.2 (continued) or more narrow-band RF pulses at a fixed frequency (214 Hz at 1.5 T) below the water peak without gradients applied, so that the RF pulses act only on the fat peak. These fat saturation pulses are applied on each pulse sequence repetition, exciting and eliminating the signal from fat prior to performing the normal SE, FSE, or gradient-echo pulse sequence.

based diagnosis primarily on the morphology of enhancing breast lesions, including their detailed shape, edge characteristics, and internal structure. Degree of enhancement was used as a secondary criterion for cancer.[1-4] This approach was typified by the rotating delivery of excitation off-resonance (RODEO) pulse sequence developed by Harms and coworkers.[5,6] RODEO acquired a unilateral 3-dimensional Fourier transform (3DFT) dataset using 128 slices with a 256×256 matrix over an 18×18 cm to obtain 1.4 mm×0.7 mm×0.7 mm voxels in an acquisition time of approximately 5 minutes each for pre- and post-contrast scans (Figure 9.3). A fundamental element of the RODEO pulse sequence was to use a special series of chemically selective radiofrequency (RF) pulses to suppress the high signal from

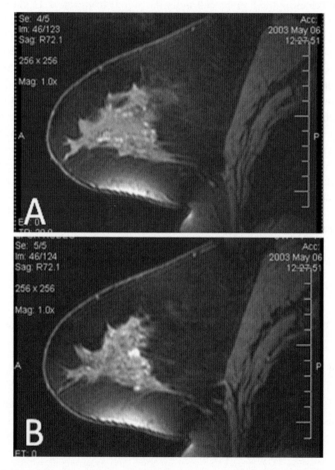

Figure 9.3 RODEO pulse sequence example. (A) Pre-contrast imaging was done using an unspoiled gradient-echo sequence with steady-state effects that made cysts bright. (B) Post-contrast sequence was done with a spoiled gradient-echo sequence that made cysts dark and enhancing lesions bright. The scan time for each was about 5 minutes.

fat on T1-weighted scans. Fat saturation minimizes bright regions of signal from fat that can confound subtle regions of contrast enhancement on post-contrast T1-weighted sequences.

A competing approach to breast MRI was to collect dynamic information about the uptake and washout of contrast agent to improve the specificity of the exam. In early implementations of dynamic CE-BMRI, either high spatial resolution or full coverage of the breasts was sacrificed so that higher temporal resolution could be obtained. For example, an approach involving very high temporal resolution by Bootes et al, was to use a turboFLASH sequence to acquire a single image every 2.3 seconds, confining image acquisition to a single 2D slice through the area of interest in the breast.[7] This required prior knowledge of the plane in the breast suspicious for breast cancer, as a temporal resolution of 2.3 s could not be achieved covering all tissue of one or both breasts. Using a definition of malignancy that included lesions enhancing within 11.5 seconds after aortic opacification, they obtained a sensitivity of 95% and a specificity of 86%.

A more typical dynamic approach, used by Kuhl et al, employed 2D FLASH imaging without fat suppression to obtain 21, 4-mm-thick contiguous transaxial slices through both breasts in an acquisition time of 42 seconds.[8] One pre-contrast and 9 post-contrast scans were obtained to provide a 10-point dynamic study of enhancement and washout. Slices were obtained in a rectangular format with a 250- to 320-mm field of view (FOV) and a 256×192 matrix, yielding voxel dimensions of approximately 1 mm (frequency) $\times 1.3$ mm (phase) $\times 4$ mm (slice). Using this technique, Kuhl et al were able to use lesion morphology combined with dynamic curve shape to obtain 91% sensitivity and 83% specificity for breast cancer.[8]

Current Approaches to Contrast-enhanced Scanning

New developments in MR gradient systems and pulse sequence techniques have made it possible to combine 3D high spatial resolution and dynamic imaging approaches so that both are obtained simultaneously over both breasts in CE-BMRI.

A goal of this chapter is to suggest some standards for high-quality breast MRI in light of these technical improvements. Because of different scanner hardware and software, the capabilities of MR scanners vary widely. This chapter provides guidance to imaging techniques that transcend specific MR scanner capabilities and provides the methods and rationale to achieve consistently high-quality CE-BMRI. The essential elements are:

1. Magnetic field strength of at least 1.5 T and high magnetic field homogeneity
2. Bilateral imaging with prone positioning using a dedicated breast coil
3. 3D gradient-echo T1-weighted pulse sequences for CE imaging
4. Good fat suppression over both breasts in CE-BMRI
5. Adequately thin image slices ($\leq$3mm, with 1 mm slices ideally)
6. Pixel sizes of less than 1 mm in each in-plane direction

7. Proper selection of the phase-encoding direction to minimize artifacts across the breasts
8. A total acquisition time for both breasts of less than 2 minutes

Each of these elements is discussed in detail below.

Magnetic Field Strength of at Least 1.5 T and High Magnetic Field Homogeneity

Above a few tenths of a Tesla, image signal-to-noise ratio (SNR) goes up approximately linearly with magnetic field strength.[9,10] Therefore, high magnetic field strength (B_o) provides high SNR for the same voxel volume, assuming appropriate pulse sequences are used. Higher SNR per unit volume means that higher spatial resolution may be obtained with adequately short scan times.

A second reason for requiring high magnetic field strength is to ensure adequately high magnetic field homogeneity over the area being imaged. High magnetic field homogeneity for breast imaging means that the static magnetic field strength should not vary significantly across a field size that includes both breasts. Since protons in water and fat differ in resonant frequencies by approximately 3.4 parts per million (ppm), magnetic field homogeneity must be significantly better than 3.4 ppm over the field-of-view of the breasts to achieve good chemically selective fat suppression; good fat suppression entails cancellation of signals from hydrogen in fat (primarily CH_2) with preservation of signals from hydrogen in water (H_2O). The standard criterion for good chemically selective fat suppression is that magnetic field homogeneity should be less than 1 ppm. Since good fat suppression is needed across both breasts, the magnetic field homogeneity should be less than about 1 ppm across a FOV that includes both breasts (30 to 35 cm). This is generally not possible for low to mid-field scanners (less than 1.0 Tesla) and is a challenge even for high-field scanners, since the locations of the breasts in prone-positioned breast MRI are not usually at the magnet's isocenter.

Bilateral Imaging with Prone Positioning

Bilateral imaging is recommended for at least four reasons. Clinically, comparing images of both breasts is as important in BMRI as it is in mammography.[11] Bilateral comparison helps identification of focal enhancement and helps prevent overcalling fibroglandular enhancement, which tends to occur bilaterally in some pre-menopausal women and some post-menopausal women on hormone replacement therapy.

Second, a few clinical studies have indicated that an asymmetric increase in total vascularity occurs in the ipsilateral breast of women with invasive breast cancer.[12,13] Such asymmetry is best seen on MIPs of subtracted early post-contrast scans of a simultaneously obtained bilateral exam. Bilateral comparison is difficult or impossible on scans where left and right breasts are imaged with different injections or with a single injection where image acquisition on the left breast is not simultaneous with image acquisition on the right breast.

Third, data from recent studies indicate that when a breast cancer occurs, mammography has a 1% to 2% chance of revealing cancer in the contralateral breast, while BMRI has an additional 3% to 5% chance of detecting a cancer in the contralateral breast.[14–20]

Finally, unilateral imaging in the transaxial or coronal plane can incur image wrap-around artifacts from the contralateral breast, especially when phase encoding is set left-to-right. While this is more likely to occur with a bilateral breast coil when the receiver coil for the contralateral breast coil is left on, some image wrap from the contralateral breast can occur even with the use of a unilateral breast coil or a bilateral breast coil with the contralateral coil turned off (see Chapter 11). Bilateral imaging with a field of view large enough to include all tissue of both breasts and phase-encoding set to be L-R is an easy way to eliminate image wrap artifacts. With no tissue extending beyond the FOV left or right of the breasts, special scan features that suppress image wrap but extend imaging time or degrade spatial resolution or SNR, such as phase oversampling or "no phase wrap," are unnecessary. When unilateral breast MRI *must* be performed, acquisition should be considered in the sagittal plane with phase-encoding set head-to-foot, so that the possibility of image wrap of the contralateral breast is eliminated.

Bilateral imaging is usually done using the body coil as the transmit coil and a prone-positioned bilateral breast coil as the receiver coil. Modern breast coils use multiple channels as receiver elements. These multichannel receiver coils measure and record signal simultaneously using multiple amplifier and analog-to-digital converter systems, but must be matched to the available receiver channels on the MR system itself. Two-channel and four-channel (quadrature) breast receiver coils and amplifier systems are common on MRI units manufactured over the last decade. Seven- and eight-channel breast receiver coils have recently been introduced (InVivo, Waukesha, WI, and GE Healthcare, Milwaukee, WI), and manufacturers are working on breast coils with 16 to 32 receiver coils.

New MR scanners are currently being manufactured with 32- or 64-channel receiver-amplifier systems. Until recently, these multiple receiver channels were all used to acquire the same dataset for image reconstruction. The development of parallel imaging, discussed later in this chapter, has enabled the simultaneous acquisition of two or more channels of data, speeding image acquisition with only a slight reduction in image quality.[21,22]

Prone positioning of the breast MRI patient in dedicated breast coils permits the breasts to hang dependently with the patient supported above and below the breasts, at the sternum, and at the outer edge of the chest. This keeps the breasts relatively stable and free from motion due to respiration and cardiac pulsation. Unlike cardiac

MRI and some body MRI applications, breast MRI does not require cardiac gating to reduce motion artifacts. Cardiac gating slows image acquisitions and makes total acquisition times vary from one series to another, features not wanted in breast MRI.

Some dedicated breast coils permit mild compression in the lateral to medial direction. This can decrease breast motion and reduce the extent of breast tissue that must be imaged in the left-to-right (lateral-medial) direction. This can be helpful when scanning in the sagittal plane by limiting the number of slices needed to cover each breast, thus shortening acquisition time for 3DFT acquisitions. Minimizing breast motion between pre- and post-contrast scans also helps minimize misregistration in subtracted images (see Chapter 11).

3D Gradient-echo T1-weighted Pulse Sequences for Contrast-enhanced Imaging

As noted previously, T1-weighted pulse sequences are used in CE-BMRI because Gd-chelates, while shortening both the T1 and T2 relaxation times of hydrogen nuclei, cause a greater fractional change in T1 than T2.[23] In gradient-echo imaging, T1 weighting is achieved by using short TR, very short TE, and a low to moderate flip angle, which depends on TR (see Chapter 5).[24] The T1 shortening caused by Gd-DTPA makes lesions brighter than most surrounding breast tissues other than fat. Thus, enhancing lesions appear bright in both fat-suppressed post-contrast scans and in properly subtracted contrast-enhanced studies, where pre-contrast images are subtracted from post-contrast images (Figure 9.4).

As discussed in Chapter 5, 3DFT sequences can have a signal-to-noise advantage over 2DFT pulse sequences in the breast because signal is acquired from a volume instead of a single plane. Thus, more signal is collected on each data measurement. 3DFT sequences require more phase encoding steps, by a factor equal to

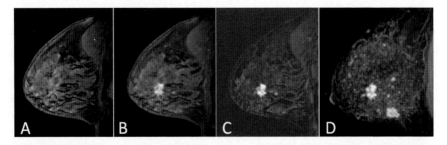

Figure 9.4 T1W gradient-echo imaging of an enhancing invasive ductal carcinoma. (A) Single slice of the pre-contrast series containing 48 2.5-mm slices. (B) Same slice location in the first post-contrast series, acquired immediately after injection ended with 2 minute acquisition time. (C) Subtracted image of (B) minus (A). (D) Maximum intensity projection of all subtracted images of the 1st post-contrast series minus the pre-contrast series showing a second cancer in the same breast.

the number of acquired slices, to resolve the volume of tissue into voxels, as described in Chapter 5. 3DFT sequences therefore require very short TR values to acquire all the necessary phase-encoding views and still keep imaging times short enough to meet the temporal resolution requirement of acquiring each series in less than 2 minutes.

Good Fat Suppression over Both Breasts in Contrast-enhanced Breast Magnetic Resonance Imaging

As mentioned above, in T1-weighted 3DFT imaging, fat suppression is achieved by applying a frequency-selective 90° saturation pulse that acts only on the hydrogen in fat. This narrow-band saturation pulse is applied to the entire volume of tissue in the body coil, without a gradient applied in any direction. If applied uniformly across both breasts, the 90° pulse effectively eliminates fat signal from the subsequent pulse sequence that follows. Fat suppression is useful, as it reduces the signal from fat in both pre- and post-contrast scans. Lack of fat suppression and even a small amount of misregistration between pre- and post-contrast scans can create artifacts in subtraction images that complicate interpretation and, in some cases, can simulate diffuse enhancing lesions (Figure 9.5). Good fat suppression has the potential to minimize the confounding effects of misregistration artifacts and to permit the detection of small or diffuse enhancing lesions.[25]

Adequately Thin Image Slices

As described in Chapter 7, slice thickness sets the limit on the smallest visible lesions. To be sensitive to a lesion of 5-mm diameter, a slice thickness of less than 5 mm should be used. Even then, partial volume averaging of the part of a

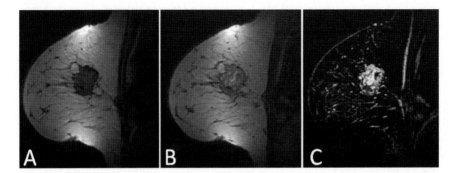

Figure 9.5 (A) Precontrast and (B) post-contrast images without fat saturation. (C) Subtracted image of (B) minus (A) showing a large enhancing lesion and other bright areas of spurious enhancement due to lack of fat suppression and misregistration of the two images due to motion.

low-contrast lesion occurring in a particular slice might make the lesion difficult to detect (see Figure 7.8). Fortunately, most enhancing breast lesions are
not low-contrast in either post-contrast images (unless fat suppression is not
used) or subtracted images, due to the shortening of T1 by gadolinium chelates
in enhancing lesions. Adequately thin slices, however, make CE-BMRI more
sensitive to small areas of distributed or diffuse enhancement in non-mass
lesions. This type of non-focal enhancement, which is characteristic of 20% to
30% of cancers, especially non-invasive cancers such as ductal carcinoma in-
situ (DCIS), is crucial to detect if breast MRI is to be sensitive to all types of
breast cancers.

To be sensitive to areas of diffuse enhancement where partial volume averaging
between enhanced and unenhanced tissues occurs, slice thickness should be 3 mm
or less for contrast-enhanced imaging. A slice thickness of 1 mm virtually eliminates partial volume averaging and permits reformatting of contrast-enhanced or
subtracted images in any plane without significant loss of spatial resolution. Thus,
a slice thickness of 1 to 3 mm is recommended, with 1 mm thickness ideal.

Pixel Sizes of Less than 1 mm in Each in-plane Direction

Smaller pixel sizes increase spatial resolution and the amount of fine detail available to the radiologist.[25,26] Smaller pixels provide better definition of lesion margins
and better visibility of lobulated and spiculated margins associated with many invasive breast cancers. Without small in-plane pixels, morphologic details essential to
raising the suspicion of cancer such as spiculations, non-smooth lesion margins,
and rim enhancement can be missed.

Pixel sizes of less than 1 mm in each in-plane direction can be achieved in bilateral imaging. If primary images are acquired in the sagittal plane, use of a 20 cm
FOV with a 256×256 matrix yields a pixel size of 0.78×0.78 mm. To avoid
excluding breast tissue in larger breasts, a field of view of up to 25 cm can be used
with a 256×256 matrix without pixels exceeding 1 mm in either in-plane direction.
This should be done, however, only if breast size requires the larger FOV to include
all breast tissue in the image.

With the phase-encoding direction selected head-to-foot (HF, also referred to as
superior-inferior or SI), it is often possible to use a rectangular FOV for sagittal
imaging, with fewer pixels needed in the head-to-foot direction than in the anterior-
posterior direction. This has the benefit of decreasing the required number of
phase-encoding steps without degrading spatial resolution. For example, in sagittal
acquisitions with a nominal 20-cm FOV and 256×256 matrix, the FOV in the HF
direction can often been reduced to be ¾ of the FOV in the A-P direction by choosing a rectangular FOV with 75% FOV in the phase-encoding direction. In this case,
256 pixels will be acquired in the A-P direction while 192 pixels (3/4 of 256) will
be acquired in the HF direction, with the same pixel size in each direction. Since
total scan time is directly proportional to the number of phase-encoding steps, scan

time will be decreased to 75% of the scan time that would have been needed with a square FOV.

If primary images are acquired in the transaxial plane, use of a 30 cm FOV with a 384×384 matrix also yields an in-plane pixel size of 0.78×0.78 mm. For larger patients, a field of view of up to 36 cm can be used, if needed, to include all breast tissue without exceeding a pixel size of 1 mm in each dimension (at 36 cm FOV with a 384×384 matrix, pixel size is 0.94×0.94 mm). It is only advantageous to use a rectangular FOV when doing so reduces the number of phase-encoding steps, since this reduces scan time. In transaxial imaging, it is seldom beneficial to use a rectangular matrix, as phase-encoding should be set left-to-right (LR, as discussed in the next section); this is usually the larger in-plane dimension, since the patient's LR width almost always exceeds the anterior-to-posterior (AP) depth of the breasts.

A common error in breast MRI is to set the FOV larger than needed to include all breast tissues. Imaging with the FOV set well beyond the extent of the breasts simply wastes pixels to image air. In addition, since the image matrix typically is fixed, spatial resolution suffers when the FOV is set larger than necessary. As a result, important details such as margins and internal structures of enhancing breast lesions are unnecessarily blurred (Figure 9.6). Technologists performing breast MRI should be instructed to set the image FOV so that it does not exclude breast tissue but also does not compromise spatial resolution within the breast (Figure 9.6). Radiologists interpreting breast MRI exams should be vigilant about "FOV creep," the tendency of some breast MR technologists to use larger FOVs than necessary so that they can be absolutely sure than no breast tissue is excluded. The price paid for FOV creep is poorer spatial resolution in all images.

Proper Selection of the Phase-encoding Direction to Minimize Artifacts Across the Breasts

The main sources of artifacts in breast MRI are vascular pulsation and breast, cardiac, and respiratory motion. Motion artifacts propagate across acquired images in the phase-encoding direction (Figure 9.7, and see Chapter 11). Therefore, it is essential to orient the phase-encoding direction to minimize motion artifacts across breast tissue, especially those from cardiac and respiratory motion. A good rule of thumb to achieve this is to put the frequency encoding direction AP. For sagittal imaging, this means orienting the phase-encoding direction HF. For transaxial imaging, this means orienting phase-encoding to be left-to-right (LR). For coronal imaging, phase-encoding can be oriented either HF or LR, since moving tissues are neither superior to, inferior to, left or right of the breasts when the patient is properly positioned; that is, with the patient's arms positioned toward her head and her head positioned posterior to the breasts. For coronal imaging, it can save time to orient the phase-encoding direction HF so that a rectangular FOV can be used with the shorter dimension in the HF direction. This reduces the FOV in the phase-encoding (HF) direction, which also reduces total scan time.

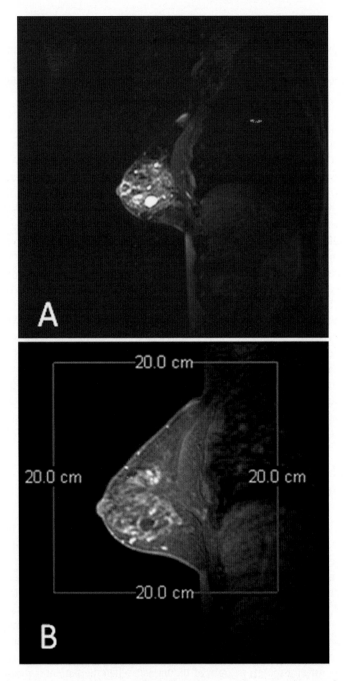

Figure 9.6 (A) One of 100 bilateral sagittal slices demonstrating a grossly excessive FOV for T2W sagittal imaging. (B) One of 104 bilateral post-contrast series slices showing a smaller, but still excessive, FOV for the pre- and post-contrast series. A box is superimposed to indicate **a** properly selected 20 cm FOV. Note that a correctly placed FOV includes all breast tissue but is biased toward the head to include as much axillary tissue as possible.

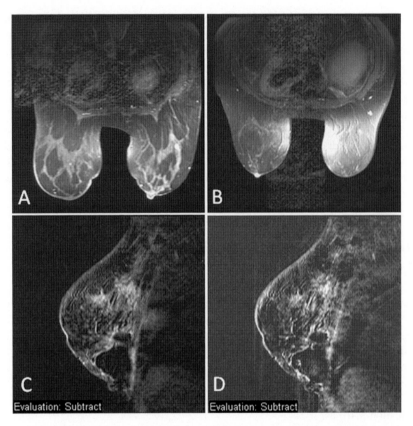

Figure 9.7 (A) For transaxial imaging, the correct phase-encoding direction is LR. (B) Incorrectly chosen phase-encoding direction for transaxial imaging is anterior-posterior (AP) causing cardiac and respiratory motion artifacts to propagate across breast tissue, especially the left breast. (C) For sagittal imaging, the correct phase-encoding direction is head-to-foot (HF or superior-inferior, SI). (D) Incorrectly chosen phase-encoding direction for sagittal imaging is AP, causing cardiac and respiratory motion artifacts across breast tissue, especially the left (see Chapter 11).

A Total 3D Fourier Transform Acquisition Time for Both Breasts of Less than 2 Minutes

As discussed in Chapter 8, the temporal resolution needed for breast MRI is determined by the time course of contrast agent uptake. Peak contrast enhancement in malignant lesions typically occurs between 1 and 3 minutes after injection, so capturing lesion dynamics accurately requires a temporal resolution of approximately 2 minutes or less. For bilateral imaging, this means that both breasts must be imaged in this time period. Typically, a single pre-contrast image set and several post-contrast image sets are acquired with identical acquisition parameters so that subtraction of pre- from post-contrast images reveals only temporal changes. This means that it is important to keep scanning parameters, including center frequency, transmitter gain, and receiver gain, identical for pre-contrast and all post-contrast scans. Allowing the MR system to re-tune or "auto-pretune" for any post-contrast sequence will defeat this requirement.

Imaging continuously with 1 to 2 minute temporal resolution for at least 6 minutes after contrast injection is long enough to determine the shape of the contrast curve and to determine whether enhancement is continuous (Type 1), plateau (Type 2), or washout (Type 3) (see Figure 8.5). As discussed in Chapter 8, collecting post-contrast data with adequate temporal resolution to portray the time course of lesion enhancement correctly is important, as it adds specificity to CE-BMRI.[7,8,25,26] This must be done with adequate SNR to permit detection of enhancing lesions and with adequate spatial resolution to depict their detailed morphology.

Meeting Temporal *and* Spatial Resolution Requirements in 3D Gradient-echo Imaging

The combined temporal resolution and spatial resolution requirements, along with the need to image all breast tissues bilaterally with adequate SNR, imposes tight constraints on CE-BMRI. The need to image both breasts in less than 2 minutes with pixel sizes less than 1 mm and a slice thickness of 1 to 3 mm demands fast 3D imaging. We now turn to a detailed discussion of how these demanding spatial and temporal resolution requirements can be met in contrast-enhanced breast MRI.

The total acquisition time of a 3D gradient-echo sequence is given in Chapter 5 (Equation 5.10) as:

$$T_{total} = (TR)(N_{slices})(N_{pe})(N_{ex}), \qquad (9.1)$$

The number of slices, FOV, and matrix requirements to cover both breasts depend on the acquisition plane. For transaxial image acquisition, 12 to 16 cm (in the head-to-foot direction) are usually sufficient to include all breast tissues including inframammary and some axillary lymph nodes. For convenience, we will assume a typical slice range of 14.4 cm. This range could be spanned with 144 1-mm thick slices, 72 2-mm thick slices, or 48 3-mm thick slices. At the same time, to maintain sub-millimeter in-plane pixels and include all breast tissue requires a FOV of 28 to 36 cm and a 384×384 (or larger) matrix. We will assume a FOV of 32 cm with a 384×384 matrix, yielding 0.83×0.83 mm pixels. This means that 384 in-plane phase-encoding steps are needed. As with most 3D imaging, we will set $N_{ex} = 1$. Thus, in Equation 9.1, $N_{slice} = 144$ (for 1 mm slices) or 48 (for 3 mm slices), $N_{pe} = 384$, and $N_{ex} = 1$. With TR = 5 ms, Equation 9.1 gives:

$$T_{total} = (TR)(N_{slices})(N_{pe})(N_{ex}) = (0.005 s)(144)(384)(1) = 276 s = 4.6 minutes$$

for acquisition of 144 1-mm slices, which exceeds our ideal maximum temporal resolution (2 minutes) by a factor of 2.3. We could easily reduce temporal resolution to 1.54 minutes by increasing slice thickness to 3 mm or be at exactly 2 minutes by changing slice thickness to 2.3 mm, as it would require only 63 2-mm slices to cover 14.4 cm. These last two options would sacrifice nearly isotropic voxels, however, so we would like to explore other ways to reduce scan time in 3D gradient echo imaging without increasing slice thickness.

Time-saving Measures in 3D Gradient-echo Imaging

Modern MR scanners provide a number of features that can be used to reduce scan time in 3D gradient-echo imaging without increasing slice thickness. The first question to pose in trying to reduce scan time on a specific scanner is: what is the shortest TR that can be used with 3D gradient-echo imaging? Newer scanners with strong gradients and short gradient rise times can make TR even shorter than 5 ms. Reducing TR to its minimum value is a simple way to decrease total scan time without adversely affecting spatial parameters. The shortest TR values achievable today are about 3.5 ms, which is not short enough to reduce total scan time by a factor of 2.3 to make temporal resolution 2 minutes or less (with 1-mm slices) in the example above. Assuming TR is made as short as possible for acquisition of 3D gradient-echo images, additional time-saving features include partial-Fourier imaging (in the in-plane phase-encoding direction), slice interpolation or partial-Fourier data collection in the slice-select direction, the use of a rectangular FOV with reduced field size in the phase-encoding direction, and parallel imaging, which uses multi-channel receiver coils to collect multiple channels of image data simultaneously. Each of these options is discussed below.

Partial-Fourier Imaging

Chapter 3 introduced the concept of image formation and described image data collection in k-space, the 2-dimensional Fourier transform of the image. A 2D MR image is a 2-dimensional matrix of signal values in x-y position space (Figure 9.8A). The discrete 2-dimensional Fourier transform of that image describes image data as an array of signal values in 2D spatial-frequency space, where k_x is the spatial frequency of image data in the x-direction and k_y is the spatial frequency of image data in the y-direction (Figure 9.8B). Each horizontal line of data in k-space is filled by measuring the signal at different time points (k_x values) with a fixed amount of phase-encoding (k_y). A full horizontal line of data in k-space is collected during a single gradient echo signal measurement (Figure 9.8C). The next gradient echo, collected after applying a different degree of phase encoding, collects a different horizontal line in k-space. Collection of each different phase-encoding "view" (to complete a different horizontal line of data in k-space) takes an additional TR of imaging time. Referring to Figure 9.8B, recall that most image contrast comes from the data collected near the center of k-space, at and

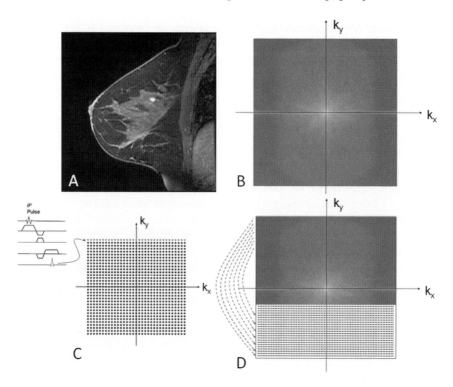

Figure 9.8 (A) A planar MR image is a 2-dimensional matrix of signal values (in x- and y-directions) represented by gray-scale intensity: the higher the pixel's signal value, the brighter the gray-scale intensity. (B) A 2-dimensional discrete Fourier transform (2DFT) of image data in x- and y- gives signal intensity as a function of k_x and k_y, spatial frequencies in the x- and y-directions, respectively. The signal intensity at each spatial frequency location represents the amount of each spatial frequency required to construct the image shown in (A). (C) The signal measured during a single gradient-echo at a given degree of phase-encoding fills out one horizontal line of k-space data. Signal measurement during a subsequent gradient-echo, acquired with a different degree of phase-encoding, fills out another horizontal line of k-space data. The degree of phase-encoding determines exactly which line is measured. (D). Half-Fourier imaging measures phase-encoding views through the center and either the top half or bottom half of k-space. Symmetry of the data around $k_y=0$ is assumed to fill out the full set of k-space data needed to reconstruct the image, thus saving nearly a factor of two in scan time by collecting only slightly more than half of the required phase-encoding views.

around $k_x=0$ and $k_y=0$, while data collected farther from the center of k-space provide fine detail to the image. Note in Figure 9.8B that the k-space data corresponding to Figure 9.8A are highly symmetric about both the $k_x=0$ and $k_y=0$ axes. Partial-Fourier imaging uses this symmetry to reduce the number of phase-encoding views collected, without sacrificing image contrast, and thus reduces scan time by collecting most, but not all, of the phase-encoding views.[27, 28]

As mentioned toward the end of Chapter 3, half-Fourier imaging is a way to speed image acquisition by nearly a factor of 2 by assuming that symmetry exists between positive and negative k_y signal values. Partial-Fourier imaging is simply a variant of half-Fourier imaging, where anywhere up to about 45% of k-space data are not measured but are assumed based on phase symmetry: that is, the signal values in k-space for a given $-k_y$ value are assumed to be equal to the measured signal values at $+k_y$ (Figure 9.8D). Instead of collecting all phase-encoding views, partial Fourier imaging collects only a fraction of the full set of phase-encoding views (usually between 55% and 99%), the specific amount prescribed by the user, and thus reduces sampling time by 45% to 1%, respectively. Each image is then constructed by taking the 2-dimensional Fourier transform of the measured and assumed k-space data.

The factor describing the fraction of phase-encoding views actually collected is called the "phase resolution factor" or "percent sampling factor." If a phase resolution factor of 75% is selected, then 25% of the most negative phase-encoding views are not measured but assumed, based on phase symmetry, yielding a 25% reduction in acquisition time.

Partial-Fourier imaging is a technique that can be used in both 2D and 3D image acquisitions. It always refers to speeding image acquisition by assuming k-space symmetry in the in-plane phase-encoding direction. Its effect on signal and noise is that SNR is reduced in proportion to the square root of the number of acquired phase-encoding steps, assuming that pixel size and slice thickness are kept constant. Therefore, if only 75% of PE views are sampled, SNR per voxel in the partial-Fourier acquired image would be $\sqrt{0.75}$ or 87% of the SNR without partial-Fourier, while image acquisition time would be 75% of the acquisition time without partial-Fourier. Furthermore, there is no loss of spatial resolution by applying partial-Fourier techniques.

Partial-Fourier in the Slice-select Direction or Slice Interpolation

The result of 3D (volume) imaging is a 3-dimensional volume of image data in position space (Figure 9.9A, and see Figure 5.9). This volume of data in position space results from the discrete 3-dimensional Fourier transform (3DFT) of a 3D dataset collected in k-space. The third dimension in k-space, as shown in Figure 9.9B, represents spatial frequencies in the slice-select (z) direction. In 3DFT data acquisitions, the phase-encoding in the slice-select (z) direction is completely analogous to the phase-encoding performed in the in-plane phase-encoding (y) direction. Thus, just as phase symmetry in the k_y-direction can be used to speed 2D image acquisitions, phase symmetry in the k_z-direction (as well as the k_y-direction) can be used to speed 3D image acquisitions. This provides another user-selectable way of reducing scan time by up to nearly 50% in 3D acquisitions, by choosing a slice resolution factor of somewhere between 100% and 50%. Assuming voxel sizes are unchanged, application of partial-Fourier techniques in the slice-select direction has the same effect on SNR as in the in-plane PE direction: resulting SNR is proportional to the square root of the number of PE steps acquired. Thus, if a slice resolution factor of 60% is selected, SNR in the resulting image would be $\sqrt{0.60}$ or 77% of what it would

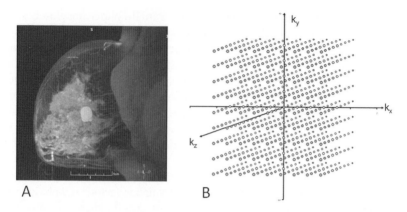

Figure 9.9 (A) A 3-dimensional volume of image data acquired in 3DFT imaging using a 3D gradient-echo pulse sequence. (B) The k-space diagram in 3-dimensions. Each point represents a signal value measured in a 3DFT (volume) image acquisition. Once all the points in 3-dimensional k-space are measured, a 3-dimensional discrete Fourier transform is performed to determine the signal in each voxel of the 3D dataset.

have been, while scan time is reduced to 60% of what it would have been, without partial-Fourier in the slice-select direction.

An alternative to partial-Fourier techniques is simple slice interpolation. This is done by using a 3D protocol to acquire contiguous slices, then interpolating one additional slice between each pair of acquired slices. For example, an axial 3D gradient-echo pulse sequence could be set up to acquire 73 2-mm slices to cover a slab 14.6 cm wide. An additional 72 interpolated slices could be calculated by averaging signal values pixel-by-pixel from each pair of adjacent acquired slices. The calculated slices would be assigned slice locations halfway between each pair of acquired slices. This would yield a total of 145 slices with effective 1-mm slice spacing (acquired with a slice thickness of 2 mm) but acquired in approximately half the time needed to obtain 145 acquired slices. The result is a dataset that can be used for multiplanar reconstructions with the smoothed appearance of 1 mm slices but with SNR higher than if 1 mm slices were acquired. Most important, these slices spaced 1 mm apart were acquired in half the scan time needed to actually acquire 1-mm slices. Most modern scanners provide a user-selectable option to acquire contiguous slices and interpolate intervening slices so that image acquisition time is reduced by nearly a factor of two. The effect on SNR per pixel of averaging adjacent slices pixel-by-pixel is to increase SNR by 41% in the interpolated slices, since signals add linearly, while noise adds in quadrature (that is, as the square root of the sum of the squares of the noise in each pixel) for each pair of adjacent pixels (see Chapter 7).

Acquiring Images with a Rectangular Field of View

Another simple way to reduce scan time is to use a rectangular in-plane FOV while maintaining square pixels, with the narrower FOV dimension in the phase-encoding direction. This only works if motion artifacts and wrap artifacts do not prevent making the phase-encoding direction smaller than the frequency-encoding direction. For example, as described above for sagittal plane acquisitions, to prevent cardiac and respiratory motion artifacts across the breast, phase-encoding is set HF (SI). Many breasts accommodate using a rectangular FOV in the sagittal plane because the breasts are narrower in the HF direction than in the AP direction (see Figure 9.10A). Thus, fewer PE steps are needed (by a factor of ¾ or 7/8), cutting scan time (to 75% or 87.5%, respectively, of what it would have been with a square FOV), while keeping the pixel size the same in the both in-plane directions. The effect on SNR of reducing the FOV in the PE direction to 75% is to reduce the SNR to $\sqrt{0.75}$ or 87% of what the SNR would have been with a square FOV.

A rectangular FOV can almost always be used in bilateral coronal scanning by setting the phase-encoding direction HF (Figure 9.10B). Wrap or aliasing artifacts should not occur with PE HF, since signal-producing tissues are not typically

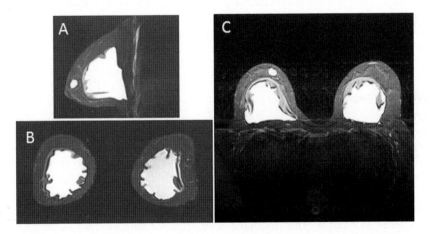

Figure 9.10 (A) Sagittal STIR image with a reduced FOV in the HF direction. This image used 75% phase sampling, cutting the field of view in the PE (HF) direction to ¾ of the FOV in the frequency-encoding (LR) direction. This also reduced the number of required PE steps (and scan time) to 75% of that required for a square FOV, without affecting spatial resolution in the PE direction, since square pixels were maintained. (B) Coronal STIR image with a reduced FOV in the PE (HF) direction. This image used 50% phase sampling, cutting the field of view in the HF direction to ½ of the FOV in the frequency-encoding (LR) direction. This reduced the number of required PE steps (and scan time) to ½ of that required for a square FOV, without adversely affecting spatial resolution, since square pixels were maintained. (C) Example of bilateral scanning in the transaxial plane, showing a STIR image of implants and cyst. Here a square FOV is used, since PE should be chosen LR to prevent cardiac and respiratory artifacts from occurring across breast tissue and the LR dimension of the breasts exceeds the HF dimension. It saves no total scan time to make the FOV in the frequency-encoding direction less than the FOV in the PE direction.

located above or below the breasts to cause image wrap or motion artifacts across the breasts. The head of the patient should be placed in an elevated position posterior to the breasts to ensure that signals from the head picked up by breast coils do not wrap into the acquired FOV causing to image wrap artifacts. The patient's arms should be positioned left and right of the breasts rather than toward the head of the patient in this case, to prevent signal from the arms picked up by breast coils from wrapping into the acquired FOV. With coronal scanning and PE selected in the HF direction, a factor of 2 (or more) in scan time can be saved by using a FOV in the HF direction that is half (or less) of the FOV in the LR direction. Reducing the FOV in the PE direction by a factor of 2 reduces SNR by $\sqrt{0.5}$ or to 71% of what the SNR would be with a square FOV, assuming voxel size is unchanged.

In bilateral transaxial scanning of the breasts, phase-encoding should be selected LR rather than AP. As a result, it is seldom possible to reduce scan time by selecting a rectangular FOV in axial scanning, since the width of both breasts far exceeds the FOV required in the AP direction. Thus, for transaxial scanning, time is saved only if the number of phase-encoding steps is reduced. In bilateral transaxial scanning, a square FOV is used, collecting more image data in the AP direction than is needed (Figure 9.10C). This makes it additionally important to select a square FOV that is not larger than necessary to include all breast tissue. In transaxial imaging, it is critically important to position the arms of the patient toward the head or, if necessary, along the sides of the patient but posterior to the breasts. This prevents signal from the arms from wrapping into the selected field of view on the opposite site and obscuring breast tissue (see Chapter 11).

Parallel Imaging

A relatively new technique called parallel imaging, which goes by acronyms such as iPAT (integrated parallel acquisition techniques) or PPA (partially parallel array), modifies conventional image acquisitions so that two or more different receiver coil and amplifier channels simultaneously acquire different image data, rather than all coils and amplifier channels collecting the same image data.[21,22,29–31] The sensitivity profiles of the different data channels are then used to combine the simultaneously acquired datasets into multi-planar 2D or 3D images. SMASH (simultaneous acquisition of spatial harmonics) and GRAPPA (generalized autocalibrating partially parallel acquisition), combine sensitivity profiles and multiple channels of acquired data to reconstruct data in spatial-frequency space (k-space). Images are then reconstructed by taking their 2D or 3D Fourier transforms. Others parallel imaging methods, such as SENSE (sensitivity encoding), mSENSE (a variant of SENSE), and ASSET (array spatial sensitivity encoding technique) take the Fourier transform of each channel's acquired data, then recombine the images in image space based on the sensitivity profiles of each coil channel. In both cases, data must be collected to measure each data channel's spatial sensitivity profile (Figure 9.11) so that post-processing can piece together the different datasets collected

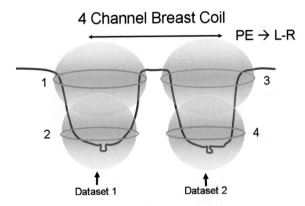

4 Channel Breast Coil

PE → L-R

Figure 9.11 Schematic of a 4-channel breast coil, each signal-measuring loop comprising a separate channel. Without parallel imaging, all four channels are used to measure the same information. With parallel imaging, each channel can be used to acquire separate information. With a nominal R factor of 2 and LR separation of datasets, two channels would acquire one dataset on the left breast, the other two channels would acquire a separate dataset on the right breast. The sensitive volume of each coil is measured to enable reconstruction of resultant image.

simultaneously by different coil elements (Figure 9.12). Parallel imaging requires more complex reconstruction software than conventional 2DFT or 3DFT techniques to combine the different simultaneously acquired datasets. Table 9.1 lists some current parallel imaging protocols for different MR manufacturers' systems.

Parallel imaging (PI) methods require acquisition of sensitivity profiles on the current coil and patient combination. Some PI techniques, such as ASSET, collect calibration data in a separate calibration sequence that is run prior to PI data collection. Other techniques, such as GRAPPA, include the calibration acquisition in the pulse sequence itself, making the pulse sequence slightly longer, but still far shorter than non-PI acquisition times. Either way, some additional image acquisition time is required. These sensitivity data can be collected at much lower resolution than conventional images (Figures 9.12D & E), keeping the additional time required to a few seconds or tens of seconds.

Parallel imaging speeds image acquisition by a factor called the acceleration factor (R). Acceleration factors equal to the number of separate channels of data, which can be 2 to 64 for modern MR scanners, are theoretically possible. For breast imaging to date, however, R values greater than 2 to 3 lead to unacceptable image artifacts and can reduce SNR to unacceptably low levels (Figure 9.13).

Parallel imaging reduces SNR by a factor equal to $1/\sqrt{R}$. Thus, parallel imaging with R=2 reduces SNR to 71% of what it would have been without parallel imaging, while reducing scan time by nearly a factor of 2 (Figure 9.13).

Prerequisites to performing parallel imaging include having an MR system with multiple channels of simultaneous data acquisition (almost all MR

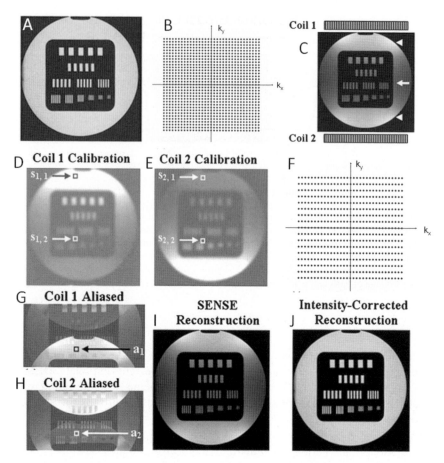

Figure 9.12 Example of parallel image acquisition on an MR phantom. (A) Image acquired without parallel imaging using a single large coil. In this case, all points in k-space were sampled, as shown in (B), and the 2DFT of that data resulted in the image shown in (A). (C) With 2 coil and amplifier channels, a loop above and a loop below the phantom, two separate channels of data can be collected. They are added together (by taking the sum of the squares of each separate image) to produce this single image. Signals in the resulting image are higher near the coils (arrowheads) than farther away from the coils (arrow). (D) and (E) In parallel imaging, low resolution calibration images are acquired separately on each coil. These images can be acquired in a few seconds. (F) With an acceleration factor of $R = 2$, each coil samples every other line in k-space. (G) 2DFT of the data acquired by coil 1 would result in a reduced FOV, aliased image. (H) 2DFT of the data simultaneously acquired by coil 2 would result in a slightly different reduced FOV, aliased image. The sampling for images (G) and (H) are shown by the k-space diagram in (F). Each of these datasets is obtained in exactly half the scan time of the image acquisition shown in (A) and (B). Post-acquisition parallel imaging reconstruction combines the two aliased images shown in (G) and (H), using the calibration images shown in (D) and (E), to result in either the SENSE image shown in (I) or the intensity-corrected image shown in (J). (Images used with permission from Glockner JF, et al., (22)).

Table 9.1 Parallel imaging techniques used by different MR manufacturers

Manufacturer	PI Method	Scheme
Generic	SMASH	k-space
Phillips	SENSE	Image space
GE	ASSET	Image Space
Siemens	GRAPPA	k-space
Siemens	mSENSE	Image space

SMASH = simultaneous acquisition of spatial harmonics
SENSE = sensitivity encoding
ASSET = array spatial sensitivity encoding technique
GRAPPA = generalized autocalibrating partially parallel acquisition
mSENSE = an autocalibrating version of SENSE

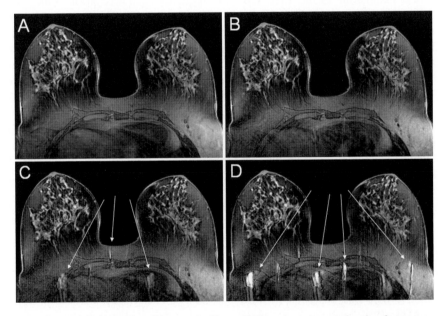

Figure 9.13 Image examples without and with parallel imaging using acceleration factors ranging from 2 to 4. (A) 3D gradient-echo bilateral transaxial image without parallel imaging. Total imaging time for a volume covering both breasts was 102 s. (B) Same pulse sequence with same spatial resolution and slice thickness as (A), with a nominal acceleration factor of R = 2. Total imaging time was 57 s. (C) Same pulse sequence with same slice thickness, spatial resolution, and coverage as (A), with nominal R = 3. Total imaging time was 42 s. (D) Same pulse sequence with same slice thickness, spatial resolution, and coverage as (A), with a nominal R = 4. Total imaging time was 34 s. Note the appearance of increasing artifacts in the posterior breast and chest as R is increased beyond 2 in C and D (arrows).

scanners have this capability), a multi-channel bilateral breast coil that is compatible with the MR system (also common), and MR system software that enables the collection and reconstruction of parallel image data (this is common only on system software introduced within the last several years). Some MR systems permit use of parallel imaging on any pulse sequence; other systems restrict use of parallel imaging to the specific coil and pulse sequence combinations for which the user is licensed. One manufacturer currently permits parallel image acquisition for only one specific pulse sequence designed for contrast-enhanced breast MRI, while other pulse sequences, such as those needed to collect T1W-NFS and T2W images are excluded from using PI. This is unfortunate, since it does not permit users to reduce patient imaging time by applying PI to non-contrast sequences.

When parallel imaging can be implemented on any pulse sequence, it not only allows users to increase the temporal resolution and improve spatial parameters for the pre- and post-contrast 3D gradient-echo pulse sequence series, but also speeds acquisition of the T1W and T2W sequences acquired prior to the contrast-enhanced series. Table 9.2 compares typical total scan times required for an efficient 1.5 T breast cancer detection protocol with and without the use of parallel imaging. As the table shows, applying parallel imaging reduces acquisition time for the contrast-enhanced portion of the protocol only slightly but reduces overall acquisition time by nearly 6 minutes, a 30% reduction in scan time. By limiting non-contrast series and using parallel imaging, total patient scan times can be made less than 15 minutes, making breast MRI a more efficient and cost-effective imaging procedure. The need to set up contrast administration and properly position the patient will extend total procedure time beyond 15 minutes, but, nonetheless, procedure time is significantly reduced by paying careful attention to the image acquisition protocol.

Table 9.2 Comparison of scan times of a bilateral cancer detection protocol with and without parallel imaging (nominal R = 2)

Pulse Sequence	Scan Time Without PI	Scan Time With PI
3 Plane Localizer	12 s	12 s
T1W-NFS – Bilat. Axial	182 s	99 s
STIR – Bilat. Axial	339 s	196 s
3D T1W FS – 1 measure Fat Sat Test	107 s	60 s

3D T1 FS – Contrast Study
    5 2-min measures without PI[*]
    7 1-min measures with PI[**]
	535 s	460 s

Total Imaging Time	19:35 m:s	13:47 m:s

Notes: m:s = minutes:seconds
[*]This series includes one 2-minute pre-contrast scan, a 40-second gap, then four 2-minute post-contrast scans
[**]This series includes one 1-minute pre-contrast scan, a 40-second gap, then 6, 1-minute post-contrast scans

Optimizing Contrast-enhanced Studies

The details of optimizing the contrast-enhanced part of a breast MRI cancer detection study depend on the details of scanner capabilities available to the user. In the preceding section, we have discussed a number of ways to reduce scan time, not all of which are necessary on most MR systems. Some general guidelines for which of these time-reduction methods to use in optimizing CE-BMRI are listed below:[25]

1. Choose a 3D gradient-echo sequence with fat saturation and the shortest available TE and TR values. Reducing TE minimizes T2*-weighting of the sequence, which counteracts T1-weighting. Reducing TR speeds image acquisition.
2. Choose parallel imaging with an acceleration factor of 2 if it is compatible with obtaining good, artifact-free images in a scan plane acceptable to the radiologist.
3. Choose a field of view that includes all breast tissue. In the sagittal plane, a 20-cm FOV is a good target; in the transaxial or coronal plane, a 30 cm FOV is a good target, increasing the FOV slightly if required to include all breast tissue on larger patients.
4. Choose a matrix that gives sub-millimeter in-plane pixel size, with square pixels. In the sagittal plane, the nominal square matrix should be at least 256×256. In the transaxial or coronal planes, the nominal square matrix should be at least 384×384.
5. Choose the frequency-encoding direction AP, so that the phase-encoding direction is not AP. In sagittal or coronal planes, the PE direction should be HF. In the transaxial plane, the PE direction should be LR.
6. For sagittal or coronal plane acquisitions, it may be possible to reduce scan time without reducing spatial resolution by using a rectangular FOV. For sagittal plane acquisitions, the phase-encoding (HF) FOV can usually be set to ¾ of the frequency-encoding FOV. For coronal plane acquisitions, the phase-encoding (HF) FOV can be set to ½ or less of the frequency-encoding FOV. This reduces the number of acquired PE steps and imaging time, while keeping pixels square (or nearly square) so that spatial resolution is unaffected.
7. Choose the slice thickness and number of slices so that scan time for a single bilateral acquisition is between 1 and 2 minutes, while making sure that slice thickness does not exceed 3 mm.
8. Isotropic or nearly isotropic imaging, with a slice thickness of 0.8 to 1.0 mm, would be ideal. If parallel imaging with an R of 2 can be used to achieve isotropic or nearly isotropic imaging with a 1 to 2 minute scan time, do so. If it is necessary to use slice interpolation to get isotropic imaging, do so. If needed, use partial-Fourier imaging in the slice-select direction and, if absolutely necessary, use partial-Fourier imaging in the in-plane phase-encoding direction to achieve the goal of 1- to 2-minute temporal resolution with isotropic sub-millimeter voxels.
9. Even with all the flexibility of modern MR scanners, some scanners will not be able to meet these temporal and spatial resolution requirements, usually due to

longer minimum TR values in 3D gradient-echo imaging. If that is the case, it may be necessary use thicker slices (up to 3 mm), which will permit reducing the number slices needed to cover both breasts and should make it possible to achieve 1 to 2 minute temporal resolution while maintaining sub-millimeter in-plane spatial resolution while imaging both breasts. Acquiring thicker slices sacrifices the ability to maintain high spatial resolution in multi-planar refor-mats and maximum intensity projections in other than the acquired plane. This is described further in Chapter 10.

10. Once temporal resolution and spatial resolution requirements (perhaps other than slices thin enough to yield isotropic voxels) are met, create a multi-series contrast-enhanced protocol with the first acquisition as the pre-contrast scan. Allow a 20 to 40 s gap between the first (pre-) and second (first post-contrast) scan for contrast agent injection and circulation of contrast agent to the breasts. A total of 5 to 7 scans (4 to 6 post-contrast scans) should be run with a scanning protocol identical to the pre-contrast scan. Post-contrast imaging should extend for at least 6 minutes after the end of contrast injection, so with 1 minute temporal resolution, a total of at least 7 scans (1 pre- and 6 post-) should be run; with 2-minute temporal resolution, a total of at least 4 scans (1 pre- and 3 post-) are needed.

11. As a final check, image quality should be evaluated to ensure that SNR is adequate to support the high temporal and high spatial resolution achieved. Adequate SNR is best evaluated by looking at subtracted images and MIP reconstructions, as described in Chapter 10.

Examples of Contrast-enhanced Scanning Protocols Meeting Temporal and Spatial Requirements

Figures 9.14 and 9.15 illustrate two different approaches to nearly isotropic 3D gradient-echo imaging. Figure 9.14 illustrates a protocol used prior to the advent of parallel imaging. It acquired two separate 3D datasets, one on each breast, in the sagittal plane at nearly isotropic spatial resolution. Table 9.3 lists the specific acquisition parameters for this protocol. Bilateral imaging was done with 91 s temporal resolution. Each 3D dataset met spatial resolution requirements by acquiring nearly isotropic voxels having an in-plane spatial resolution of 0.70 mm (frequency) × 0.70 mm (phase) with 1-mm slice thickness. One disadvantage of this approach was that the 3D datasets acquired on right and left breasts were acquired separately and sequentially rather than simultaneously. That is, the right breast dataset was acquired in the first 45.5 seconds, then the left breast dataset for the following 45.5 seconds, for a total temporal resolution for both breasts of 91 seconds. This was less efficient than collecting 3D data simultaneously on both breasts, as is done in a single 3D volume or with parallel imaging, and some images acquired with this protocol exhibited SNR that was at the lower edge of acceptability. The protocol also had the disadvantage of not collecting data on both

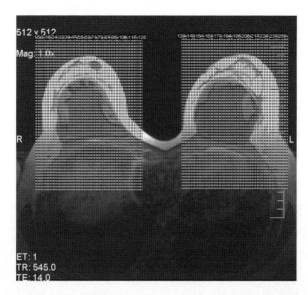

Figure 9.14 The slice localizer for the contrast-enhanced series consisting of one pre-contrast and four post-contrast series acquired in the sagittal plane as separate volumes on each breast. Figures 8.4A and B show one slice of 128 1-mm thick pre- and first post-contrast sagittal slices identically acquired on each breast. The FOV was 18×18 cm with a 256×256 matrix, yielding displayed voxels 0.70×0.70×1.0 mm in size. A post-processed MIP image for this breast is shown in Figure 10.11D.

breasts simultaneously, so that enhancement patterns in left and right breasts could be compared directly, as it can in simultaneously acquired bilateral imaging.

Figure 9.15 illustrates our current breast MRI protocol, which consists of parallel image acquisition of 140 to 160 1-mm slices in the transaxial plane. The full list of protocol parameters is given in Table 9.4. This protocol is more efficient in terms of SNR than the protocol described above in that this protocol collects 3D data on both breasts simultaneously. This is more efficient that collecting two separate 3D datasets, one after the other. As a result, SNR in this newer protocol is quite acceptable. Simultaneously acquiring data on both breasts in the transaxial plane also has the advantage of simplifying bilateral comparison. Temporal resolution in this protocol is exactly 1 minute, while spatial resolution for a 30 cm FOV is 0.67 mm (frequency)×0.67 mm (phase)×1 mm, yielding nearly isotropic voxels.

Examples of Deficient Contrast-enhanced Protocols

Figure 9.16 illustrates the contrast-enhanced portion of a breast MRI protocol that fails to meet temporal and spatial resolution requirements. The CE protocol consisted of one pre-contrast and one post-contrast 2D T1W SE pulse sequence on each breast. Pulse sequences were run separately for the left and right breasts. Hence, no dynamic information was obtained in this protocol and post-contrast scans were obtained at different phases of contrast uptake on left and right breasts. Based on time stamps for individual pulse sequences, there was a delay of nearly 6 minutes between the end of the pre-contrast scan and start of the post-contrast scan for the right breast, and a delay of 14 minutes for the left breast. This allowed considerable time for motion to occur between pre- and post-contrast scans, which would make image subtraction more likely to have motion-induced misregistration.

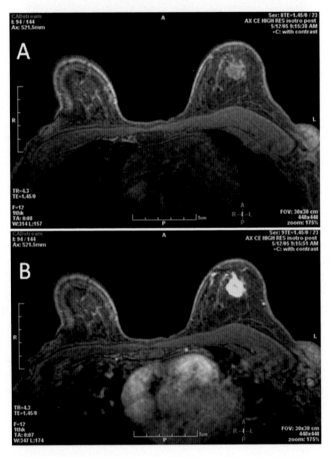

Figure 9.15 (A) One of 160 1-mm thick pre-contrast transaxial images acquired using parallel imaging. The FOV was 30×30 cm with a 448×448 matrix, yielding displayed voxels 0.70×0.70×1.0 mm in size. (B) An identically acquired first post-contrast transaxial image displaying a 2-cm enhancing lesion in the right breast. Post-contrast series were acquired bilaterally (and simultaneously on both breasts) with 1-minute temporal resolution. A post-processed transaxial MIP of subtracted images is shown in Figure 10.10B.

Table 9.3 Scanning parameters used in the CE bilateral sagittal scanning protocol shown in Figures 9.14 and 8.4

Scan Parameter	
Sequence:	3D – Gradient echo
Special Features:	Slice interpolation (× 2 acquisition speed)
Parallel Imaging:	No
TR:	3.78 ms
TE:	1.77 ms
Flip Angle:	25°
N_{ex}:	1
Slice Plane:	Sagittal
Slice Thickness:	2 mm acquired – 1 mm spacing after slice interpolation
Number of Slices:	256 – 128 on left, 128 on right in 2 3D blocks (see **Figure 9.14**)
Phase Encoding Dir.:	HF (SI)
Nominal Scan Matrix:	256 × 256
Phase Scale Factor:	73.83%
Field-of-View:	18 × 18 cm
Nominal Pixel Size:	0.70 × 0.70 mm
Total Scan Time:	91 s = (0.00378 s)*(256*0.7383)*(256)*(1)/2, the factor of 2 in the denominator due to slice interpolation

Table 9.4 Scanning parameters used in the CE bilateral axial scanning protocol shown in Figure 9.15

Pulse Sequence Scan Parameters	
Sequence:	3D – Gradient echo
Special Features:	Slice interpolation (× 2 acquisition speed)
Parallel Imaging:	Yes, GRAPPA (R = 1.8)
TR:	4.3 ms
TE:	1.45 ms
Flip Angle:	12°
N_{ex}:	1
Slice Plane:	Transaxial
Slice Thickness:	2 mm acquired – 1 mm spacing after slice interpolation
Number of Slices:	160 – 1 mm slices
Phase Encoding Dir.:	LR
Nominal Scan Matrix:	448 × 448
Phase Scale Factor:	69.92%
Field-of-View:	30 × 30 cm
Nominal Pixel Size:	0.67 × 0.67 mm
Total Scan Time:	60 s = (0.0043 s)*(448*0.6992)*(160)*(1)/((2)*(1.8), the factor of 2 in the denominator is due acquiring every other slice, the factor of 1.8 in the denominator is the parallel imaging acceleration factor, R.

Scan parameters indicate that the scanner was being retuned between pre- and post-contrast scans so that a readjustment of transmit and receive gain settings occurred, further complicating potential subtraction of pre- from post-contrast scans. As a result of these scan protocol deficiencies, image post-processing such subtractions and MIPs were not performed at this site.

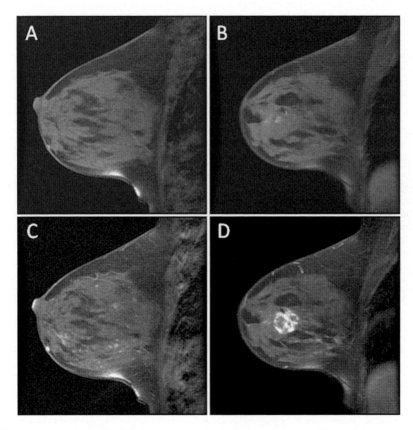

Figure 9.16 Example of a deficient CE breast MRI protocol on a case of invasive breast cancer. Example T1W and STIR images for this study were shown in Figure 8.1. (A) Left and (B) right pre-contrast fat-saturated T1W sagittal 2D SE images acquired with 5-mm slices (no gap), 256×192 matrix, and 18 cm FOV, resulting in 0.70×0.93×5 mm voxels. (C) Left and (D) right post-contrast fat-saturated T1W sagittal 2D SE images acquired with the same spatial parameters as (A) and (B). Deficiencies of the contrast-enhanced portion of this protocol are detailed in the text.

In-plane spatial resolution was adequate, since a 256 (frequency)×192 (phase) matrix was used with an 18-cm FOV, yielding 0.70 mm (frequency)×0.94 mm (phase) in-plane pixels. Slice thickness, however, was higher than recommended at 5 mm, and 2D rather than 3D image acquisitions were used. Thicker slices increase partial volume effects and, as will be shown in Chapter 10, render multi-planar reformatting unsatisfactory. Surprisingly, including pre-contrast series, this protocol took 40 minutes of scan time.

Another deficient breast MRI protocol is shown in Figure 9.17. This protocol performed over 11 separate pulse sequences, took 64 minutes of scan time, and resulted in a large number of substandard images. A T1W-NFS, T2W, and CE series are shown in Figure 9.17. A common error in breast MRI, which occurred

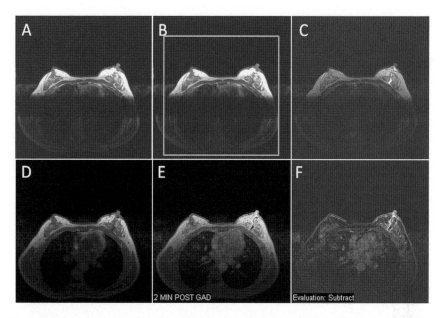

Figure 9.17 Another deficient breast MRI protocol. (A) One of 56 T1W NFS SE images acquired with 3-mm thick slices, 256×256 matrix, and 36×36 cm FOV, yielding 1.4×1.4×3 mm voxels. A horizontal saturation band has been applied to suppress cardiac signal, but does so only partially and obscures some axillary tissue. (B) Same image as (A) with smaller FOV superimposed to illustrate that a 30×30 cm FOV would have been adequate to include all breast tissue. (C) One of 56 T2W FS SE images acquired with the same spatial parameters as (A), also with a horizontal saturation band. Only partial fat-saturation occurred. (D) Pre-contrast and (E) post-contrast series, each acquired as one of 54 T1W 3D gradient-echo slices without fat saturation as part of the contrast series. All images in the contrast series were acquired with the same spatial parameters as A-C. (F) Subtracted image of E-D. Note that limited spatial resolution compromises identification of edges of enhancing structures, and significant LR cardiac motion artifacts obscure posterior breast tissue. The unnecessarily large FOV compromised spatial resolution in all images.

in all images in this case, is setting the FOV larger than necessary: a 36-cm FOV was used when a 30-cm FOV would have been ample to include all breast tissue (Figure 9.17B). The matrix selected for all imaging was 256×256, resulting in pixel sizes of 1.4×1.4 mm. Slice thickness was 3 mm for all images. Fat was only partially saturated on T2-weighted scans, with fat slightly brighter than fibroglandular tissues (Figure 9.17C).

The acquired CE scans shown in Figure 9.17D-F were acquired without fat saturation, which makes identification of small areas of enhancement somewhat more difficult. More important, if motion occurs, misregistered fat can simulate contrast-enhancement, confounding interpretation. In spite of larger voxels, SNR was low in all acquired CE images, resulting in noisy subtracted images, as shown in Figure 9.17F. Positioning of the breasts was suboptimal also, as cardiac motion artifacts propagating LR obscured an appreciable amount of axillary breast tissue.

Chapter Take-home Points

We summarize the take-home points for this chapter on breast MRI acquisition protocols by listing seven requisites of an optimal MRI protocol:

- Using a scanner with a magnetic field strength of 1.5 T or greater
- Acquiring images bilaterally on women who have both breasts
- Acquiring T2W and contrast-enhanced (CE) images, both pre-and post-contrast, with fat suppression
- Acquiring CE images with pixel sizes in either in-plane direction of 1 mm or less
- Acquiring CE images with slice thickness of 3 mm or less
- Acquiring CE images with dynamic information at a temporal resolution of 1–2 minutes.

References

1. Heywang SH, Hahn D, Schmidt H, et al. MR imaging of the breast using Gd-DTPA. J. Comput. Assist. Tomogr. 1986; 10: 615–620.
2. Heywang SH, Bassermann R, Fenzl G, et al. MRI of the breast: histopathologic correlation. Eur J Radiol 1987; 7: 175–182.
3. Heywang-Koebrunner SH, Haustein J, Pohl C, et al. Contrast-enhanced MRI of the breast: comparison of two dosages. Radiology 1994; 191: 639–646.
4. Runge VM, Nelson KL. Contrast agents. In DD Stark and WG Bradley, eds. Magnetic Resonance Imaging, 3rd Edition. St. Louis: C. V. Mosby Publishing Co., 1999, 257–275.
5. Harms SE, Flamig DP, Hensley KL, et al. MR imaging of the breast with rotating delivery of excitation off-resonance: clinical experience with pathologic correlation. Radiology 1993; 187: 493–501.
6. Harms SE. Staging for breast cancer treatment. In DD Stark and WG Bradley, eds. Magnetic Resonance Imaging, 3rd Edition. St. Louis: C.V. Mosby Publishing Co., 1999; 321–333.
7. Bootes C, Barentsz JO, Mus RD, et al. MR characterization of suspicious breast lesions with a gadolinium-enhanced turbo-FLASH subtraction technique. Radiology 1994; 193: 777–781.
8. Kuhl CK, Mielcarek P, Klaschik S, et al. Dynamic breast MR imaging: are signal intensity time course data useful for differential diagnosis of enhancing lesions? Radiology 1999; 211: 101–110.
9. Edelstein WA, Glover GH, Hardy CJ, et al. The intrinsic signal-to-noise ratio in NMR imaging. Magn. Reson. Med. 1986; 3: 604–618.
10. Haacke EM, Brown RW, Thompson MR, et al Magnetic Resonance Imaging: Physical Principles and Sequence Design. New York: John Wiley & Sons, 1999, p. 378.
11. Friedman PD, Swaminathan SV, Herman K, et al. Breast MRI: the importance of bilateral imaging. AJR 2006; 187: 345–349.
12. Mahfouz AE, Sherif H, Saad A, et al. Gadolinium-enhanced MR angiography of the breast: is breast cancer associated with ipsilateral higher vascularity. Eur Radiol 2001; 11: 965–969.
13. Sardanelli F, Iozzelli A, Fausto A, et al. Gadobenate dimeglumine – enhanced MR imaging breast vascular maps: association between invasive cancer and ipsilateral increased vascularity. Radiology 2005; 235: 791–797.
14. Fischer U, Kopka L, Grabbe E. Breast carcinoma: effect of preoperative contrast-enhanced MR imaging on the therapeutic approach. Radiology 1999; 213; 881–888.

15. Liberman L, Morris EA, Kim CM, et al. MR imaging findings in the contralateral breast of women with recently diagnosed breast cancer. Am. J. Roentgenol., 2003; 180: 333–341.

16. Lee, S.G., et al., *MR imaging screening of the contralateral breast in patients with newly diagnosed breast cancer: preliminary results.* Radiology, 2003. 226(3): p. 773–8.

17. Lehman, C.D., et al., *Added cancer yield of MRI in screening the contralateral breast of women recently diagnosed with breast cancer: results from the International Breast Magnetic Resonance Consortium (IBMC) trial.* J Surg Oncol, 2005. 92(1): p. 9–15; discussion 15–6.

18. Slanetz, P.J., et al., *Occult contralateral breast carcinoma incidentally detected by breast magnetic resonance imaging.* Breast J, 2002. 8(3): p. 145–8.

19. Viehweg, P., et al., *MR imaging of the contralateral breast in patients after breast-conserving therapy.* Eur Radiol, 2004. 14(3): p. 402–8.

20. Lehman CD, Gatsonis C, Kuhl CK, Hendrick RE, Pisano ED, et al. MRI evaluation of the contralateral breast in women with recently diagnosed breast cancer. N Engl J Med 2007; 356:1295–1303.

21. Dietrich O, Nikolaou K, Wintersperger BJ, et al. iPAT: Application for fast and cardiovascular MR imaging. Electromedica 2002; 70: 133–145.

22. Glockner JF, Houchun HH, Stanley DW, et al. Parallel imaging: a user's guide. Radiographics 2005; 25: 1279–1297.

23. Hendrick RE, Haake EM. Basic physics of contrast agents and maximization of image contrast. J. Magn. Reson. Imaging 1993; 3: 137–148.

24. Frahm J, Haenicke W. Rapid scan techniques. In DD Stark and WG Bradley, eds. Magnetic Resonance Imaging, 3rd ed. St. Louis: C.V. Mosby Publishing Co., 1999; 87–124.

25. Rausch D, Hendrick RE. How to optimize clinical breast MR imaging practices and techniques on your 1.5 T system. RadioGraphics 2006; 26:1469–1484.

26. Kuhl CK, Schild HH, Morakkabati N. Dynamic bilateral contrast-enhanced MR imaging of the breast: trade-off between spatial and temporal resolution. Radiology 2005; 236: 789–800.

27. Perman WH, Heiberg EV, Herrmann VM. Half-Fourier, three-dimensional technique for dynamic contrast-enhanced MR imaging of both breasts and axillae: initial characterization of breast lesions. Radiology 1996; 200: 263–269.

28. Frahm J, Haenicke W. Rapid scan techniques. In: Stark DD, Bradley WG, eds. Magnetic Resonance Imaging, 3rd edition. New York: C.V. Mosby Publishing, 1999: 87–124.

29. Hutchinson M, Raff U. Fast MRI data acquisition using multiple detectors. Magn. Reson. Med. 1988; 6: 87–91.

30. Carlson JW, Minemura T. Imaging time reduction through multiple receiver coil data acquisition and image reconstruction. Magn. Reson. Med. 1993; 29: 681–687.

31. Pruessmann KP, Weiger M, Scheidegger MP, et al. SENSE: sensitivity encoding for fast MRI. Magn. Reson. Med. 1999; 42: 952–962.

Chapter 10
Image Post-processing Protocols

This chapter describes image post-processing protocols. Image post-processing is designed to provide the radiologist with all necessary supplemental data for image interpretation beyond primary acquired images. These additional data should include subtracted images, maximum intensity projections (MIPs) of subtracted data, and time-enhancement curves for suspicious lesions. Image post-processing may also include image reconstruction in orthogonal planes, enhancement maps, and image overlays that provide additional dynamic information or mark suspicious lesions in the breast.

Image post-processing can be done at the MR acquisition console, although this is usually a time-consuming and inefficient use of scanner time, since it involves MR technologist interaction to control post-processing and often delays starting the next patient. Where possible, it is more efficient to perform most or all image post-processing on an independent console, review workstation, or computer-aided diagnosis (CAD) workstation that is directly available to the radiologist. Current CAD workstations can perform most required post-processing automatically as long as acquisition protocols are standardized and labeled so that breast MRI exams and image acquisition formats can be recognized and processed. It is helpful for the radiologist to have direct hands-on interaction with the CAD or review workstation, so that suspicious lesions identified during interpretation can be evaluated in greater detail. This chapter will discuss and illustrate image post-processing techniques that can be automated or prescribed on every breast MRI exam and those that can be performed electively by the radiologist on selected lesions.

Automated or Prescribed Post-processing Techniques

Automated or prescribed post-processing techniques consist of image reconstruction and analysis that can be performed on every contrast-enhanced breast MRI exam. On CAD workstations and on some MR scanners, these tasks can be automated and performed on every breast MRI exam. On other scanners, independent consoles, or review workstations, these image reconstruction tasks can be prescribed on every exam, but may require manual control of post-processing by a technologist, radiologist assistant, or radiologist. These automated or prescribed post-processing features consist of the following possible tasks:

1) Image subtraction, if possible with re-registration of pre- and post-contrast images
2) Maximum intensity projections of subtracted data
3) Multiplanar image reconstructions (MPRs)
4) Creation of enhancement maps based on multiple time point acquisitions
5) Creation of time-enhancement curves for suspicious enhancing lesions
6) Lesion evaluation for degree of suspicion.

Of these six steps, the first two should be performed routinely on contrast-enhanced image data. The others are optional, although creating enhancement curves for suspicious lesions based on dynamic imaging is standard at many sites. Breast MRI "CAD systems" routinely provide the first five items on the list. No commercial system to date provides the last, a quantitative evaluation of degree of suspicion based on both lesion morphology and dynamics, although the capability to provide the radiologist with that information is currently the subject of considerable research.[1-3] The first five items on the list are discussed and illustrated below.

Image Subtraction and Re-registration

Image subtraction involves subtracting pre-contrast images from each post-contrast image, pixel by pixel. Thus, subtracted images represent the change in image data due to contrast administration, which should occur between the pre-contrast and first post-contrast acquisition. Figure 10.1 illustrates image subtraction of a bilateral transaxial acquisition in a patient with an invasive breast cancer. In this case, one pre-contrast and five post-contrast series were obtained. A subtracted image set is constructed consisting of one subtracted image for each image in each post-contrast series.

To date, there are four manufacturers with FDA approved breast MRI CAD workstations: CADStream™, (Confirma, Inc., Kirkland, WA) DynaCAD™ (InVivo, Inc., Wakesha, WI), OnCAD™ (Penn Diagnostics, Rockville, MD), and *f*TP™ Software (*f*TP™ stands for "full-time-point", CAD Sciences, White Plains, NY). All of these MRI CAD systems provide automatic image registration of pre- and post-contrast scans to help correct for patient motion. With all systems, the user has the choice of viewing original or re-registered images. Simple re-registration algorithms shift one image relative to the other globally in the acquired plane. That is, if one pixel shifts by a given amount in the in-plane (x-y) direction, all pixels in the image shift by the same amount to align the pre- and post-contrast slices. More sophisticated re-registration algorithms, such as those on breast MRI CAD systems, correct for voxel displacement elastically, so that different pixels shift by different amounts to help align image data. Some re-registration algorithms also include voxel shifts in the third, slice-select (z-) direction to register pre- and post-contrast images, since motion of the breast is not restricted to the in-plane direction. Figure 10.2 illustrates the effect of image re-registration on subtracted images in a typical breast MRI case.

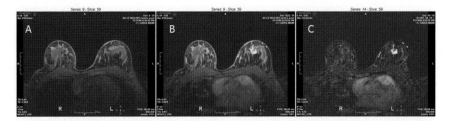

Figure 10.1 One of 128 transaxial pre-contrast (A) and first post-contrast (B) slices acquired using a T1W gradient-echo series. (C) A subtracted image resulting from B minus A, showing an enhancing invasive breast cancer and vessels. A total of 5 post-contrast series were acquired and one subtracted image was calculated for each slice in each post-contrast series by subtracting the corresponding pre-contrast slice from each post-contrast slice pixel by pixel.

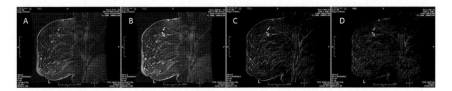

Figure 10.2 One of 96 fat-suppressed sagittal pre-contrast (A) and 5th post-contrast (B) slices acquired in a contrast-enhanced study. (C) Subtracted image of B minus A without image registration. (D) Subtracted image of B minus A with automated image registration prior to subtraction. Note the elimination of some artifacts in D compared to C due to automated image registration.

Errors that can occur in subtracted images include the following:

1. Subtracting one post-contrast series from another rather than subtracting pre-contrast from post-contrast scans (Figure 10.3). This will typically fail to demonstrate the most suspicious enhancing lesions, since enhancement is often greatest in the first post-contrast series, with decreasing signal thereafter. Subtracting the first post-contrast from subsequent post-contrast series will result in negative signal values from lesions that peak in the first post-contrast series and decrease in signal thereafter, which are typically the most suspicious lesions. Most subtracted image display algorithms will not distinguish between negative and zero signals, displaying both as black. Thus, the most suspicious lesions might be missed altogether if post-contrast scans were subtracted from one another and only subtracted images were reviewed. Subtracting post-contrast from pre-contrast images (rather than the reverse) is another error that will result in any enhancing area having negative or zero signals and thus be black in subtracted images. This is easily perceived in subtracted images, as neither vascular nor cardiac enhancement will be seen, even though contrast agent uptake is evident in unsubtracted post-contrast images.

2. Displaying subtracted images with different window widths and window levels. This makes difficult the visual assessment of degree of enhancement and enhancement curve shape. This can be corrected by displaying all subtracted images with

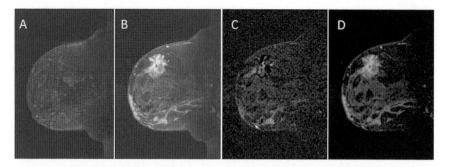

Figure 10.3 Pre-contrast (A) and first post-contrast (B) sagittal images of a case of invasive ductal carcinoma. In performing automated subtractions, the system was incorrectly set to subtract the first post-contrast series from second post-contrast series (not shown) resulting in the subtracted image shown in (C). Proper image subtraction should have taken B - A, resulting in (D).

the same window width and window level and by constructing time-enhancement curves on all suspicious lesions.

3. Displaying subtracted images on an improper gray scale. On some image post-processing systems, it is possible to display subtracted images on a gray scale that displays both positive and negative signals. This method is sometimes useful for displaying the effects of motion, but is less useful for displaying enhancing lesions, as setting zero signals at a median gray level displays enhancing lesions with reduced contrast (Figure 10.4).

4. Motion between pre- and post-contrast scans. As described in Chapter 9, this can lead to spurious enhancement due to mis-registration of data in pre- and post-contrast scans, especially when pre- and post-contrast images are not fat-suppressed or re-registered (Figure 10.5).

5. Allowing the scanner to re-tune between pre- and post-contrast scans. This resets the center frequency, transmitter coil gain, and receiver coil gain between pre- and post-contrast scans. Because contrast agent makes signals from some tissues in post-contrast scans higher than signal from pre-contrast scans, re-tuning will often reset the received signal gain to make the baseline signals of post-contrast images lower than those of pre-contrast images. As a result, mild enhancement may not be displayed at all and time-enhancement curves will not demonstrate the correct degree of enhancement when re-tuning occurs between pre- and any post-contrast scans (Figure 10.6).

Maximum Intensity Projections of Subtracted Data

Maximum intensity projections (MIPs) take a stack of planar images and create a post-processed view that shows one or more projections of the 3D dataset based on the brightest objects in that image stack. The MIP algorithm takes a set of parallel

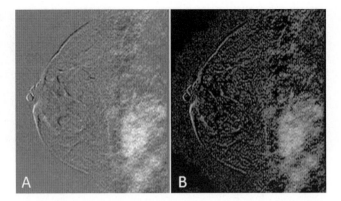

Figure 10.4 (A) Subtracted image of first post-contrast minus pre-contrast image, in which zero signal was set to a median gray scale so that both positive and negative signals could be displayed. This results in reduced image contrast. Note that motion between pre- and post-contrast images resulted in a black-white line at tissue interfaces, yielding both negative (darker) and positive (brighter) signals in the subtracted image. (B) Result of the same two images subtracted and displayed so that only positive signals are bright in the subtracted image.

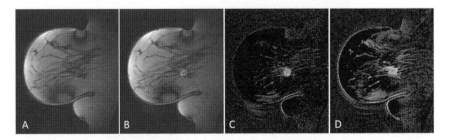

Figure 10.5 (A) One of 80 pre-contrast slices acquired using T1W gradient-echo where the applied fat-saturation failed. (B) The same slice as in A of 80 first post-contrast T1W gradient-echo slices. (C) Subtracted image of B - A showing an invasive breast cancer. (D) Subtracted image of pre-contrast from last (4th) post-contrast scan showing blooming of the invasive breast cancer and areas of spurious enhancement due to the combination of motion between pre- and last post-contrast scan and failure to fat-suppress primary images (A and B).

rays through the 3D dataset and assigns a pixel value to a 2D image that is the highest signal value along each ray (Figure 10.7). In MIPs, rays passing through non-enhancing or mildly enhancing areas are typically displayed as zero signal or black, while rays passing through strongly enhancing pixels will be displayed as high signal values (bright). As a result, MIPs look different than 3D backprojection images that sum the signals from each pixel along each ray projection.

MIPs typically are performed only on subtracted images where signals of unenhanced tissues are set to zero. MIPs provide an excellent overview of subtracted image data and can steer the radiologist to suspicious lesions in the breast. They have limitations, however, in displaying lower signal internal structures within

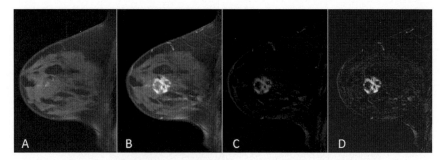

Figure 10.6 A single slice from (A) a pre-contrast series and (B) a post-contrast series showing a large invasive cancer acquired with re-tuning between A and B, the same case shown in Figure 9.23. (C) Subtraction of A from B shows the background and areas within the breast as having zero signal, indicating that image A was acquired with a different (higher) gain factor than image B. (D) Subtraction of A from B after rescaling image B to match background levels of image A yields a more normal looking subtracted image. It is not possible to fully recover the information in subtracted images lost by retuning between pre- and post-contrast scans.

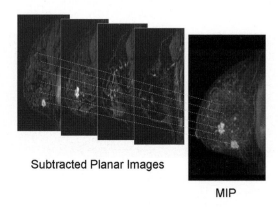

Subtracted Planar Images

MIP

Figure 10.7 Maximum intensity projection (MIP) image is constructed by taking a set of parallel rays through a 3D dataset, assigning a pixel value to the 2D MIP image that is the highest signal value found along each parallel ray. By rotating the angles of projection, multiple MIP images can be generated from the same 3D dataset.

enhancing lymph nodes or lesions, rim-enhancing lesions, necrosis within lesions, and septations within fibroadenomas (Figure 10.8). To examine details of enhancing nodes or lesions, primary or subtracted planar images should be examined in addition to MIP images.

As demonstrated in Chapter 9, MIPs in planar projections other than the primary acquisition plane are best done on 3D (rather than 2D) datasets and are best done with isotropic or nearly isotropic 3D data (rather than 3D data with thicker slices). When MIPs of 2D data are done in planes other than the primary acquisition plane, enhancing vessels often appear as dotted lines due to the Gaussian profile of 2D slices. When thicker slices are MIPed into other planar projections (eg, sagittally acquired images MIPed into the transaxial plane),

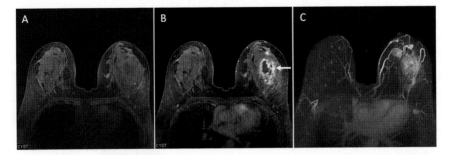

Figure 10.8 One of 80 1.5 mm thick transaxial slices from (A) pre-contrast and (B) first-post-contrast series. A large area of enhancement with non-enhancing center is evident (arrow). (C) Transaxial MIP projection of the subtracted 3D dataset (B - A). Three lesions are visible in the MIP image. Note that the largest lesion's dark necrotic center, easily visible in B, is not apparent in the MIP reconstructed image. The three largest enhancing lesions were biopsied under ultrasound guidance. Pathology showed organizing abscess and inflammatory change, but no malignancy.

blurring occurs in proportion to the slice thickness and to the cosine of the angle of projection relative to the plane of acquisition. That is, projections made at near 90° relative to the acquired plane have little blurring, while projections more parallel to the acquired plane have greater blurring due to thicker slices (Figure 10.9).

Properly windowed MIPs of subtracted image datasets provide a good estimate of image quality in contrast-enhanced scans. Even in patients without enhancing lesions, blood vessels usually can serve as a surrogate for enhancing lesions in the breast and provide a simple way to assess image quality. By looking at MIPs of subtracted images in the acquired plane (ie, a sagittal projection for sagittally-acquired images or a transaxial projection for axially-acquired images), one gets a qualitative estimate of image quality by assessing the smallest visible blood vessels. Figure 10.10 demonstrates this with MIPs of subtracted 3D contrast-enhanced acquisitions of varying quality. Problems that can affect the quality of MIPs include inadequate contrast uptake, motion during image acquisition or between pre- and post-contrast images, low SNR, and excessively thick slices that "partial volume away" small vessels and diffuse lesions. One caveat to using blood vessels in MIP images as an way to assess image quality is that some breasts have larger vessels than others. In particular, post-radiation breasts and surgically reconstructed breasts may have smaller vessels than normal breasts and therefore may look less vascular on MIP reconstructions. On the other hand, breasts containing cancers may have larger vessels and more of them than normal breasts.[4,5]

Multiplanar Image Reconstruction

Reformatting 3D datasets into multiplanar reconstructions (MPRs) orthogonal to the primary acquisition plane is a good way for the radiologist to pinpoint the location of enhancing lesions in the breast and examine lesion internal structure and margins from a different perspective. Image reformatting of 3D data takes advantage

Figure 10.9 MIP projections of 3D datasets, with slices thicker than the in-plane pixel size, have higher spatial resolution when projected perpendicular to the acquired slice plane (90° angle), less spatial resolution when projected at oblique angles (eg, 45°), and worst spatial resolution when projected parallel to the acquired plane (0°). Blurring is proportional to the slice thickness and the cosine of the angle of projection relative to the acquired slice plane.

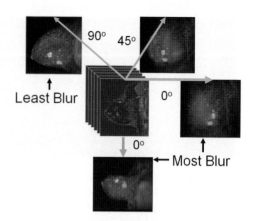

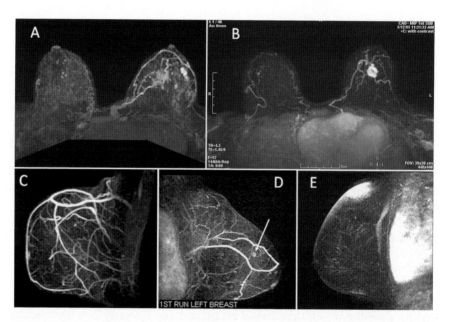

Figure 10.10 (A) MIP of subtracted transaxial CE study revealing an invasive breast cancer located centrally in the breast on the right (planar transaxial image shown in Figure 10.1) and a multilobulated area of DCIS located laterally in the breast on the right. Note that vascularity is increased in the cancer breast shown on the right and that vessels in the breast serve as a good metric for detection of enhancing lesions. (B) MIP of the invasive cancer case shown as planar images in Figure 9.22, showing good vascularity in both breasts and increased vascularity in the cancer breast shown on the right. (C) High quality MIP of subtracted sagittal images in one breast of a study negative for breast cancer. (D) MIP of a breast containing a 4-mm grade 3 infiltrating ductal carcinoma (arrow). Planar images for this case were shown in Figure 9-21. This MIP demonstrates some small vessels, but has lower SNR than MIPs shown in A-C. (E) Low-quality MIP of subtracted 3D CE data, due to both motion, suggested by the bright signal due to misregistration of skin at the top of the breast, and by low SNR, resulting in few vessels displayed.

of the true three-dimensional nature of MRI, an advantage not available in planar imaging such as mammography and most ultrasound exams. Reformatting can be done on pre-, post-, or subtracted images.

The effect of acquired slice thickness on MPRs is similar to the effect of acquired slice thickness on MIPs reconstructed in planes orthogonal to the primary acquisition plane. 3D data acquisitions with thin slices, so that spatial resolution is isotropic or nearly so, result in far better MPRs than 3D datasets with thicker slices (Figure 10.11). When isotropic data are collected, image reformatting can be done without loss of spatial resolution.

Creation of Enhancement Maps Based on Multiple Time Point Acquisitions

In dynamic contrast-enhanced breast MRI, since signal from each pixel in each plane is measured at multiple time points, it is possible to create color maps that

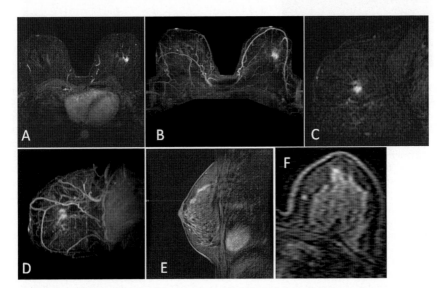

Figure 10.11 (A) Single subtracted 1-mm thick transaxial slice of the first-postcontrast series in a case of invasive breast cancer in the breast shown on the right. (B) MIP of the subtracted first-postcontrast dataset. (C) A single sagittal slice through the enhancing cancer reconstructed from the subtracted first post-contrast transaxially-acquired data. (D) A sagittal MIP from the transaxially-acquired data. Note that because the 3D dataset, acquired transaxially, was nearly isotropic (due to 1-mm thick slices), both MPRs and MIPs in orthogonal planes have high spatial resolution, demonstrating lesion extent and margins nicely. (E) A different case than A-D showing a 3-mm thick sagittal first-postcontrast image with an enhancing lesion near the nipple and extending away from the nipple. (F) Example of a transaxial MPR at the location shown by the dotted line in (E). The MPR is blurred in the left-to-right direction due to the 3-mm thickness of acquired sagittal slices, making the enhancing lesion near the nipple poorly seen.

represent the degree of enhancement, degree of washout, or curve shape, pixel by pixel. Since slowly enhancing pixels are of little interest, most enhancement maps add color only to tissues that enhance at or in excess of a pre-specified amount relative to pre-contrast signal values (eg, 50% or 100%). Because curve shape appears to add greater specificity than other enhancement properties such as degree of enhancement,[6] most enhancement maps assign color according to curve shape. For example, for pixels meeting the degree of enhancement threshold (50% to 100%, calculated based on Equation 8.3), CADStream™ assigns one of three colors to distinguish type 1, type 2, and type 3 curves (Figure 10.12). This color overlay can be applied to planar, MPR, or MIP images.

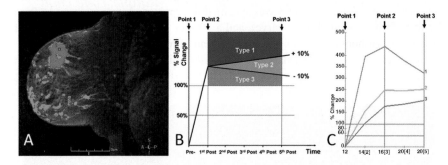

Figure 10.12 (A) The invasive breast cancer case described in Figure 10.3 with a color map overlay from CADStream™. Colors were assigned only to tissues enhancing by at least 100% between pre- and 2nd post-contrast series. Note the manual placement of 3 ROIs in the image, to illustrate the three curve (and color) types. (B). Schematic illustrating assignment of color using a 100% enhancement criterion. The specific criterion is user-selectable, but most users choose a fixed criterion between 50% and 100% signal increase for color maps. In this example, all tissues enhancing by at least 100% between Point 1 (pre-contrast) and Point 2 (here the 2nd post-contrast series, but ideally assigned to be the point of maximum post-contrast enhancement within the first 3 minutes of injection, which is usually the 1st post-contrast series) are assigned color. The specific color assigned to each pixel or voxel depends on curve behavior between point 2 and point 3. Pixels with curves continuing to increase by at least 10% between point 2 and point 3 are assigned blue indicating a type 1 curve (continuous uptake). Pixels with curves decreasing by at least 10% between point 2 and point 3 are assigned red indicating a type 3 curve (uptake followed by washout). Pixels that are nearly level between point 2 and point 3 (± 10%) are assigned green indicating a type 2 curve (plateau). Other CAD systems can use different criteria for percent increase or decrease for color assignment. For example, the DynaCAD™ system typically uses ± 20% (C). Actual time-enhancement curves for the 3 ROIs placed in A, illustrating assignment of blue to tissues exhibiting Type 1 behavior (continuous uptake of contrast agent), green to tissues exhibiting Type 2 behavior (plateau), and red to tissues exhibiting Type 3 behavior (washout). In this automated program (CADStream™), the user specifies the post-contrast series to be used to determine degree of enhancement and curve shape. In this particular example, series 12 was designated as the pre-contrast series (point 1), series 16, the second post-contrast series, was designated as point 2, and series 24, the last post-contrast series, was designated as point 3. These series numbers were not continuous because data for left and right breasts were accumulated into separate series and subtractions were done automatically and assigned separate series numbers for each breast between assigned series. This complicated scheme of automated subtractions done by the scanner was dropped once CADStream™ was implemented into routine clinical use.

To determine curve shapes using automated CAD systems, users typically prescribe which pulse sequence series (time points) will be used to determine pre-contrast (point 1), maximum post-contrast (point 2), and final post-contrast (point 3) signal values. Point 1 is specified to be the baseline signal value (at $t = 0$). Usually, the first or second post-contrast series is prescribed to be point 2, which along with point 1 is used to determine the degree of enhancement (the vertical solid line in the center of Figure 10.12C indicates that the second post-contrast series was prescribed as point 2). One of the subsequent post-contrast series is specified to be point 3, the final curve shape point, which along with points 1 and 2 is used to determine curve shape. In this example, the final post-contrast series was used as Point 3, which is typical. Users can also specify the range of increase or decrease between point 2 and point 3 that separates the three curve shapes. In this example, a 10% or greater increase from point 2 to point 3 was specified to separate continuous uptake (Type 1 curve) from plateau (Type 2 curve), and a 10% or greater decrease was specified to separate washout (Type 3 curve) from plateau (Type 2 curve).

Errors that can be made with color overlays include the following:

1. Mis-setting the degree of enhancement criterion so that enhancing lesions are excluded from the color map. Using a lower degree of enhancement criterion (eg, 50%) usually avoids this error, but at the cost of including more spurious enhancing tissues in the color map. Consistent enhancement maps depend on using a consistent criterion for degree of enhancement, and also depend on using consistent contrast agent quantity (based on body mass; eg, 0.1 mmol/kg) and injection rate. Basing the quantity of Gd-chelate contrast agent on body mass and using a consistent injection rate add reliability, but care must be taken by the MR technologist to ensure that contrast agent is actually injected into the venous system of each breast MRI patient and does not end up on the table or extravasate at the injection site.

2. Selecting inappropriate pulse sequences for the pre-, maximum post-, and final post-contrast sequences (points 1–3). If incorrect sequences are selected for any of these, color maps will misrepresent the true curve shape. Since the pulse sequence for each time point is prescribed globally (ie, for all cases), not just case by case, inappropriate selection can affect color maps on all cases.

3. Mistaking vessels for tumor. Color maps show all pixels or voxels meeting a specified enhancement criterion. Vessels larger than 1-2 mm often meet this enhancement criterion. The radiologist must distinguish between vessels and lesions in interpreting color maps and suspicious enhancement curves (Figure 10.13).

Other alternatives for color maps are certainly possible, but it makes sense to use color only to represent a diagnostically important criterion that is not evident from grayscale images. While systems providing color maps claim to be "CAD" systems, this is only partly true. A true CAD system would mark lesions above a certain level of suspicion or better yet, would provide a degree of suspicion of cancer for each enhancing lesion above some user-specified enhancement criterion. Such CAD systems are in development, but are not currently available for clinical use.

Figure 10.13 Color map overlying
the MIP image shown in Figure
10.10A of transaxially-acquired
subtracted first post-contrast 3D
dataset (Figure 10.1) revealing both
invasive breast cancer centrally and
DCIS laterally in the breast shown
on the right. Note that the color map
highlights vessels as well as
enhancing lesions.

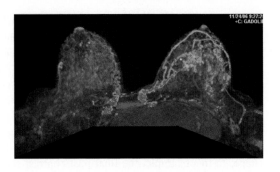

Creation of Time-enhancement Curves for Suspicious Enhancing Lesions

Time-enhancement curves display lesion signal (before and after administration of contrast agent) versus time or series number, and have been previously described in Chapter 8. Time-enhancement curves can be constructed manually or automatically using breast MRI post-acquisition analysis or CAD software. Manual construction of time-enhancement curves typically requires the user to specify a region-of-interest (ROI) on a planar image of an enhancing lesion and the range of pulse sequences to be included in the curve analysis. Software then evaluates the mean signal within the same ROI location in the same slice for each pulse sequence time point and graphically constructs a time-enhancement curve. Figures 10.12A and C illustrate manually selected ROIs and their resulting time-enhancement curves.

Time-enhancement curves should be constructed from originally acquired images, not from subtracted images. Use of originally acquired images allows software to determine percent signal increase relative to pre-contrast signal. Subtracted images give only the signal difference between pre- and post-contrast images, with no basis for comparison to pre-contrast signal, making it more difficult to distinguish significant from insignificant enhancement.

Time-enhancement curves should be based on the most strongly and rapidly enhancing pixels in a lesion. Hence, it is best to use an early (first or second post-contrast) subtracted image to determine placement of the ROI, even though the analysis is done using primary, unsubtracted images. An ideal ROI includes 3-10 pixels representing the most strongly enhancing, non-vascular pixels. Use of too large an ROI tends to underestimate degree of suspicion by averaging over both strongly and less strongly enhancing tissues.

The main concern of the radiologist or technologist in manually selecting an ROI for time-enhancement curve analysis is to exclude vessels and include only the most strongly enhancing lesion tissue. As Figures 10.13 shows, vessels often have highly suspicious enhancement curves. Some breast MRI CAD systems automatically select and present the time-enhancement curve from the single voxel with the most suspicious curve shape within a specified lesion, showing the user the location of that voxel. The radiologist needs to confirm that the most suspicious voxel's curve represents lesion rather than vessel.

CAD systems also typically show the user the breakdown among Type 1-3 curves in a specified lesion (Figure 10.14). This breakdown of curve shape may be useful in determining degree of suspicion of morphologically benign lesions. Morphologically suspicious lesions, however, should not be discounted as being suspicious for cancer based the presence of, or higher distribution of, benign curve shapes.[3] Often, curve shapes merely add confidence in rating morphologically suspicious lesions as highly suspicious for cancer.

It has been demonstrated that there is a high degree of variability in curve shape estimates from manually-placed ROIs. An unpublished study at Northwestern University showed that radiologists had a relatively low agreement rate (60%) when

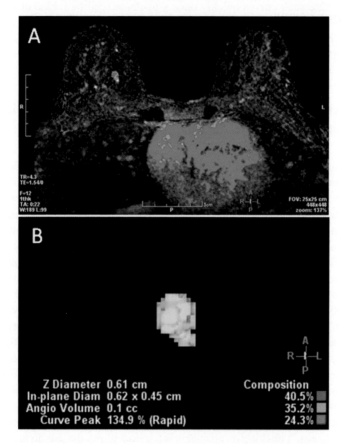

Figure 10.14 (A) Color map overlay of a transaxial scan showing a small focal enhancing lesion that contains pixels of all three curve types. (B) After post-processing, by clicking on the enhancing lesion, the radiologist can generate a 3D display and automated measurement of the lesion's x, y, and z dimensions. The distribution of curve types among voxels in the automatically selected lesion volume is shown under "Composition" in the lower right hand corner of B.

estimating curve shape based on manually-placed ROIs.[7] The agreement rate improved to 73% when ROIs were automatically selected using a breast MRI CAD system.[8]

A practical issue in interpreting MRI exams is that curve shapes are useful during interpretation, but the radiologist usually needs to review the exam to determine which lesions require time-enhancement curves. At sites where time-enhancement curves must be generated manually at the MRI scanner or independent console, this requires the radiologist to conduct at least 2 reviews of the same study, with a time gap in between. It also requires the radiologist, technologist, or some knowledgeable third party to draw ROIs and generate time-enhancement curves based on the radiologist's request. This makes interpretation of breast MRI exams time consuming and cumbersome.

A more efficient approach is to interpret the exam at a CAD or review workstation that automatically generates time-enhancement curves or permits the radiologist to generate such curves quickly once a lesion is specified. One of the biggest assets of breast MRI CAD workstations is eliminating the need for the radiologist to review the case twice by allowing the radiologist to identify suspicious lesions and generate time-enhancement curves easily.

Breast Magnetic Resonance Imaging Computer-aided Diagnosis Workstations

All FDA-approved breast MRI CAD workstations automate post-processing of acquired breast MRI exams. Users can prescribe subtractions, MIPs, and MPRs of primary or subtracted images to be constructed automatically on every breast MRI. Color map overlays are automatically constructed for each planar image summarizing dynamics pixel by pixel. Color maps can be toggled on or off over pre-contrast, post-contrast, subtracted or MIPed images. As described above, only tissues meeting a user-specified degree of enhancement from pre- to a specified post-contrast series (usually the first post-contrast series) are assigned color, with specific colors representing the three curve types based on the dynamics of contrast uptake (Figures 10.12). Subtle differences exist between the different breast MRI CAD systems. For example, CADStream™ assigns three different colors of constant intensity to pixels meeting the degree of enhancement criterion, one color for each of the three curve shapes, as shown in Figure 10.12. DynaCAD™ assigns a spectrum of colors ranging from cool (blue) to hot (red) colors to pixels meeting the degree of enhancement criterion. In addition, color intensity is modulated to reflect faster rates of enhancement for those meeting the threshold enhancement criterion.

All breast MRI CAD systems offer software to further analyze suspicious lesions. With CADStream™, clicking on an enhancing lesion allows the user to automatically determine lesion boundaries, lesion volume, and analyze for the most suspicious enhancement curve within that three-dimensional volume. The system even provides a graphic of lesion volume with 1 cm margins beyond the enhancing lesion in each direction to aid surgery or treatment planning. With DynaCAD™, lesion volume can be determined automatically, but the user manually selects ROIs for curve analysis by placing a cursor in the lesion, guided by the more detailed color map. Both systems provide a histogram or distribution of curve types for voxels within the selected lesion, to aid in assessing the lesion's degree of suspicion.

While not complete CAD systems, these breast MRI-specific analysis systems are immensely helpful to most radiologists interpreting breast MRI by providing image post-processing and consolidating display and analysis functions. They can make interpretation of breast MRI exams faster and, some believe, more reliable than interpretation from PACs or film. They also provide summary reports consistent with ACR Breast MRI-BIRADS™ and enable the radiologist to select and attach key images to the report that help summarize findings.

It is only a matter of time before breast MRI CAD systems add the ability to estimate probability of malignancy for enhancing lesions. Image analysis programs are being developed to combine time-enhancement data such as degree of enhancement and curve shape with morphologic features important to the radiologist, such as lesion margin shape, presence of rim enhancement, and details of tissue heterogeneity, to estimate probability of malignancy. As with mammography, research evaluating the accuracy of breast MRI CAD programs in the hands of the radiologist will be important for establishing their clinical utility.

Chapter Take-home Points

- Contrast-enhanced (CE) breast MRI post-processing should include image subtraction, regardless of whether fat-suppression was used in acquisition
- Subtracted images should be reviewed with a black background and with the same window width and level settings from series to series
- Maximum intensity projection (MIP) reconstructions of subtracted images provide a useful summary of CE study data
- Presence of vessels in properly windowed MIP images can serve as a qualitative measure of image quality in CE breast studies
- Time-enhancement curves of enhancing lesions can help improve the specificity of breast MRI
- Enhancement maps can provide a useful summary of time-enhancement curves
- Some cancers will not meet criteria for inclusion in enhancement maps and will not have highly suspicious curve types, so radiologists should not rely solely on CAD markings.

References

1. Deurloo EE, Muller SH, Peterse JL, et.al. Clinically and mammographically occult breast lesions on MR images: potential effect of computerized assessment on clinical reading. Radiology 2005; 234: 693-701.

2. DeMartini W, Lehman C, Peacock S, et. al. Computer-aided detection applied to breast MRI: assessment of CAD-generated enhancement and tumor sizes in breast cancers before and after neoadjuvant chemotherapy. Academic Radiology 2006; 12: 806-814.
3. Mitchell D. Schnall MD, Blume J, Bluemke DA, et. al. Diagnostic architectural and dynamic features at breast MR imaging: multicenter study. Radiology 2006; 238: 42-53.
4. Mahfouz AE, Sherif H, Saad A, et.al. Gadolinium-enhanced MR angiography of the breast: is breast cancer associated with ipsilateral higher vascularity. Eur Radiol 2001; 11: 965-969.
5. Sardanelli F, Iozzelli A, Fausto A, et.al. Gadobenate dimeglumine – enhanced MR imaging breast vascular maps: association between invasive cancer and ipsilateral increased vascularity. Radiology 2005; 235: 791–797.
6. Kuhl CK, Peter Mielcareck P, Klaschik S, et. al. Dynamic breast MR imaging: are signal intensity time course data useful for differential diagnosis of enhancing lesions? Radiology 1999; 211: 101–110.
7. Gabriel H, Miller L, Roberson S, et.al. How reliable are time-signal intensity curves in breast MR interpretation. (Abstract). The Radiological Society of North America 89th Scientific Assembly and Annual Meeting, p. 289, Chicago, IL, December 2003.
8. Gabriel H, Barke L, Wolfman J, et.al. Do automated methods of contrast kinetic analysis (CADstream™) improve interobserver variability in breast MRI contrast kinetic analysis: a comparison study between automated and manual ROI determination. (Abstract). The Radiological Society of North America 91st Scientific Assembly and Annual Meeting, Chicago, IL November 30, 2005.

Chapter 11
Artifacts and Errors in Breast Magnetic Resonance Imaging

Artifacts

Like other breast imaging modalities, breast MRI can have image artifacts. Breast MRI artifacts may sometimes mimic pathology, at other times obscure pathology, and often reduce the reliability of the diagnosis. The complexity of MRI sometimes makes artifacts more difficult to recognize and their causes more obscure than in mammography.[1,2] Once recognized, it is often possible to reduce or eliminate artifacts for future patients. Here is a list of image artifacts occurring in breast MRI and discussed in this chapter:

1. Ghost artifacts
2. Aliasing artifacts
3. Truncation artifacts
4. Chemical shift artifacts
5. Metallic artifacts including biopsy marker clip artifacts
6. RF transmission artifacts
7. Reconstruction artifacts
8. Other randomly occurring image artifacts

We will demonstrate these artifacts, describe their causes, and discuss ways to reduce or eliminate them in breast MRI. In addition, we will discuss and illustrate some common equipment errors.

Ghost Artifacts

Ghost artifacts in acquired images are almost always patient-induced due to motion of signal-producing tissues during data acquisition. Motion produces not just blurred images, but also ghosts of bright moving structures (Figure 11.1A). Ghost artifacts appear as structured noise patterns propagating in the phase-encoding (PE) direction, regardless of the direction of motion of bright tissues. They occur due to misregistration of image data or changing signal values of fixed structures acquired in different PE views. They propagate in the PE direction

R.E. Hendrick (ed.), *Breast MRI: Fundamentals and Technical Aspects.*
© Springer 2008

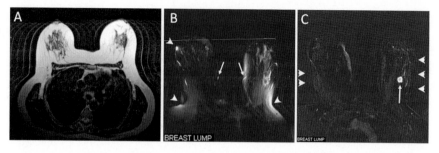

Figure 11.1 (A) T1W transaxial image without fat-saturation showing motion ghosting of fat outside and inside the breasts. Phase-encoding is left-to-right. (B) T2W fat-saturated transaxial images of a different patient with a newly discovered breast mass showing signal flare due to tissue near receiver coil elements distally and near the chest wall (short arrows). Motion ghosting artifacts due to the combination of bright blood in T2W images and vascular pulsations in larger vessels (longer arrows) appear as repeating bright artifacts duplicating the vessels and displaced in the PE (LR) direction. Other effects of non-uniform fat suppression and motion are visible throughout this image. (C) Subtracted T1W gradient-echo image of the same section of the same patient as B shows an enhancing lesion, which was invasive ductal carcinoma (long arrow). Slight mis-registration and motion artifacts are visible at the lateral aspect of each breast (short arrows). The bright-dark regions medially in the breast on the right are also due to image mis-registration. Note that the cancer in C is partially obscure in B due to motion ghosting across the lesion.

because the time gap from one PE view to the next (TR) is much longer than the time gap from one frequency-encoding (FE) sampling to another, which is the total sampling time (T_s) divided by the number of FE samples (N_{FE}). In 2D SE or FSE, TR is half a second to several seconds, while the time gap from one FE sample to another is a few microseconds. Hence, there is more likelihood of misregistration of data between different PE views than between different FE views.

One way to minimize patient motion and resulting ghost artifacts is to immobilize the breasts. Immobilizing the breasts is important, as they can move due to patient respiration or by the patient shifting position during scanning, either randomly or to cope with discomfort. When the breasts entirely fill the breast coil, for example, motion is less likely to occur, but this can lead to signal flaring where breast tissues are directly adjacent to receiver coil elements (Figure 11.1B). Some breast coils have compression plates that permit mild compression to help immobilize breasts during scanning. For example, coils with lateral and medial compression plates that can be adjusted during patient positioning are useful to minimize patient motion. Such coils are more helpful if scanning occurs in the sagittal plane, as mediolateral (ML) compression reduces the number of slices needed in each breast. ML compression reduces motion if scanning in other planes, but at the expense of spreading breast tissue in the head-to-foot (HF) direction, requiring more slices or thicker slices to cover the breasts when transaxial plane imaging is performed.

Breasts smaller than the coil volume can be immobilized by filling unoccupied portions of the coil with foam or cloth pads. Ideally, a facility would have a set of foam pads to comfortably support and immobilize any breast size smaller than the coil volume. The technologist positioning the patient would select the appropriate sized foam pads to best immobilize the breasts without deforming them. This can significantly decrease motion artifacts due to motion of the breasts themselves.

The number of ghosts and their spacing is related to the frequency of tissue motion relative to the pulse sequence repetition time, TR. Ghosting is more pronounced in pulse sequences where blood is bright, such as T1W gradient-echo with contrast agent (Figure 11.1A) or T2W SE or FSE without contrast agent (Figures 11.1B and C). Even when the breasts are completely immobilized, cardiac and vascular pulsations can cause motion artifacts. Periodic motion of brighter tissues (cardiac or vascular pulsations in T2W images or in post-contrast or subtracted T1W images) results in ghost artifacts that recur at regular intervals along the PE direction (Figure 11.2).

Motion during or between pre- and post-contrast scans can cause image misregistration in subtracted images (Figure 11.1C). The steps taken to minimize patient motion during scanning also minimize motion between scans. In addition, subtraction artifacts can be reduced by minimizing the time gap between pre- and post-contrast scans, thereby minimizing the time for patient motion. Technologists can also help minimize misregistration by preparing the patient for the contrast series prior to scanning the pre-contrast sequence and not talking to the patient during the time gap between pre- and post-contrast scanning, while injection is occurring. It is much easier to do this with automated injection, where the technologist injects from the scanner console, than with manual injection, where the technologist enters the room to inject.

On some scanners, software permits setting up a multi-sequence scan run for contrast-enhanced scanning, where the same pulse sequence is repeated automatically without time gaps, unless prescribed by the user. For breast MRI, the first measure is the pre-contrast series. A 20–40 second pause is prescribed for contrast injection, saline flush, and to allow time for the contrast agent to get to the breast. Then, 3–6 post-contrast series are run continuously for 6–8 minutes. The patient can be instructed prior to initiation of the pre-contrast scan not to move during this entire pre- and post-contrast multi-series set. This procedure, along with mild compression or padding of the breasts, is usually sufficient to minimize breast motion.

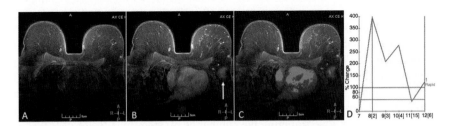

Figure 11.2 Single slice of (A) pre-contrast and (B) first post-contrast images of a study absent of enhancing lesions. B shows artifactual enhancement of the left breast (on the right) due to cardiac pulsation (arrow). (C) The color map of tissues enhancing by at least 100% indicates that the artifactual enhancement shown in B has significant signal change from the unenhanced image. (D) The most suspicious curve generated from the artifactually enhanced region. The zig-zag curve shape is characteristic of vascular enhancement. In this case it is notable because it is caused by the combination of high cardiac signal in post-contrast images and cardiac pulsation artifacts.

Most modern MRI systems have improved MR pulse sequence designs that attempt to minimize motion artifacts. These include automated motion-suppression techniques such as gradient-moment nulling and reordering of k-space acquisitions.[2,3] Some motion-reducing options such as cardiac triggering and prospective gating reduce motion artifacts, but extend scan time or cause scan time to vary. This renders these techniques incompatible with dynamic, high-resolution contrast-enhanced breast imaging, where maintaining a fixed temporal resolution of 1–2 minutes is important for interpretation of results.

Motion is only one cause of ghost artifacts. Ghost artifacts also can be caused by equipment instabilities in the MR scanner itself, such as mechanical vibrations within the gradient coils, fluctuations of the magnetic field during scanning, and temporal variations in receiver coil sensitivity.[2] Any of these sources of ghost artifacts other than patient motion that occur intermittently or consistently should be corrected by the MRI system service engineer.

Aliasing Artifacts

Aliasing artifacts (also known as "wraparound" or "image wrap" artifacts) occur when signal-producing tissues exceed beyond the prescribed field-of-view in either the FE or PE direction. Aliasing occurs because MRI requires collection of a discrete number of signal values in each direction to form an image; that is, a fixed number of FE and PE steps. Having a discrete number of pixels means that 2D or 3D reconstruction cannot distinguish between properly assigned signal-producing tissues within the scan field-of-view (FOV) and corresponding signal-producing tissues outside the scan FOV (Figure 11.3). This causes signals from tissues outside the prescribed FOV to be added to signals from pixels within the FOV on the opposite side of the image. Aliasing artifacts add structured noise that can obscure details in the breast and can occasionally simulate pathology.

Aliasing artifacts more commonly occur in the PE direction than in the FE direction (Figure 11.4). That is because MR manufacturers implement techniques that automatically suppress image wrap in the FE direction, including applying frequency filters that suppress signal from tissues just beyond the selected FOV and oversampling the number of data points in FE direction. Recall that to resolve 256 pixels in the FE direction, at least 256 data point measurements must be made at slightly different time points during each signal echo. Oversampling in the FE direction is done by intentionally sampling enough data to reconstruct a larger matrix (eg, 512 pixels) in the FE direction, but only presenting the central 256 pixels to the viewer. Oversampling the number of FE steps by a factor of two suppresses image wrap from signal-producing tissues within one FOV on either side of the prescribed FOV and, thus, eliminates most artifacts. The combination of frequency oversampling and a low-pass frequency filter that suppresses signal just beyond the selected FOV is sufficient to eliminate all aliasing in the FE direction.

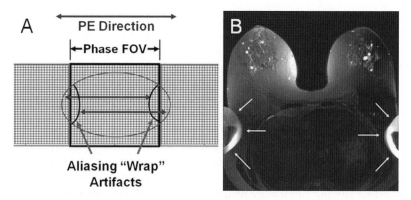

Figure 11.3 (A) Schematic illustrating aliasing in the PE direction (LR). The center matrix (dark outlin) represents the selected FOV with body tissue extending beyond the prescribed FOV to the left and right. Because only a discrete number of PE steps are used to acquire the image, reconstruction cannot distinguish between pixels within the prescribed image and corresponding pixels in image matrices repeating to the right and left, and other matrices repeating infinitely in both directions (not shown). When signal-producing tissues extend beyond the prescribed FOV in the PE direction, pixels outside the FOV to the left add to the signal from pixels on the right side of the image, as shown by the upper horizontal arrow. Similarly, pixels outside the prescribed FOV to the right add to the signals from pixels on the left side of the image exactly one image width away, as shown by the lower horizontal arrow. Thus tissues wrap or "alias" to the far side of the prescribed FOV. (B) T2W (STIR) image with patient's arms by her side and too anterior, causing exterior portions of each arm to wrap into the opposite side of the image (arrows), partially obscuring axillary breast tissue.

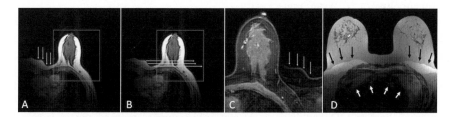

Figure 11.4 (A) Transaxial localizer acquired with a large FOV. The white box indicates the FOV chosen for unilateral CE scanning. Signal producing tissues lying outside the selected FOV in the PE direction (horizontal), but within the sensitive volume of the unilateral breast receiver coil (arrows), cannot be distinguished from corresponding pixels within the selected FOV. (B) Aliasing in the PE direction (LR) causes the signals from corresponding pixels inside and outside the FOV (separated by a distance equal to the width of the image, as shown by the horizontal arrows) to be added together in the smaller FOV image (C), a T1W gradient-echo image. The tissues visible below the vertical arrows in C are primarily aliasing artifacts. More subtle aliasing artifacts are also visible within the breast due to signal-producing tissues one image width away wrapping into the acquired image. (D) 3D acquisition of a non-fat-suppressed T2W image on a different subject showing image wrap in the slice-select PE direction (perpendicular to the image plane). Subcutaneous fat from outside the selected 3D volume in the slice-select direction is aliased across both breasts (dark arrows) and abdominal tissue is aliased into lung fields (white arrows).

Automatically suppressing image wrap in the PE direction is not so easily achieved, since there is usually a price to be paid. Some systems permit users to specify a fixed amount of oversampling (1–100%) in the PE direction to cope with the situation where signal-producing tissue outside the specified FOV is unavoidable (eg, cardiac MRI). This can eliminate or reduce aliasing artifacts, but at the price of extending total scan time. If 20% phase oversampling is selected, scan time will be 20% longer than without oversampling.

Other systems provide users with an option called "no phase wrap" (NPW), where the number of PE steps is automatically doubled. This would normally double imaging time, but at least one vendor (GE) automatically shifts to half-Fourier imaging along with doubling the number of PE steps when NPW is selected. The result is that aliasing artifacts are reduced or eliminated and scan time is essentially unchanged. Signal-to-noise ratio (SNR) is also essentially unchanged since the same number of PE steps is acquired. That is, the $\sqrt{2}$ loss in SNR due to half-Fourier imaging is offset by the $\sqrt{2}$ increase in SNR due to doubling the number of PE steps to expand the phase FOV.

For bilateral breast MRI, it is usually possible to pick the in-plane PE direction so that no signal-producing tissue lies outside the selected FOV. Chapter 9 discussed and illustrated rules for avoiding aliasing artifacts by selecting the PE direction LR for transaxial scanning, HF for sagittal scanning, and either LR or HF for coronal scanning. One key to avoiding aliasing artifacts is to position the patient's arms so that they do not wrap across the breasts with any selected scan plane (Figure 11.3B). Placing the arms above the head or by the side, but posterior to all breast tissue, minimizes arms wrapping into the image and obscuring lateral axillary breast tissue. The other key is to make sure the selected FOV includes all signal producing tissue in the PE direction. If that is done, then options such as phase oversampling or NPW are unnecessary.

3D acquisitions have two PE directions, one in-plane and the other perpendicular to the selected slice plane, the slice-select direction. Hence, 3D acquisitions with tissues outside the selected volume in either PE direction will experience aliasing artifacts (Figure 11.4D). This makes it important to ensure that the selected 3D volumes extend to the edge of all signal-producing tissues in both in-plane PE and slice-select directions, so that aliasing does not wrap tissue outside the selected FOV onto the breasts. 2D acquisitions do not suffer image wrap in the slice-select direction.

In 3D gradient-echo imaging in the transaxial plane, it is not possible to eliminate phase wrap in the slice-select direction. With good positioning, body tissues outside the selected volume in the slice-select direction only wrap onto other body tissues within the selected volume, not across breast tissue. Fat suppression also eliminates a primary source of bright signals in the body that might wrap in the slice-select direction, as in Figure 11.4D. Still, when interpreting incidental findings in the chest, the radiologist should be aware that image wrap can occur in the slice-select direction, which is head-to-foot in transaxial 3D acquisitions.

Truncation Artifacts

Truncation artifacts, also known as "Gibbs", "edge", or "ringing" artifacts are another result of the finite sampling occurring in MRI. Truncation artifacts tend to occur adjacent to high-contrast, sharp interfaces, as illustrated in Figure 11.5. Because of finite sampling of the image in each in-plane direction, image reconstruction with a discrete number of samples tends to overshoot the true signal changes across sharp interface and produce ringing artifacts beyond the interface. This overshooting is called the Gibbs phenomenon, which enhances contrast across the interface, and the ringing associated with it is responsible for the light and dark banding occurring adjacent to sharp interfaces and falling off as the distance from the interface increases. One way to decrease truncation artifacts is to use a higher matrix, but scan time must be increased to increase matrix size in the PE direction.

Truncation artifacts are common in the spine due to sharp signal changes between cord and cerebrospinal fluid (CSF). They also sometimes occur just within the skull in head MRI because of sharp signal changes between air, skin, bone, and brain. Fortunately, there are rarely sharp interfaces in the breast to produce truncation artifacts. When truncation artifacts do occur in the breast, such as just inside the skin line, they tend to be mild, seldom obscuring breast pathology (Figure 11.5C). Choosing a matrix and FOV that produce sub-millimeter pixels in both in-plane directions is usually sufficient to minimize truncation artifacts. Moreover, in

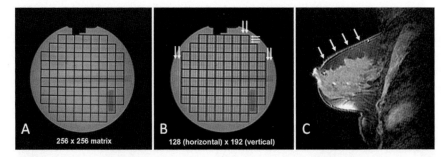

Figure 11.5 (A) Grid section of the ACR MRI Phantom imaged with a 256 × 256 matrix using a T1W pulse sequence. There are mild truncation artifacts visible as finely space light and dark lines in the signal-producing fluid between grid sections. (B) The same section of the same phantom imaged with a 128 (horizontal) × 192 (vertical) matrix. Note the more prominent truncation artifacts in B than in A, visible as more prominent light-dark bands between grid interstices and at the edges of the phantom (arrows). Truncation artifacts are more prominent when sharp boundaries are present and a lower matrix is used. This is evident as more prominent bands running vertically (double arrows) due to only 128 matrix elements being selected in the horizontal direction. The bands running horizontally (triple arrows) are less prominent than the vertical bands, but more prominent than in A, due to 192 matrix elements being selected in the vertical direction. (C) Truncation artifacts are visible at the superior edge of the breast as parallel light and dark bands near the sharp black-white interface at the edge of the breast. Truncation artifacts decrease in magnitude as distance from the sharp interface increases. Signal flare due to breast tissue adjacent to a receiver coil element is visible in the lower part of the breast.

the absence of motion, truncation artifacts tend to be the same in pre- and post-contrast scans and are often eliminated in subtracted images.

Chemical Shift Artifacts

Chemical shift artifacts occur because hydrogen nuclei in fat resonate at a slightly different frequency than hydrogen nuclei in water, as illustrated in Figure 9.2C. The resonant frequency of water is 3.35 parts per million higher than that of fat, which amounts to 214 Hz at 1.5 T (3.35 ppm × 42.6 MHz/T × 1.5 T = 214 Hz). This leads to two different kinds of chemical shift artifacts. Chemical shift artifacts of the first *kind* occur in all MR images due to the application of a frequency-encoding gradient during signal measurement. Because a FE magnetic field gradient is always applied during signal readout, there is a shift in the location of the "fat image" relative to the "water image" along the FE direction in any MR image containing both tissues. At a magnetic field strength of 1.5 T, the amount of position shift in terms of pixels depends only on the frequency shift from one pixel to the next, called the pixel bandwidth. In the images shown in Figure 11.6A and B, the pixel bandwidth was 122 Hz/pixel. Hence, the resonant frequency difference between water and fat of 214 Hz amounts to a position shift of 1.8 pixels between the water image and fat image (out of 256 pixels in the FE direction). This chemical shift between the two images always occurs in the FE direction.

One way to decrease image noise is to decrease the bandwidth of the image, which for a fixed number of FE steps means decreasing pixel BW. This has the unwelcome effect of increasing chemical shift artifacts by spreading them over more pixels. For example, if BW is decreased by a factor of 7, from 122 Hz/pixel to 17.4 Hz/pixel, the chemical shift between water and fat will increase by a factor of 7, from just under 2 pixels to more than 12 pixels (Figure 11.6C and D).

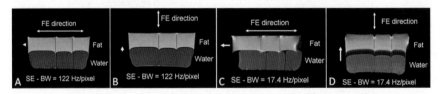

Figure 11.6 SE images of a fat-water phantom demonstrating chemical-shift artifacts of the first kind. The phantom contains canola oil floating on top of a highly dilute suspension of Gd-DTPA in water, with two straight plastic septa running vertically to help assess chemical shift. All images acquired with TR = 150 ms, TE = 15 ms, 256 × 256 matrix, 16 cm FOV, for 0.625 × 0.625 mm pixels. (A) Frequency-encoding horizontal, bandwidth (BW) = 122 Hz per pixel. Chemical shift artifact (of the first kind) has caused fat to shift to the left relative to water by 1.8 pixels or 1.1 mm. (B) Same as A, but with FE vertical instead of horizontal. Chemical shift artifact has shifted fat upward relative to water by 1.8 pixels or 1.1 mm. (C) Same as A, but with BW = 17.4 Hz per pixel. Note that the chemical shift artifact has displaced fat to the left by about 12 pixels or 9 mm. (D) Same as C, but with FE vertical instead of horizontal.

Figure 11.7 illustrates the effect of chemical shift artifacts in non-contrast T2W images without fat suppression. Because both fat and water are bright, where chemical shift causes fat and water to overlap, signals are extremely bright. In the gap created on the opposite side of the vessel by separation of water and fat, there is a signal void. Chemical shift artifacts are seldom apparent when fat-saturation is performed, simply because the signal from fat is no longer bright, so there is little signal to add to or subtract from the water signal.

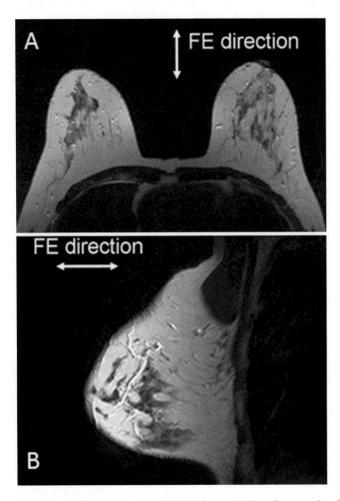

Figure 11.7 (A) Transaxial and (B) sagittal T2W SE images without fat-saturation. Frequency-encoding was AP in both images. Chemical shift artifacts of the first kind cause vessels to have a black-white appearance because fat is shifted upward relative to water in A, to the left relative to water in B. Dark pixels (signal voids) result where fat and water are shifted apart along the FE direction due to chemical shift. Bright pixels occur where fat signal and water signal add because of overlap along the FE direction due to chemical shift.

Chemical shift artifacts of the second kind occur when fat and water overlap (due to chemical shift of the first kind) in gradient-echo images. Just after the $\theta°$ excitation pulse in gradient-echo imaging (ie, at TE = 0), hydrogen nuclei in fat and water are in-phase. Because proton magnetic dipoles in fat and water have slightly different precessional frequencies, they go out-of-phase and in-phase every (3.3 ms·T) /B_0, where B_0 is given in Tesla. That is, when B_0 = 1.5 T, protons in water and fat are exactly out-of-phase at a TE of 2.2 ms ((3.3 ms·T) /(1.5 T) = 2.2 ms) and back in-phase at TE = 4.4 ms. This out-of-phase and in-phase pattern continues as TE is increased (Figure 11.8A). When in-phase, signals from overlapping fat and water add, producing a bright line at overlapped fat-water interfaces (Figure 11.8B). When out-of-phase, signals from overlapping fat and water cancel one another, producing a dark line at overlapped fat-water interfaces (Figure 11.8C). These chemical shift artifacts of the second kind occur in addition to those of the first kind, which are responsible for displacing the fat image from the water image and creating signal voids where the two tissues separate.

At 3.0 T, precession of hydrogen nuclei in fat and water is twice as fast, so the two tissues are out-of-phase at TE values of 1.1 ms, 3.3 ms, 5.5 ms, etc, while overlapping fat and water add constructively at TE values of 2.2 ms, 4.4 ms, 6.6 ms, etc. If bandwidth per pixel is reduced, a wider band of artifacts of the second kind (either black or white) will occur on one side of the fat-water interface and a wider dark band will occur on the other side due to the greater separation of the two tissues.

Chemical shift artifacts of the first kind are always present regardless of the pulse sequence used. Chemical shift artifacts of the second kind occur only in gradient-echo images. When fat-suppression is applied successfully, chemical shift artifacts are of minor importance in breast MRI. The one pulse sequence where chemical shift artifacts occur routinely is a T1W-NFS sequence. If SE or FSE sequences are used, only chemical shift artifacts of the first kind occur, as shown in Figure 11.7. If a gradient-echo sequence is used for T1W-NFS imaging, then chemical shift artifacts of both the first and second kind are present, as shown in Figures 11.8B and C. In such cases, it is best to set TE to be near an even multiple of (3.3 ms·T)/B_0. (that is, near 4.4 ms, 8.8 ms, 13.2 ms, etc., at 1.5 T) so that fat and water signals are in-phase rather than out-of-phase. This prevents signal voids on one side of water-fat interfaces. Both types of chemical shift artifacts can be minimized by keeping bandwidth per pixel reasonably high. This is done at the price of a slight decrease in image SNR, since higher bandwidth means that a wider range of noise frequencies contribute to the image.

Metallic Artifacts

Metallic artifacts occur when pieces of metal in or near the scanner perturb the magnetic field in the image field. Ferromagnetic metals, which include iron, nickel, and cobalt, have the unique property that their atomic magnetic dipole moments (due to unpaired electrons) have a lower energy state when aligned.[4] This means that within a certain area of the crystal domain, that includes millions of metal atoms, they exhibit a net magnetism. When not placed in a magnetic field, different

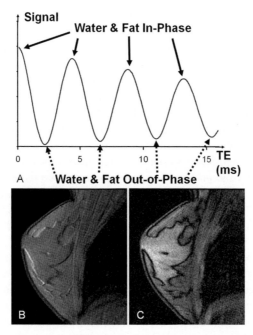

Figure 11.8 In gradient-echo imaging, chemical shift artifacts of both the first and second kind occur. Chemical shift artifacts of the second kind are due to the phase relation between hydrogen dipoles in water and those in fat, which is determined by TE. When water and fat overlap due to chemical-shift artifacts of the first kind, signals from the two tissues can be in-phase, resulting in signals from water and fat adding, or out of phase, resulting in signals from water and fat canceling one another, depending on TE. (A) A graph of the signal from overlapping water and fat versus TE. At 1.5 T, water and fat are in-phase at TE = 0, 4.4, and 8.8, 13.2 ms (solid arrows) and other integer multiples of 4.4 ms. Water and fat are out-of-phase, resulting in dark line interfaces, at TE values of 2.2, 6.6, 11.0, and 15.4 ms (dashed arrows). (B) A 1.5 T gradient-echo image of a normal volunteer acquired with TR = 200, TE = 4.4 ms, 256 × 256 matrix, pixel bandwidth of 81.4 Hz, so that the water-fat image shift corresponds to 2.75 pixels due to chemical-shift artifacts of the first kind. Frequency-encoding is LR. The water-fat shift creates dark bands due to signal voids just inside the skin line and on the right-hand side of the fibroglandular (primarily water-based) tissue in the center of the breast. Because of the TE setting of 4.4 ms at 1.5 T, water and fat are in-phase so that where superimposed due to chemical shift of the first kind, signals from water and fat add. This results in the bright band on the left hand side of fibroglandular tissue at the center of the breast. (C) The same gradient-echo image acquisition as B, but with TE = 7 ms, all other acquisition parameters the same as in B. In this image, chemical shift artifacts of the second kind produce a dark line on the left side of glandular tissue because water and fat are nearly out-of-phase, causing their signals to cancel one another where the two tissues overlap.

crystal domains have different magnetic fields pointing in different directions, making the net magnetization approximately zero. When placed in a strong magnetic field, however, different domains align, magnetizing the material. The unique aspect of ferromagnetic materials is that this magnetization remains, even when the strong magnetic field is removed. This leads to net magnetization which is retained by the ferromagnetic material, making it possible to use magnetized ferromagnetic materials as permanent magnets, compass needles, etc.

Ferromagnetic materials strongly perturb the main magnetic field (B_0) of an MRI system whenever they occur in the bore of the scanner, either as loose objects or within the patient. As a result, ferromagnetic objects cause sizeable image artifacts.[5] These are typically evident as magnetic field distortions producing warped images or signal voids, possibly also with flaring of bright signals, in the vicinity of any piece of ferrous metal outside or inside the human body. These artifacts are caused by an abrupt change in the magnetic field due to the added magnetic fields contributed by the ferrous material, which leads to misallocation of measured signal.

Stainless steel comes in a number of forms, some of which are ferromagnetic, others of which are not. Stainless steel used for breast biopsy marker clips, and titanium used for the same purpose, are non-ferromagnetic (Table 11.1), but can still cause MRI-visible artifacts due to distortion of magnetic fields in their immediate vicinity (Figures 11.9 and 11.10)[5]. Artifacts caused by non-ferrous materials tend to be smaller in size and effect than artifacts from ferrous metals.[6] Biopsy marker clips should be visible under mammography, ultrasound, and breast MRI, but produce small artifacts on MRI. Depending on clip design and composition, their appearances can vary widely on standard breast MRI pulse sequences[6] (Figures 11.10).

The appearance of metallic artifacts can differ between gradient-echo and SE or FSE pulse sequences, as shown on the right side of Figure 11.10. Metallic artifacts in gradient-echo images tend to cause signal voids, while SE and FSE sequences typically cause signal flares in addition to signal voids. As demonstrated by Figure 11.10, the size of clip artifacts does not differ significantly between gradient-echo and SE or FSE sequences. Some clips, such as the MammoMark™ (Artemis Medical, Hayward, CA) produce minimal artifacts with any typical MRI pulse sequence. Ideal marker clips are those that can be seen under mammography, breast ultrasound, and breast MRI, but do not cause artifacts so large that they obscure breast lesions on follow-up MRI[6,7] (Figure 11.11).

Radiofrequency Transmission Artifacts

Radiofrequency (RF) transmission artifacts typically occur due to incomplete RF shielding of the MRI exam room. RF shielding is provided by a Faraday cage that

Table 11.1 Characteristics of the six breast biopsy marker clips shown in Figure 11.10

Clip Manufacturer	Clip Name	Clip Composition	Shape	Length	Width	Thickness
SenoRx	Ultracor ™	Stainless Steel	S	2.7	1.0	~0.2
SenoRx	Gelmark ™	Stainless Steel	Ω	3.2	1.4	~0.2
SenoRx	Gelmark Ultra ™	Stainless Steel	Ω	3.2	1.4	~0.2
Artemis	Mammomark ™	Titanium	α	1.4	1.4	~0.2
Inrad	Ultraclip ™	Stainless Steel	γ	3.0	1.7	~0.2
Ethicon	Micromark ™	Stainless Steel	See Images	2.0	1.6	~0.2

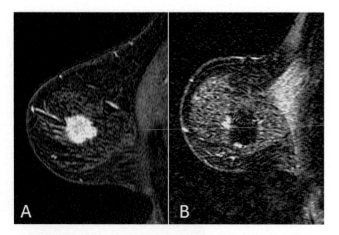

Figure 11.9 (A) Fat-suppressed contrast-enhanced sagittal image showing a rapidly-enhancing 2-cm invasive ductal carcinoma. (B) Same pulse sequence of the same lesion after placement of an Inrad clip (see **Table 11.1**) and neoadjuvant therapy. The large signal void caused by the clip limited the assessment of lesion size and characteristics after therapy. The bright area anterior to the clip artifact was interpreted as residual tumor. (Courtesy of Dr. Wendie Berg, Principal Investigator, ACRIN 6666 and Staff Radiologist, American Greensprings – Johns Hopkins University, Greensprings, MD, Reprinted with permission from Amirsys, Inc.).

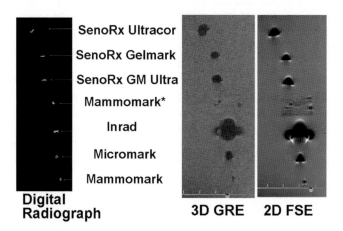

Figure 11.10 Comparison of digital radiograph (left) and 3D gradient-echo (right) and 2D FSE (far right) MR images of 6 different breast biopsy marker clips suspended in a uniform water-based medium consisting of double-strength Knox™ gelatin. One clip (MammoMark™, Artemis Medical, Hayward, CA) was included twice, once with and once without its collagen plug. Note the wide variation in the size of artifacts depending on the clip size, shape, and composition. Note also that artifacts in the gradient-echo image tend to be signal voids, while artifacts in 2D FSE tend to include a signal flare component.

Figure 11.11 Reasonable sized clip artifact (arrow) in a T1W fat-saturated 3D gradient-echo image. TR = 6.5 ms, TE = 3.2 ms, flip angle was 10°, and pixel bandwidth was 244 Hz. Hence, chemical shift artifacts were slightly less than one pixel.

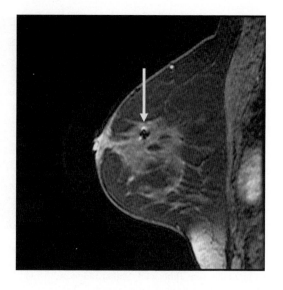

consists of a wire mesh shell built into the inside walls, windows, and doors of the MRI scan room. If the door is left ajar or if there is a break in the RF shield, radio transmissions at one or more discrete frequencies near the Larmor frequency (63.6–63.9 MHz) can appear as a distinct line in the image.[8] Such RF transmission artifacts are fixed in location along the FE direction, but smear in the PE direction due to having different measured amplitudes in different PE views (Figure 11.12).

Other sources of line artifacts include RF feedthrough from transmit coils to receive coils and sources of RF interference within the scanner room. Sources of line artifacts include faulty lighting fixtures and patient monitoring equipment within the MRI scan room. These usually produce broad spectrum RF interference that appears as one or more broad lines running across the image in the PE direction.[2] These artifacts can be isolated by acquiring phantom images with the lights turned on, then off, or with peripheral electrical equipment in the scan room turned on, then off or removed from the scan room, until line artifacts are eliminated. If such artifacts persist on images when the door is tightly shut and possible sources inside the scan room have been eliminated, the MRI system service engineer should be contacted to investigate the integrity of the RF shielding.

Reconstruction Artifacts

Reconstruction artifacts usually appear as a repeated pattern of lines or dots at fixed periodicity (spatial frequency) in planar images (Figure 11.13). These usually occur because of corrupted data being measured during signal acquisition or altered prior to 2DFT or 3DFT image reconstruction. Looking at the k-space representation of image data can sometimes reveal, and permit correction of, corrupted data.

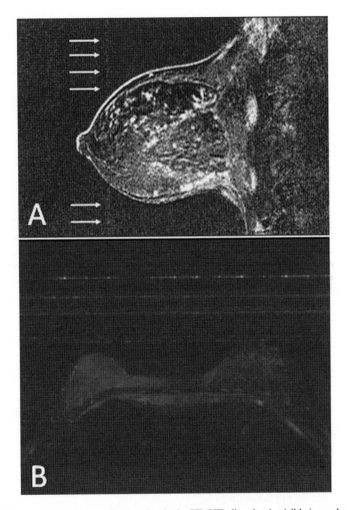

Figure 11.12 (A) Vertical line artifact running in the PE (HF) direction is visible in a subtracted contrast-enhanced 3D gradient-echo image. Such lines are characteristic of RF transmissions leaking into the scan room due to improper RF-shielding. (B) Multiple horizontal lines artifacts running in the PE (LR) direction are visible in this transaxial image due to broadcast radio transmissions into the scan room. In this case, the technologist did not shut the scan room door completely during scanning. (B Reprinted with permission from Harvey JA, Hendrick RE, Coll J, et al. Breast MR imaging artifacts: how to recognize and fix them. RadioGraphics 2007; 27: In Press)[8].

Other Randomly Occurring Image Artifacts

There are a myriad of other MRI artifacts due to equipment malfunctions. If these artifacts occur repeatedly, it is important to seek correction of the problem by a qualified MRI service engineer. Keeping a log of identified problems, including artifacts and equipment errors, and service correction of those problems is an important aspect of quality assurance in breast MRI, just as it is in mammography.

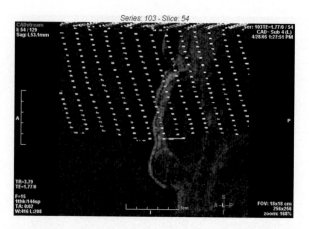

Figure 11.13 Reconstruction artifacts visible as a repetitive set of white dots in diagonal patterns, like due to a single spike in acquired k-space data. A log of this kind of reconstruction error should be kept by the MR technologist. If this type of reconstruction artifact appears in more than one image or series or in other studies, an example should be saved and shown to the MR system service engineer to correct the problem.

Other Equipment and User Errors

In Chapters 8 and 9, we described and illustrated a number of equipment errors and user errors including:

1. Using the body coil as the receiver coil rather than the breast coil
2. Choosing the PE direction incorrectly
3. Choosing too large a FOV in either bilateral or unilateral imaging
4. Incomplete fat suppression
5. Excessive slice thickness
6. Excessive pixel size
7. Inadequate SNR
8. Failure to collect both pre- and post-contrast images
9. Failure to collect or analyze dynamic information
10. Incorrectly selecting ROIs for dynamic analysis
11. Mistaking vascularity or pulsation artifacts for enhancing lesions
12. Failure to inject the proper dose of contrast agent into the patient

An additional error that can be made is to select too small a FOV (Figure 11.14). The selected FOV in any plane should include all breast tissue and be large enough to exclude all other tissues from aliasing across the breasts.

Other equipment problem errors are described below.

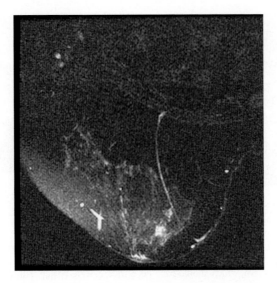

Figure 11.14 A 15 × 15 cm FOV was selected for this unilateral transaxial T2W fat-saturated multislice 2D acquisition. The field of view is too small to include all breast tissue. In addition, fat-saturation is incomplete, as show by the higher signal from fat at the distal and lateral (left) edge of the breast. The bright curved line is the aliased signal from the opposite breast.

Poor Magnetic Field Uniformity or Magnetic Gradient Linearity

Occasionally, artifacts can reveal other equipment problems besides the artifacts themselves. Figure 11.15A shows a repetitive bright signal due to vascular pulsation. This recurring artifact propagates in the PE direction, which in a properly shimmed magnet with linear gradients would be exactly vertical. In this example, the line of recurrent bright dots is not straight, but warped, as are the edges of all images acquired on the same MRI system (Figure 11-15B and C). Distortions such as those of the ghost artifact and image edges indicate that the magnet is not properly shimmed or that the magnetic field gradients are not linear. Such problems lead to reduced image quality, image distortions, and inaccuracies in measurements of lesion size and location from MR images. They can pose serious problems if MR images are used for treatment planning.

Another example of poor magnetic field shimming revealed by artifacts is the occurrence of Moire pattern artifacts (Figure 11.16). This artifactual light-dark banding occurs due to both image wrap and poor magnetic field shimming. Image wrap causes tissues outside the field of view to superimpose the image, while poor shimming causes a varying phase relationship between signals inside and signals outside but wrapping into the selected FOV. The phase difference between tissues inside and outside the FOV causes the combined signals to alternately go in-phase

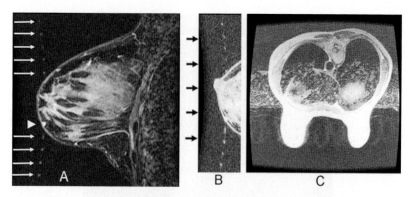

Figure 11.15 (A) Sagittal STIR image of a breast with prominent vascular pulsation causing ghosting of bright blood in the PE direction. The fact that ghosting does not run vertically may indicate that the magnet is poorly shimmed. (B) When windowing was altered to reveal the image background, the left edge of the background noise pattern was bowed similarly to the ghost artifacts (arrows). (C). When windowing was altered on transaxial images, all edges of the image background noise pattern, which should have been square, were bowed. All of these features can indicate poor static magnetic field shimming or non-linear gradients.

(bright) and out-of-phase (dark), yielding the Moire interference pattern banding across the image. The bands always change from light to dark along the PE direction and are reasonably uniform along the FE direction. These artifacts can often be corrected for the patient at hand by adding oversampling in the PE direction. Their presence suggests that the static magnetic field should be re-shimmed by the MRI system service engineer.

Radiofrequency Receiver Coil Problems

Figure 11.17 illustrates a problem with a four-channel RF receiver coil used for breast imaging. The breast receiver coil was intermittently yielding lower signal on the right breast (arrow) than the left. The signal difference was evident on some (Figure 11.17A), but not all (Figure 11.17B) clinical images. Identical uniform phantoms were placed in left and right breast coils, and SNR was measured (Figure 11.17C). SNR in the right breast coil (arrow) was measured to be approximately one-half that in the left coil, suggesting that one of the two channels used for the right breast was not functioning. Through further phantom testing, the problem was identified to be a defective wire for a single channel at the connection exiting the breast coil. When the wire was re-positioned, the defective coil channel would sometimes function properly (Figure 11.17D). The breast coil was returned to the manufacturer for repair.

Awareness of image artifacts is the first step toward improved image quality. It is helpful for the MR technologist to keep a log of identified artifacts. This log should be shared with the MRI service engineer to aid in correcting image quality

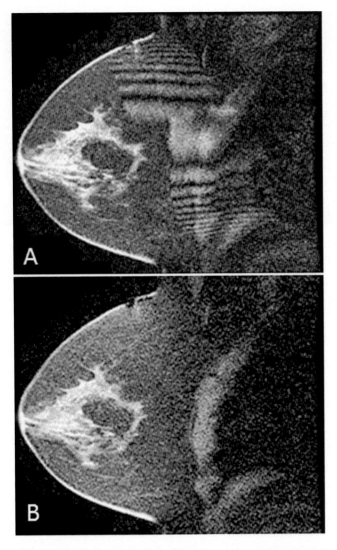

Figure 11.16 (A) 3D gradient-echo image acquired with in-plane PE selected HF. No precautions were taken to prevent phase-wrap. The combination of phase-wrap HF and poor shimming resulted in the Moire pattern artifact shown. (B) Same plane of the same pulse sequence and volunteer as in A, but with no-phase-wrap (NPW) selected. This doubled the scanned FOV in the PE (HF) direction, simultaneously switching to half-Fourier image acquisition. This eliminated the Moire pattern artifact.

problems. Recurrent RF transmission artifacts indicate problems with the MR systems RF shielding. Problems such as Moire artifacts or image distortion indicate that the static magnetic field may need re-shimming or that magnetic field gradients may need to be re-calibrated by the service engineer.

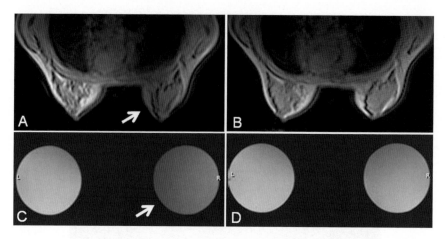

Figure 11.17 (A) 3D gradient-echo transaxial image showing reduced signal in the right breast (arrow) compared to the left breast. (B) A different gradient-echo image acquired on the same volunteer after identifying and correcting the coil problem. (C) Identical, uniform phantoms in each breast coil, showing SNR reduced by a factor of two in the right coil (arrow). The signal is lower medially than laterally for the right breast coil (D). Same phantoms imaged after correcting the breast coil problem, indicating similar SNR on both sides of the coil.

Chapter Take-home Points

- Artifacts in breast MRI have many different appearances: ghosts, image super-positions, lines, dots, signal voids, shading, and geometric distortions.
- Ghosts due to patient or physiologic motion are the most common source of artifacts in breast MRI.
- Motion artifacts propagate in the PE direction, regardless of the direction of motion that causes them.
- Motion and aliasing artifacts can obscure pathology and occasionally simulate pathology.
- Aliasing artifacts occur most commonly in the PE direction.
- Aliasing can be minimized by ensuring that no signal-producing tissues lie outside the selected FOV in the PE direction.
- Chemical shift artifacts of the first kind shift fat relative to water along the FE direction.
- Chemical shift artifacts of the second kind occur only in gradient-echo images, causing water signals and fat signals to add or subtract depending on B_0 and TE values.
- Bandwidth per pixel determines the extent of chemical shift between fat and water.
- Truncation artifacts are minor in breast MRI, usually occurring at the edge of the breast.

- Metallic artifacts are usually due to surgical clips or breast biopsy marker clips causing signal voids, sometimes accompanied by signal flares.
- Line artifacts are usually due to RF transmission into the scan room or RF interference caused by a source in the scan room.
- Poor magnetic field shimming or mis-calibrated magnetic field gradients can result in non-linear motion artifacts, image edges, or Moire artifacts when aliasing also occurs.
- Keeping a log of artifacts and equipment errors aids in their correction.
- Recurrent artifacts or image distortions should prompt service correction of identified problems.

References

1. Hendrick RE, Russ PD, Simon J. *MRI: Principles and Artifacts*, Raven Press, 1993.
2. Wood ML, Henkelman RM. Artifacts. In Stark DD, Bradley WG, eds. Magnetic Resonance Imaging, 3rd Edition, 1999. St. Louis: Mosby Publishing Co., Vol 1, Ch. 10, p. 215–230.
3. Pattany PM, Phillips J, Chiu LC, et.al. Motion artifact suppression technique (MAST) for MR Imaging. J. Comput. Assist. Tomogr. 1987; 11: 369–377.
4. Purcell EM. Electricity and magnetism. Berkeley Physics Course – Volume 2. New York: McGraw-Hill Book Co. 1965, p. 394–399.
5. Berg W, Birdwell R. Diagnostic Imaging: Breast, Salt Lake City: Amirsys, Inc. 2006, p. IV-7-18 to 23.
6. Genson CC, Blane CE, Helvie MA, et.al. Effects on breast MRI of artifacts caused by metallic tissue marker clips. AJR 2007; 188: 372–376.
7. Chen X, Lehman CD, Dee KE. MRI-guided breast biopsy: clinical experience with 14-gauge stainless steel core biopsy needle. AJR 2004; 182:1075–1080.
8. Harvey JH, Hendrick RE, Coll J, et.al. Breast MR imaging artifacts: how to recognize and fix them. Radiographics, to be published November/December 2007.

Chapter 12
Magnetic Resonance Imaging Safety and Patient Considerations

Safety is crucial at every MRI site.[1-5] Most hospitals and outpatient facilities have established safety procedures for MRI; breast MRI is just one of many MR examinations falling under such procedures. MR safety issues may be less familiar to breast imaging centers that have added dedicated breast MRI to their imaging procedures. In either case, the safety of patients, site workers, and visitors entering the MRI suite is a major concern.

The American College of Radiology's Guidance Document for Safe MR Practices: 2007 points out that a system for quality improvement of MR safety should be in place at every MR facility.[3] The system should include written policies and procedures for MR safety, review of those procedures on a regular basis, an MR medical director who ensures that safe practice guidelines are established and maintained, and a process for reporting adverse events, MR "incidents", and near-incidents to the MR medical director in a timely manner, so that continuous quality improvement can occur.[3]

Everyone entering a MRI scan room must be screened for carried or implanted objects that could pose a hazard to themselves or others in the room. Deaths and serious injuries have resulted from improper screening for foreign objects in MRI patients and site workers.[6] In the strong magnetic field of an MR scanner, objects that are normally innocuous can become potentially lethal. This chapter provides an overview of MRI safety issues, with a special focus on issues important to breast MRI.

There are a number of valuable resources available to deal with both general and specific questions about MRI safety.[3-5] One of the best free resources is a website developed by Dr. Frank Shellock, a well-known expert on MRI safety.[5] This website provides information on every aspect of MR safety, including a patient screening form for use by MRI sites. This website lists MRI information of over 1,500 objects, ranging from a 357 magnum to breast biopsy marker clips. If an MRI site has any question about the safety of a specific object or implanted medical device in the scan room, Dr. Shellock's list usually provides the answer.

Safety issues in breast MRI can be divided into three distinct categories: effects of static magnetic fields, effects of magnetic gradients, and effects of radiofrequency (RF) fields. Each of these three areas is discussed below, in each case beginning with U.S. Food and Drug Administration (FDA) guidelines.[7]

R.E. Hendrick (ed.), *Breast MRI: Fundamentals and Technical Aspects.*
© Springer 2008

Static Magnetic Fields

One concern with static magnetic fields is that either brief or long-term exposure might cause long-term biological effects. While there are numerous studies of the effects of static magnetic fields on cells and lower life forms, there is no clear deleterious effect of short-term or long-term exposure of humans to high magnetic fields.[1,2,8–10] The latest guidelines from the U.S. FDA advise that clinical MR systems with static magnetic fields up to 8.0-Tesla are considered a "non-significant risk" for adult patients.[7] The main risks are those cited below from introducing patients with implanted metal devices or from patients, visitors, or site personnel inadvertently carrying ferromagnetic objects into the strong static magnetic field of the MRI system.

Magnetic Shielding

Early clinical MR installations often used passive shielding of MRI scanners. Passive shielding encloses the scan room with a high permeability metal, called μ (mu)-metal, that helps contain magnetic field lines within the room. Shielding was added to ensure that magnetic fields extending outside the scan room were less than 5 gauss (1 gauss = one ten-thousandth of one Tesla), which is about 10 times the naturally-occurring magnetic field at the earth's surface. At 5 gauss or less, magnetic fields may affect sensitive electronic instruments such as electron paths in cathode ray tubes, linear accelerator beams, or electron-beam CT scanners, but do not alter the performance of cardiac pacemakers or other implanted medical devices. Five gauss is well below the level of magnetic fields that will damage analog watches or erase magnetic strips on credit cards. This requires several hundred gauss, a field strength that occurs inside the scan room a few meters from the scanner bore.

Modern MR scanners are typically actively shielded. Active shielding is achieved by adding superconducting coils at the ends of solenoidal magnets. Active shielding confines external magnetic field lines to occur within or near the scanner itself and reduces fringe magnetic fields away from the scanner. Active magnetic shielding eliminates the need for heavy and expensive μ-metal room shielding, but makes the static magnetic field gradients at the ends of the scanner bore even stronger, potentially increasing the risks of ferromagnetic objects brought into the scan room being accelerated into the scanner. Short-bore magnets tend to have stronger magnetic field gradients at the ends of the scanner bore than long-bore magnets. And of course, higher field clinical scanners such as 3 T systems have much stronger fringe fields at each end of the scanner bore than lower field systems.

Metallic Objects in the Scan Room

One of the greatest hazards with MRI occurs when ferromagnetic objects are inadvertently brought into the MRI scan room. Ferromagnetic objects (those that can be attracted by a bar magnet) experience two kinds of effects in the presence of the main magnet's static magnetic field: translational attraction and torque.[2,5] Static magnetic fields cause these effects on any ferromagnetic object, such as wrenches, screwdrivers, scissors, IV poles, fork lift tines, or others. Some tools are specifically designed to be acceptable for use in the MR environment (non-ferromagnetic), such as those used by a MR service engineer, but the assumption should be that any metal object is ferromagnetic until proven otherwise. The torque exerted on a ferromagnetic object by the MR magnet's static magnetic field can easily twist a loosely held object out of the grasp of unsuspecting site personnel.

In addition, the static spatial magnetic field gradient that exists near each end of the MR scanner attracts ferromagnetic objects into the scanner, thus, causing translational attraction. This attractive force is due to the increasing magnetic field at closer distances to the solenoidal scanner bore (Figure 12.1). The combination of strong torque and attraction at closer distances to the scanner can abruptly pull metal objects out of the hands or pockets of those approaching the magnet and then accelerate those objects into the bore of the magnet, whether a patient is present or not (Figure 12.2).

It is these twisting and accelerating forces due to the static magnetic field that cause most MR-related injuries. The FDA maintains a list of MR-related adverse events and most are accidents that occurred because someone inadvertently entered the MR scan room without proper screening. These accidents include:[6]

- Death or serious injury caused by ferromagnetic portable oxygen tanks carried into the scan room being abruptly accelerated into the scanner bore and striking the patient lying on the scan table in the bore of the magnet.
- Blindness or vision problems caused by iron filings or metal objects in or near the eyes undergoing torques and linear forces, due to placement of the patient in the scanner. RF fields can cause heating of these small foreign bodies, as well.
- Ferromagnetic IV poles, scissors, scalpels, and other objects being pulled into the bore of the scanner with a patient on the scan table, causing patient injuries, some serious.

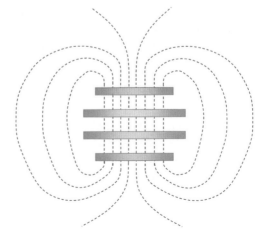

Figure 12.1 Schematic top view of an MRI unit showing superconducting magnet coils and resulting lines of constant magnetic field (dashed lines). Note that the magnetic field is uniform inside the solenoidal bore of the magnet, but weakens with increasing distance from each end of the magnet's bore, as shown by the diverging magnetic field lines at either end of the magnet's bore.

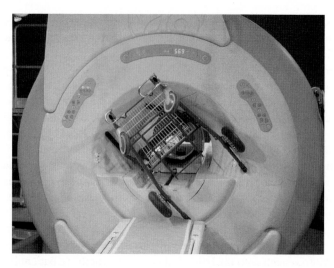

Figure 12.2 Placing any ferromagnetic object near the ends of the magnet risks rapid acceleration of the object into the scanner bore. In this case, a patient was brought into the room on a
ferromagnetic wheeled basket chair. After moving from the chair to the scan table, the patient
pushed the chair aside and it was pulled up against the magnet by the static magnetic field gradient near the bore. The technologist called a transport employee to help remove the chair and in
trying to remove the chair lifted it, causing it to be pulled into the scanner bore itself. The chair
was removed by a crew using a wench apparatus the next day. The patient was not hurt, but there
was damage to the scanner shroud and head coil, which was positioned in the scanner bore as the
patient was taken into the room. (Reprinted with permission from www.simplyphysics.com, courtesy of Moriel NessAiver, Ph.D.).

- Steel tines from a fork lift, weighing 80 pounds each, being accelerated into the
  scanner and striking site personnel standing between the fork lift and the scanner
  bore, knocking him over 15 feet and causing serious injury.

Many of these accidents occurred because those involved did not know that the static
magnetic field of a superconducting magnet is always on, even when the MRI system
is not scanning a patient. Often, site personnel unfamiliar with MRI, such as nurses,
construction workers, cleaning workers, or emergency personnel enter a scan room
when an MR-technologist is not present, unaware that the static magnetic field is on. To
prevent such accidents, signs posted outside MRI areas should be revised to read:

DANGER!
THIS MAGNET IS ALWAYS ON!

In addition, since MRI technologists cannot be present 24 hours a day to screen
site staff cleaning or maintenance personnel entering the scan room, everyone who
has access to the scan room after hours needs to be educated about the potential
dangers of the strong magnetic fields associated with a MRI system.

In addition to the potential for personal injury and site liability, MRI accidents
such as these are disruptive to the site even when a patient is not present in the
scanner. Accidents often require the site to close the scanner and ramp down the

superconducting magnet, which can take days, to permit removal of larger metal objects from the bore of the scanner. This costs the typical MRI site an average of $10,000 per day in technical income. It also inconveniences patients who have to reschedule appointments.

I have personally witnessed two potentially serious accidents involving metallic objects inappropriately taken into the scan room. The first occurred in 1984 and involved a patient brought to an outpatient imaging center from a nearby hospital. The patient had been placed on an MR-compatible stretcher at the hospital. Unbeknownst to the site's MRI technologist, a portable oxygen tank had been placed between the patient's legs and a blanket was covering the patient's lower torso and legs, along with the oxygen tank. The patient was brought from a hospital by a transport team on an MR-compatible stretcher and placed directly on the scan table. The patient and stretcher were placed head-first on the scan table at the end of the magnet. After positioning the supine patient in a head coil outside the scanner, the technologist started moving the table into the scanner bore. After a few inches of motion, the table and patient were abruptly pulled into the scanner due to the accelerating force of the static magnetic field gradient on the ferromagnetic oxygen tank a meter or two away from the entrance to the scanner bore. No injury occurred, primarily because this happened in 1984 on a 0.15 T magnet. Had this been one of today's 1.5 T or 3.0 T (superconducting) magnets, the patient likely would have been seriously injured.

A second incident occurred while training personnel to perform MR-guided breast biopsies. A patient had just been positioned in the breast biopsy coil, head-first and prone, with her head just outside the bore of the magnet. An attending physician involved in the procedure inadvertently entered the room with a pair of sharp-pointed small metal scissors in her hand. While standing near the bore of the magnet and leaning forward to inspect the biopsy device, the scissors were abruptly pulled out of her hand and toward the opening of the scanner bore. The scissors were stopped by a pillow that was beneath and, fortunately, puffed up around the side of the patient's head. The scissors that were accelerating into the scanner were stopped by the pillow a few inches from the eyes of the patient. The scissors were quickly grabbed and removed from the scan room. By luck, a serious accident was narrowly averted.

MRI-guided breast biopsies provide new opportunities for adverse events to occur in the MRI scan room. All personnel involved in these procedures need to be educated about the hazards of introducing ferromagnetic objects into strong magnetic fields and carefully screened for metal objects that could harm other medical personnel or the patient. Metal objects used in MR-guided breast biopsy procedures need to be tested beforehand with a bar magnet to assess their acceptability in the MR environment before being permitted in the scan room.

In addition, everyone entering the scan room should be screened for watches, credit cards, cameras, ID badges, cell phones, PDAs and other electronics, as those items can be damaged or erased by the high magnetic fields near the bore of the scanner. Like patients, medical personnel should also be screened for pens, paper clips, jewelry that contains ferromagnetic components, and other metal objects that can be drawn into the bore of the magnet. And like patients, personnel should be screened for implanted metal objects such as pacemakers, heart valves, aneurysm clips, shrapnel, iron filings in or near the eyes, dental implants, and other metallic implanted objects (see the screening forms and checklists in the Appendix of this book).

Gradient Magnetic Fields

Magnetic field gradients are switched on and off hundreds of times during performance of a single MR pulse sequence. Even though weaker than the static magnetic field by a factor of about 1000, the switching on and off of magnetic field gradients induces electric fields and weak electrical currents in the human body, just as precessing magnetization induces a weak current in a loop of wire. These currents in the human body cause an insignificant amount of tissue heating compared to the pulsed RF fields described later. At higher gradient levels or more rapid rates of change than are used in current clinical protocols, switched magnetic field gradients can cause neurostimulation. Neurostimulation is first evident to the patient as a tingling or tapping sensation, but at higher gradient strengths and switching rates, neurostimulation can be painful.

The main concern of the FDA with regard to pulsed magnetic field gradients is that their strength and rate of change may cause discomfort or painful nerve stimulation.[7] No specific numerical value is given by the FDA for the maximum rate of change of magnetic fields per unit time (dB/dt) for MRI gradients.

When studies are done with dB/dt values that exceed those of modern MR scanners by a factor of 1.5 to 2.0, peripheral nerve stimulation occurs at a number of different anatomical sites depending on the specific gradient used.[11-14] High level x-gradients (see Chapter 3 and Figure 3.5) cause neurostimulation in the bridge of the nose, the left side of the thorax, the iliac crest, the left thigh, buttocks, and lower back. High level y-gradients cause neurostimulation in the scapula, upper arms, shoulder, right side of the thorax, iliac crest, hip, hands, and upper back. High level z-gradients cause neurostimulation in the scapula, thorax, xyphoid, abdomen, iliac crest, upper and lower back. Peripheral nerve stimulation sites tend to occur at bony prominences, probably because bone is less conductive than soft tissues.[14] As a result, higher current densities occur in the narrower soft tissue areas at bony prominences. Neurostimulation and other adverse effects of magnetic gradients should not occur from the pulse sequences currently used for breast MRI.

Acoustic Noise During MR Scanning

Acoustic noise is the most obvious effect of magnetic field gradients turning on and off during scanning. Rapid pulse sequences such as 3D gradient-echo are louder and knocking sounds occur more frequently (due to the more rapid switching of magnetic gradients) than slower pulse sequences such as 2D spin-echo. Acoustic noise is the result of mechanical stresses experienced by gradient coils as they are turned on and off. For example, when two parallel loop coils carry current in opposite directions to produce a z-gradient, the magnetic field produced by one coil links the other current-carrying coil. As a result, each current-carrying coil exerts a repelling force on the opposite coil that must be resisted by supporting structures surrounding the bore of the scanner. As the gradient coils flex against their supports, acoustic noise occurs. Typically, measures taken to increase a scan's spatial resolution (thinner slices, smaller FOV) or temporal resolution (shorter TR, faster gradient rise times) increase the acoustic noise levels in the scanner.

FDA recommendations for noise levels within MR scanners are that they should be less than a peak unweighted sound pressure level of 140 decibel (dB) or a weighted root-mean-square (rms) sound pressure of 99 dB, with hearing protection in place.[2,15] Within the bores of MRI scanners, ambient rms sound pressures of 65–95 dB have been measured. This is within FDA guidelines for recommended noise levels, but is loud enough to cause temporary hearing loss unless hearing protection is used. In a study of patients undergoing MRI without hearing protection, 43% of subjects reported a temporary hearing loss.[16] Of greater concern is that MR gradients might cause permanent hearing loss in patients who are particularly susceptible to the effects of loud noises.[16,17] Some newer scanners have new gradient coil designs that reduce noise to very low levels for all pulse sequences.

Providing the patient with hearing protection during scanning can avoid the problem of temporary hearing loss.[16,17] Having all patients wear disposable earplugs is a simple and inexpensive way to minimize the effects of acoustic noise on patients. Another option is to use noise-muffling earphones. One drawback to either of these approaches is that they make verbal communication between the technologist or radiologist and patient more difficult. Another alternative is to use noise canceling earphones, which measure ambient noise and produce a pattern of destructive interference to cancel outside noise. These have been safely implemented in MR scanners. As with monitoring devices, care must be taken with earphones to ensure that these devices are MR-compatible and that wires to the earphones do not pass through the bore of the magnet, as this can significantly degrade image quality. Both muffling and noise-canceling earphones facilitate communication between technologist and patient through the patient intercom system. Noise-canceling earphones are not desirable if communication is needed in the room, such as during MR-guided breast localizations and biopsies.

Radiofrequency Fields

Radiofrequency (RF) waves are sent into the patient by transmitter coils at least once during each repetition of the basic MR pulse sequence. For gradient-echo imaging, an RF pulse is sent in once per measured echo, for spin-echo twice, and for inversion-recovery 3 times. For fast-spin-echo and multi-echo sequences, an additional RF pulse is used for each additional echo formed. A reasonable fraction of the RF energy sent into the patient is absorbed in tissue, generating heat. The resulting heating of tissues within the sensitive volume of the RF transmit coils is of concern.

RF power deposition in tissue is quantified by a quantity called the specific absorption rate (SAR). SAR is the average rate at which RF power is deposited in tissue, normalized by the volume of tissue. SAR is given in units of watts per kilogram (W/kg). SAR is a complex function of the number of RF pulses per unit time, the flip angle of each pulse, the type of RF transmit coil used, the volume of tissue within the transmit coil, the configuration of anatomy within the transmit coil, and the resistivity of tissue. The amount of RF radiation absorbed by tissue depends on the wavelength of RF radiation, which is determined by the Larmor frequency.

FDA requirements for RF energy deposition are that the SAR should be less than:[2,7]

- 4 W/kg averaged over the whole body for any period of 15 minutes
- 3 W/kg averaged over the head for any period of 10 minutes
- 8 W/kg in any gram of tissue in the head or torso, or 12 W/kg in any gram of tissue in the extremities, for any period of 5 minutes.

SAR for specific MR pulse sequences is reported in the DICOM header files of each slice. The SAR reported is the same for each slice in the pulse sequence. For breast MRI, the body coil is almost always used as the transmit coil, so energy is deposited in a broad area of the torso centered on the breasts in the head-to-foot direction. Therefore, for breast MRI, the upper limit of 4 W/kg averaged over the whole body for 15 minutes applies. The SAR for current pulse sequences specific to breast MRI typically varies from 0.5 to 1.5 W/kg for 2D T1W and STIR sequences, from 1.0 to 2.7 W/kg for T2W FSE sequences, and from 0.25 to 1.1 W/kg for 3D gradient-echo sequences. 3D gradient-echo sequences have lower SAR values because they have only one RF pulse per excitation and use small flip angles (typically 8–20°), in spite of having much shorter TR values than 2D T1W, T2W, and STIR sequences. All of these SAR values are such that tissue heating should not be an issue in current breast MRI protocols.

Other Patient and Personnel Safety Considerations

Patients, Visitors, or Site Personnel with Metallic Implants and Devices

Every person entering the scan room must be screened for the presence of implanted medical devices such as cardiac pacemakers, heart valves, intravascular coils, filters, stents, aneurysm clips, dental devices, ocular implants, orthopedic implants, otologic implants, vascular ports, breast expanders, and other metallic objects. For certain implants and devices, static magnetic fields cause torque and translational displacement than can dislodge the metallic implant. Changing magnetic gradients and RF fields used during scanning can induce spurious electrical currents that might improperly activate or deactivate implanted electrical devices such as a pacemaker. These changing fields can also cause substantial heating of certain implanted metal devices or wires.

Some MRI adverse events involving implanted medical devices reported to the FDA include:

- Patients with implanted cardiac pacemakers dying during or shortly after MRI scanning due to MRI-induced malfunction of the pacemaker.
- Patients with implanted intracranial aneurysm clips dying due to shifting of the clip as a result of being placed in an MR scanner. The staff claimed to have obtained information indicating that the clip could be scanned safely.
- Burns occurring on patients' hands and arms caused by an electrically conductive wire lead being looped and placed against the patient's bare skin.
- Implanted insulin infusion pumps ceasing to function after the patient was placed in an MR scanner.

If a patient or site worker reveals the presence of implanted medical devices, the MR compatibility of the specific device must be determined before allowing the person to enter the scan room (inside the 5 Gauss line). It should not be assumed that a medical device deemed safe at one magnetic field strength is necessarily safe at another field strength, especially at higher magnetic field strengths such as 3 or 4 T.

Pregnant Patients or Technologists

Pregnant Patients

There are two concerns with pregnant patients. One is exposure of the fetus to the static magnetic field, magnetic gradients, and RF fields of the MR scanner, the other is exposure of the fetus to contrast agent administration. Since gadolinium-chelate contrast-agent administration is essential for breast cancer detection, both effects must be considered.

It is known from studies in primates that gadolinium-based MRI contrast agents administered in clinical doses cross the blood-placental barrier and appear in the fetal bladder within 11 minutes of intravenous administration. Enhancement of the primate placenta was detectable up to two hours after administration. Hence, it must be assumed that the fetus is exposed to Gd-based contrast agents administered to the pregnant patient, clearing, but also being reabsorbed, via the amniotic fluid. No data are available on the rate of clearance of gadolinium chelates from amniotic fluid. Moreover, adequate studies on the effects of gadolinium based contrast agents on the fetus are not available.[3] As a result, the ACR's Guidance Document for Safe MR Practices: 2007 recommends that all women of reproductive age be screened for pregnancy prior to admitting them to the MR environment. If pregnancy is established, the potential risks and benefits of the study should be assessed to determine if the woman could wait until the end of pregnancy to perform the test.

ACR guidance recommends that pregnant patients at any stage of pregnancy be informed of the risk-benefit ratio for the performance of an MR scan, with or without contrast media. The final decision about an MR examination should be made on a case-by-case basis by a MRI-qualified radiologist after assessing the risk-to-benefit ratio for the patient and fetus. If the decision is made to scan the pregnant patient, with or without contrast agent, the radiologist should consult with the referring physician and document: 1) that the information desired from the scan cannot be obtained from some other non-ionizing imaging technique, such as ultrasound, 2) that the data needed from the MR scan is needed during the pregnancy, and 3) that the referring physician does not feel that it is prudent to wait until after pregnancy to perform the MR scan.[3]

One consideration in breast MRI of the pregnant or post-partum patient is that lactating fibroglandular tissues can cause spurious enhancement patterns similar to those of invasive breast cancers (see Chapter 8). Pregnant patients undergoing MRI should provide written informed consent acknowledging that they understand the risks and benefits of MRI (with or without contrast), that they understand the alternative diagnostic options, and that they wish to proceed with the MRI procedure.[3]

Pregnant Technologists

MR technologists who are pregnant are permitted to work in all areas of the MR suite, including the scan room.[18] They can inject contrast agent, position patients, and enter the scan room in case of emergency. They should avoid entering the bore of the magnet or the scan room during data acquisition.[18, 3]

Cryogens and Quenches

Superconducting magnets are kept at temperatures below 15° Kelvin (that is, within 15° Centigrade of absolute zero or at about −430° Fahrenheit) so that electricity flows through the niobium-titanium (Nb-Ti) solenoidal coils without electrical resistance. Since liquid helium has a boiling point of 4.2°K, as long as the Nb-Ti coils are bathed in liquid helium, they remain superconducting. This requires approximately 1000 liters of liquid helium held inside a cryostat, a giant annular-shaped thermos enclosing the scanner coils and secondary coils used for active shielding. A faint pumping noise that is sometimes audible in the scan room is the refrigeration system that keeps the liquid helium below its boiling point.

Under normal operating conditions, having a small amount of liquid helium boil off and vent through an escape valve is of no consequence. If the superconducting coils heat to a temperature above about 15°K, then they stop being superconductive. When this occurs, electrical current flows with resistance. Once that happens, the magnet coils heat up rapidly, quickly causing liquid helium to boil off into gaseous helium. This process is called a magnet "quench".

All MRI suites are designed to have a venting system that carries boiled-off gaseous helium out of the scan room and vents it outside in case of a quench. If the venting system fails, the scan room may fill with gaseous helium. In addition to being cold and foggy, liquid helium filling a scan room will displace oxygen and can asphyxiate anyone left in the scan room for more than a few minutes. In the case of a quench and improper venting of a scan room with a patient in the room, the technologist or other personnel should remove the patient and anyone else from the room as quickly as possible. Unless previously tested and known to be MR-compatible, oxygen tanks should never be brought into a scan room, even in the case of a magnet quench.

In case of an emergency, such as a patient going into cardiac arrest, it is never a good idea to quench the magnet in an attempt to eliminate the static magnetic field and make the room safe for emergency personnel who may not have been screened for metal and implanted objects. Quenching the magnet takes several minutes and, as described above, increases the risk of asphyxiation to anyone in the scan room. Instead, it is best to remove the patient from the scan room as quickly as possible, so that emergency personnel can access the patient without entering the scan room.

Chapter Take-home Points

- Every MRI site should have a written policy and procedures manual for MRI safety.
- Every MRI site should have an MR medical director who ensures that safe practice guidelines are established and maintained.
- Every technologist and all site personnel should be trained on MRI safety and procedures, including a review of the site's policy and procedures manual.
- Every patient, visitor, or site employee who enters the scan room should be screened for ferromagnetic objects, implanted medical devices, surgical clips, metal fragments in or near the eyes, and other metallic objects.
- FDA guidelines state that:
  - static magnetic fields less than 8 T pose an insignificant risk to MRI adult patients.
  - the rate of change of pulsed magnetic field gradients should be low enough not to cause patient discomfort or painful nerve stimulation.
  - the specific absorption rate (SAR) should be less than 4 W/kg averaged over the whole body for any period of 15 minutes.

- In general, pregnant patients should not be given Gd-chelate contrast agent, but if deemed a medical necessity, pregnant patients undergoing MRI or receiving contrast agent should provide written informed consent.

References

1. Shellock FG, Crues JV. MR procedures: biologic effects, safety, and patient care. Radiology, 2004;232:635–652.
2. Shellock FG. Magnetic Resonance Procedures. Health Effects and Safety. CRC Press, Boca Raton, FL, 2001.

3. Kanal E, Barkovich AJ, Bell C, et.al. ACR Guidance Document for Safe MR Practices: 2007. Am. J. of Roentgenology 2007; 188: 1–27.
4. Radiology Websites: MRI Safety Websites: http://www.refindia.net/rlinks/reviewedlinks/ MRI_safety.htm, last accessed 2/1/07.
5. Shellock FG. http://www.mrisafety.com/ is an invaluable website for MRI safety, last accessed 2/1/07.
6. Shellock FG. Reference Manual for Magnetic Resonance Safety and Implants: 2007 Edition. Biomedical Research Publishing Group, Los Angeles, CA, 2007.
7. U.S. Department of Health and Human Services, Food and Drug Administration, Center for Devices and Radiological Health, Guidance for Industry and FDA Staff. Criteria for Significant Risk Investigations of Magnetic Resonance Diagnostic Devices, July 14, 2003.
8. Schenck JF. Health effects and safety of static magnetic fields. In: Shellock FG, ed. Magnetic resonance procedures: health effects and safety. Boca Raton, FL: CRC Press, 2001; pp. 1–30.
9. Schenck JF. Safety of strong, static magnetic fields. J Magn Reson Imaging 2000; 12; 2–19.
10. Schenck JF, Dumoulin CL, Redington RW, Kressel HY, Elliott RT, McDougall IL. Human exposure to 4.0-Tesla magnetic fields in a whole-body scanner. Medical Physics 1992; 19: 1089–1098.
11. Shellock FG. Bioeffects of gradient magnetic fields. Available at http://www.mrisafety.com/, last accessed 2/1/07.
12. Abart J, Eberhardt K, Fischer H, et al. Peripheral nerve stimulation by time-varying magnetic fields. J Comput Assis Tomogr 1997; 21: 532–538.
13. Bourland JD, Nyenhuis JA, Schaefer DJ. Physiologic effects of intense MRI gradient fields. Neuroimaging Clin North Am 1999; 9: 363–377.
14. Schaefer DJ, Bourland JD, Nyenhuis JA. Review of patient safety in time-varying gradient fields. J Magn Reson Imaging 2000; 12: 20–29.
15. FDA (USDHHS), Center for Devices and Radiologic Health, Office of Device Evaluation, Division of Reproductive, Abdominal, Ear, Nose, Throat and Radiological Devices, Computed Image Device Branch, 1997 (http://www.fda.gov/cdrh/ude/magdev.html).
16. Brummett RE, Talbot JM, Charuhas P. Potential hearing loss resulting from MR imaging. Radiology 1988; 169: 539–540.
17. Shellock FG, Kanal E. Policies, guidelines, and recommendations for MR imaging safety and patient management. J. Magn. Reson. Imaging 1991; 1: 97–101.
18. Kanal E, Gillen J, Evans JA, et al. Survey of reproductive health among female MR workers. Radiology 1993; 187: 395–399.

Chapter 13
New Developments in Breast Magnetic Resonance Imaging

This chapter describes some of the new developments in breast MRI including higher field systems, dedicated breast MRI systems, and imaging and spectroscopic techniques that attempt to improve the specificity (and possibly sensitivity) of breast MRI. Those include diffusion-weighted breast imaging, perfusion imaging, hydrogen spectroscopy and spectroscopic imaging.

Higher Field Systems

Clinical MRI systems at 3.0 T are now available from several major MRI manufacturers including GE, Phillips, and Siemens. The GE HDx Excite®, Phillips Achieva and Intera®, and Siemens Magnetom Trio® are all 3 T systems used extensively for neuro and body MRI, on which breast MRI can be performed. Since coils are built to resonate at specific frequencies, it is not possible to interchange breast receiver coils between 1.5 T and 3 T systems. Coils compatible with these high-field systems are now being sold commercially, either by the MRI manufacturer or by third-party coil companies such as InVivo (Invivo, Inc, Orlando, FL, see: www.intermagnetics.com).

The potential advantage of 3.0 T is that they have higher signal-to-noise ratios (SNR) per unit time. Theoretically SNR should double in going from 1.5 T to 3 T.[1-3] Figure 13.1 compares SNR measurements on the same uniform phantom acquired at 1.5 and 3 T using the same pulse sequence and receiver coil design (a 4-channel InVivo coil in each case). In our phantom testing, SNR at 1.5 T was 1.5–2.0 times higher at 3 T than at 1.5 T. Tissue T1 values are about 20% longer at 3 T than at 1.5 T, which means that recovery of longitudinal magnetization is less for a given TR values, which slightly lowers the full factor of two improvement in SNR for the same pulse sequence TR values. Nonetheless, the improved SNR at 3 T can be traded for higher spatial resolution, higher temporal resolution, or both. Figure 13.2 illustrates the image quality achievable with 3 T systems in contrast-enchanced breast MRI.

Kuhl, et. al. compared contrast-enhanced breast MRI at 3 T to 1.5 T in the same 37 patients, using higher resolution techniques at 3 T.[4] They found that overall image quality scores were slightly higher at 3 T, and differential diagnosis of enhancing lesions was made with greater confidence at 3 T, as shown by larger areas under the ROC curve.[4]

R.E. Hendrick (ed.), *Breast MRI: Fundamentals and Technical Aspects.*
© Springer 2008

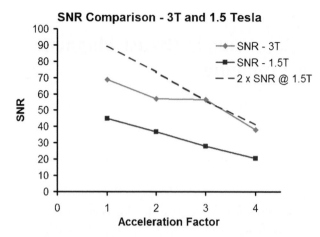

Figure 13.1 Signal-to-noise ratio (SNR) measurements in a uniform phantom at 1.5 T and 3 T for parallel imaging (GRAPPA) using identical 3D gradient echo pulse sequences with acceleration factors (R) ranging from 1 to 4 (plotted on the x-axis). The theoretical expectation is that SNR at 3 T would be double that at 1.5 T at any R value, as shown by the dashed line. Measured SNR at 3 T ranged from 1.54 to 2.03 of those at 1.5 T.

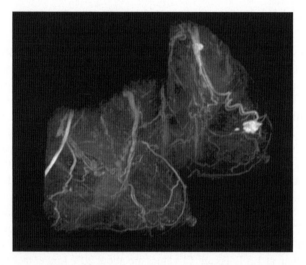

Figure 13.2 A maximum-intensity projection (MIP) image reconstructed in the left mediolateral oblique (MLO) projection of subtracted 3D gradient echo image data acquired in the transaxial plane approximately 90-seconds after the end of contrast injection on a Siemens Trio™ 3 T system. The image displays an enhancing invasive ductal carcinoma with irregular margins in the left breast. (Image provided by Dr. Nanette DeBruhl, Professor, Department of Radiology, David Geffen School of Medicine, UCLA Healthcare, Los Angeles, CA).

Figure 13.3 compares images acquired on the same volunteer at 1.5 T and 3.0 T systems using the same 4-channel coil design and pulse sequence. In this comparison, less image noise is apparent at 3 T than at 1.5 T, but fat-suppression is not as uniform

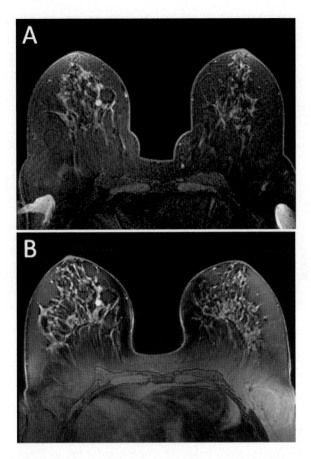

Figure 13.3 Comparison of images acquired on the same volunteer at (A) 1.5 T and (B) 3.0 T using the same 4-channel bilateral breast coil design and pulse sequence in each case. Note that fat saturation is more uniform in A, SNR is higher in B.

at 3 T as at 1.5 T due to greater difficulty in shimming the 3 T magnet. To date, the added costs, additional technical issues such as getting good fat-suppression, and the limited availability of breast coils, have limited the adoption of 3 T systems for breast MRI. New techniques mentioned later in this chapter, such as hydrogen spectroscopy, would also benefit from the use of 3 T systems in terms of increased spectrum resolution and higher SNR.

Dedicated Breast Magnetic Resonance Imaging Systems

One company (Aurora Imaging Technology, Inc., North Andover, MA, see: www. auroramri.com) has pursued the goal of manufacturing a dedicated breast MRI system for the past decade. A decade ago their goal was to build a lower-cost, mid-field

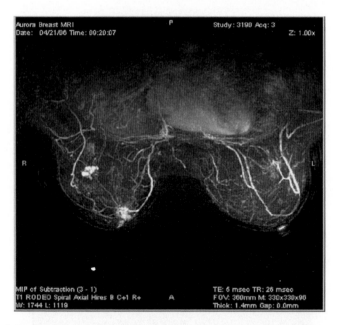

Figure 13.4 Subtracted transaxial MIP image acquired using Spiral RODEO™ on the Aurora dedicated breast MRI system showing two enhancing invasive ductal carcinomas in the right breast. 3D fat-suppressed Spiral RODEO images were acquired with TR = 26 ms, TE = 5 ms, with a 36 cm FOV, 330 × 330 matrix, 96 1.4-mm slices, for voxel sizes of 1.09 × 1.09 × 1.4 mm. (Courtesy of Dr. Steven Harms, Director of Breast Imaging, The Breast Center of Northwest Arkansas, Fayetteville, Arkansas.).

(0.5 T) scanner. They recently released a new clinical product: a 1.5 T dedicated breast MRI system capable of performing bilateral dynamic scanning using a new technique called Spiral RODEO™. Spiral RODEO combines spiral sampling of k-space[5] (Chapter 5) with the high-resolution 3D technique of RODEO (Chapter 9),[6] developed in the early 1990's, to achieve bilateral high-resolution scans with a temporal resolution of about 2 minutes (Figure 13.4). The system also has a unique positioning table specifically for breast MRI that places the breasts at the isocenter of the magnet, which should help make fat suppression more uniform. The system uses dedicated transmit and receive coils. The table and coils are designed to enhance access to the breasts for MRI-guided breast biopsies.

Dedicated Breast Magnetic Resonance Imaging Table and Coils

Another company (Sentinelle Medical, Inc., Toronto, ON, Canada; see www.sentinellemedical.com) has developed a dedicated breast MRI table and breast coils for use on GE 1.5 T breast MRI systems.[7] The 8-channel coils provide parallel imaging capabilities. The table and coils are designed to enable breast intervention

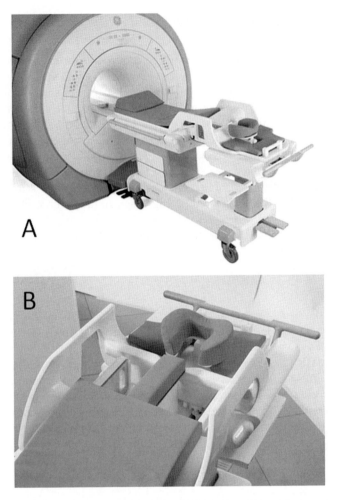

Figure 13.5 (A) The Sentinelle Medical dedicated breast imaging and intervention table and breast coils, shown with a GE 1.5 T MRI system. (B) Top view of table and coils.

with both medial and lateral access to either breast. (Figure 13.5). The table system comes with its own disposable biopsy plates and guidance software.

Novel Techniques to Improve the Specificity of Breast Magnetic Resonance Imaging

Several new techniques beyond contrast-enhanced breast MRI have been investigated to try to improve the specificity of breast MRI. Some of the most promising are described briefly below: diffusion imaging, perfusion imaging, measurement of the choline peak in proton spectroscopy, and spectroscopic imaging.

Diffusion-weighted Breast Imaging

Molecular diffusion is a physical phenomenon defined as the net action of matter, due to its thermal motion, to minimize a concentration gradient. Diffusion occurs within cells to equalize distribution of cell components. For small enough molecules, diffusion occurs across cell membranes to equalize their extracellular and intracellular concentration. MRI can be used to measure the diffusion of water in-vivo.[8] Diffusion-weighted MR pulse sequences measure the apparent diffusion coefficient (ADC) of water in tissue voxels. Diffusion-sensitizing gradients can be applied in one, two, or three directions to weight the pulse sequence by the ADC of water. In the one-dimensional measurement, a pair of gradients is applied along a single axis to alter the signal of diffusing water. In the absence of diffusion or other motion, the signal is unaffected by the pair of gradients. In the presence of diffusion or motion along the selected direction, signal is reduced exponentially in proportion to the ADC:

$$S_{measured} = S_0 e^{-b_g(ADC)},$$ (13.1)

where, S_0 is the signal without diffusion and b_g is a term determined by the diffusion gradient strength and time duration.[9] The ADC is determined by repeating the pulse sequence at least twice, using two or more different known values of b_g and using the measured signals to calculate the ADC in each voxel. While the measured ADC is affected by diffusion, it is not identical to the diffusion coefficient measured in water-containing tissues in a test tube, which depends entirely on the random thermal motion of water. In-vivo measurements of the ADC have the complicating effects of blood flow, tissue vibrations caused by systolic motion, and subject motion.

Typically, to remove directionality, the average ADC in x, y, and z, known as the diffusion trace, is measured by separately determining the diffusion coefficients along the x, y, and z directions and combining them to obtain:

$$ADC_{trace} = ADC_{xx} + ADC_{yy} + ADC_{zz}.$$ (13.2)

In-vivo measurement of ADC depends on having pulse sequences fast enough to reduce the effects of physiologic motion. This typically has been done using echo-planar techniques, which collect all phase-encoding views by repeating signal measurements using multiple spin-echoes, each with a different amount of phase-encoding, immediately after a single 90° pulse (see Chapter 6).[10] While echo-planar imaging is fast, it typically lacks the high spatial resolution of CE-BMRI and suffers some geometric distortion. Echo-planar images typically require larger FOVs (20–25 cm) and limited matrix sizes (128 × 256 is typically maximal), yielding larger pixel sizes than state-of-the-art CE-BMRI.

Measurements of ADC by Sinha, et.al., showed a distinction between mean ADC_{trace} values for fibroglandular tissues (2.37×10^{-3} mm^2/s), cysts (2.65×10^{-3} mm^2/s), benign lesions (2.01×10^{-3} mm^2/s), and malignant lesions (1.60×10^{-3} mm^2/s).[9,11] Some overlap existed between ADC_{trace} values for different tissues, however, and the number of measurements in each tissue type was limited: 16 measurements in normal tissue, 6 in cysts, 6 in benign lesions, and 17 in malignant lesions. Nonetheless, this method holds promise for providing adjunctive information that might help separate benign from malignant enhancing lesions.

Perfusion Imaging of the Breast

Perfusion imaging can be performed with or without a contrast agent. Without a contrast agent (endogenous perfusion imaging), perfusion is measured by using spin labeling that saturates incoming intravascular protons in water.[12] The measurement of the subsequent blood signal combines the effect of the saturated blood (which should produce no signal) with unsaturated blood (which has maximum signal). The measured signal is the combined effect of black blood and visible blood, which gives information about the perfusion of the saturated into the unsaturated blood pool. This method does not require contrast agents, but produces relatively small effects, especially in tissues like breast lesions, where blood volumes in vessels and perfusion in lesions is small.

Perfusion measurements *with* a contrast agent require very high temporal resolution (on the order of a few seconds) to be sensitive to the rapid changes in signal that occur as contrast agents enter the pre-selected region of interest, in this case an enhancing breast lesion. The basic concept is that during the first bolus of perfusing contrast agent, the magnetic susceptibility ($T2^*$) of protons in the blood is shortened, thus decreasing the signal observed in $T2^*$-weighted imaging sequences. To be sensitive to the effect of Gd-chelates on magnetic susceptibility, either gradient-echo or gradient echo-planar imaging techniques are used. Voxels with more signal loss on $T2^*$-weighted sequences during the Gd-chelate bolus would indicate areas with greater vascular perfusion.[13,14]

Kuhl, et.al., compared $T2^*$-weighted perfusion imaging of the breast to T1-weighted CE-BMRI in a study of 18 subjects.[15] They found that malignant lesions showed a strong perfusion-related signal loss due to $T2^*$ shortening on gradient-echo imaging compared to benign lesions such as fibroadenomas. An animal study in rats demonstrated that $T2^*$-weighted first pass perfusion imaging allowed differentiation between implanted fibroadenomas and breast carcinomas, where T1-weighted dynamic CE-BMRI sequences failed to reveal a difference between the two lesion types.[16]

A larger clinical study by Kvistad, et.al., involving 130 subjects, compared the effect of Gd-DTPA-BHA (Omniscan™, Nycomed Amersham, now GE Healthcare) on separation between benign and malignant lesions using both T1W gradient-echo and T2*W gradient-echo sequences.[17] Using separate injections of 0.1 mmol/kg followed by 20 ml of saline, they found that the average T1W signal increase was 83% ± 74% for benign lesions and 179% ± 87% for malignant lesions. This yielded a significant difference in average signal changes between benign and malignant lesions (p<0.001), but there was significant signal overlap between the two groups. When the same lesions were studied with first pass perfusion T2*W imaging, the mean signal loss was 9% ± 7% for benign lesions and 31% ± 15% for malignant lesions. This difference was also highly significant (p<0.001), and signal change between benign and malignant lesions had less overlap with T2*W perfusion imaging than with T1W CE-BMRI. Plus or minus one standard deviation error bars were distinct for T2*W first pass perfusion imaging, but were not distinct for T1W CE imaging.

The time scale of signal increase in breast cancers using T1W sequences was on the order of 1–2 minutes after contrast agent administration, while the time scale of signal loss in breast cancers using T2*W perfusion sequences was within 15–20 seconds of contrast agent administration.[17] The authors concluded that two different biological processes were at work. The signal increase of cancers on T1W sequences was attributed to Gd-chelates entering the extravascular spaces in the vicinity of breast cancers due to leaky vessels. The signal decrease of cancers on T2*W sequences was due to magnetic susceptibility effects of Gd-chelates within the vascular beds of cancers. This difference in biological process (extravascular vs. intravascular) may explain the longer time scale of T1 effects compared to T2*-effects.

Another recent study by Delille, et.al., used gradient echo-planar imaging on 13 subjects to measure blood flow and blood volume.[18] They found that both blood flow and blood volume were increased in malignant lesions compared to normal breast tissues, but they did not report the improvement in specificity from this technique by comparing its results on both benign and malignant lesions.

Choline Peak in Hydrogen Spectroscopy

An interesting new technique that appears to increase the specificity of CE-BMRI is measurement of the choline peak in hydrogen spectroscopy. It is well established that phosphocholine (PC) and total choline (tCho) are elevated in prostate, liver, brain, and breast cancers. In vitro ^{1}H and ^{31}P spectroscopy have demonstrated high levels of PC in tissue extracts from breast cancers, while low levels were measured in extracts from normal and benign breast tissues. For example, Gribbestad, et al, analyzed human breast tissue extracts using ^{1}H spectroscopy, finding PC levels of 0.79 ± 0.55 millimolar (mM) in cancer tissue extracts, compared to 0.029 ± 0.027 mM in normal breast tissue extracts.[19] Total choline from ^{1}H spectroscopy was 1.19 ± 0.64 mM in breast cancer extracts, compared to 0.082 ± 0.062 mM in normal breast tissue extracts. ^{31}P spectroscopy has been used to measure PC, phosphoehanolamine (PE), and phosphomonoesters (PME) at elevated levels in breast cancer extracts compared to normal breast tissues.[20,21]

The increase in total choline signal measured in ^{1}H spectrospcopy, is believed to be the result of a switch in the phenotype of phosphocholines that occurs as cells become malignant. Studies using human breast cell lines indicate that the glycerophosphocholine (GPC) in normal cells is transformed to PC as cells become malignant, with a stepwise increase in PC as tissues progress through the stages of invasive breast cancer.[22] As PC increases, the total choline peak increases, as measured by ^{1}H spectroscopy. [31]P spectroscopy measures a change in the levels of phosphomonoesters (PME) and phosphodiesters (PDE), but ^{31}P spectroscopy measuring PME and PDE appears to be less sensitive to changes between benign and malignant cells than ^{1}H spectroscopy measuring tCho. Moreover, ^{1}H spectroscopy can be performed with the same receiver coils and narrowband RF amplifiers used for proton imaging, while ^{31}P spectroscopy requires separate RF coils and separately tuned RF amplifiers or broadband RF amplifiers that are less commonly available with MRI systems.

A number of in vivo ^{1}H spectroscopy studies have been performed to assess the sensitivity and specificity of choline spectroscopy to breast cancer.[23-30] Almost all have been performed at 1.5 T using single-voxel spectroscopy with minimum voxel sizes of 1 cm on a side. At 1.5 T, most researchers used the criterion of a discernable choline peak as the indicator of malignancy. Most were performed on small study groups that included larger than average breast lesions. Table 13.1 presents a summary of clinical ^{1}H spectroscopy studies performed prior to 2002, along with their sensitivities and specificities. The paper by Katz-Brull, et al, summarized the data from the previous 7 studies listed in Table 13.1.[31]

Advances in acquisition methods using variable TE and spatial-spectral selective pulses show that artifacts produced by large lipid signals can be reduced significantly.[32,33] As spectroscopic techniques improve, quantitation of in vivo spectra can be done more reliably.[34,35] This may permit replacement of the criterion of seeing or not seeing a choline peak with quantitative criteria for judging a breast lesion to be malignant.

Quantitative criteria were used in a more recent study by Bartella, et al, to assess the benefit of ^{1}H spectroscopy at 1.5 T for lesions larger than 1 cm in diameter.[36] A total of 56 patients with 57 suspicious lesions going to biopsy or biopsy-proven lesions were examined by single voxel spectroscopy. Shimming and collection of the ^{1}H spectrum took approximately 20 minutes initially, falling to about 10 minutes toward the end of accrual. Following a previous study,[37] a choline peak located at 3.2 ppm with a SNR greater than 2 was used as the criterion for a positive finding by ^{1}H spectroscopy (Figure 13.6). Physicists analyzing spectroscopic SNR values

Table 13.1 Summary of ^{1}H choline peak studies prior to 2002

Author (Yr Pub)	Number of Subjects	Sensitivity	Specificity
Roebuck et al[24] (1998)	17	70%	86%
Gribbestad et al[25] (1998)	12	(cancer cases only)	
Kvistad et al[26] (1999)	22	82%	82%
Yeung et al[27] (2001)	30	92%	83%
Jagannathan et al[28] (2001)	67	78%	86%
Thomas et al[29] (2001)	8	67% (only 2 benign lesions)	
Cecil et al[30] (2001)	38	83%	87%
Katz-Brull et al[31] (2002)*	153	83%*	85%*
		(92%)**	(92%)**

Notes: * summary of all previous studies listed
** summary results with technical failures excluded
Source: Adapted from Katz-Brull R, et al., (31).

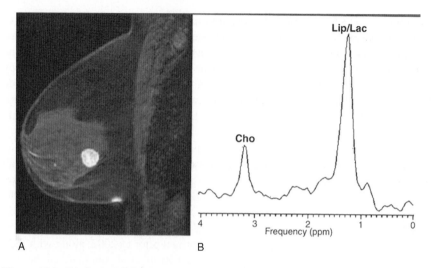

Figure 13.6 (A) Sagittal T1W MRI showing a contrast-enhanced mammographically-detected and biopsy-proven invasive ductal carcinoma in a 52 year old woman. (B) ^{1}H single-voxel spectrum of the enhancing lesion showing a distinct choline peak (marked Cho) with SNR > 2 at 3.2 parts per million (ppm). The large peak to the right of the choline peak is a lipid and lactate peak. (Reprinted with permission from Bartella L, et al. (36)).

were blinded to the cancer status of subjects. Of the 31 malignant lesions included in the study, all had a positive choline peak, for a sensitivity of 100%. Of the 26 benign lesions, 3 had a positive choline peak, for a specificity of 88%. In the 40 lesions of unknown histology, if biopsy had been performed only on lesions with a positive choline peak, 58% (23 of 40) would have been spared biopsy and none of the cancers in this series would have been missed. This is an extremely promising result on the benefit of ^{1}H spectroscopy, which needs confirmation in a larger, multi-center study.

Yeung, et.al, investigated the use of a choline peak in ^{1}H spectroscopy at 1.5T to evaluate the presence of metastatic cancer in axillary lymph nodes in 39 patients.[38] Using a choline peak SNR > 2 as a marker of metastatic cancer in lymph nodes gave a sensitivity of 69% and a specificity of 100% for lymph node metastasis, compared to histopathology after nodal dissection.

To test the benefit of adding single-voxel ^{1}H spectroscopy to CE-BMRI, Meisany, et al, performed both examinations at 4T on 55 patients going to breast biopsy.[39] Performing ^{1}H spectroscopy added about 9 minutes to the CE-BMRI study. Focusing on the lesion in question, four radiologists independently interpreted each case in two ways: first, based on CE-BMRI alone, using both morphology and dynamic information; next based on CE-BMRI and quantitation of the choline peak relative to the water peak. Radiologists were advised of the choline peak level that gave the best separation of benign from malignant lesions. In each reading, each radiologist gave a BI-RADS score and estimated probability of breast cancer. ROC curve areas based on probability of cancer improved significantly ($p \leq 0.05$) for all four readers when the choline peak information was added.

The surprising feature of this analysis was that both specificity *and* sensitivity improved when choline peak information was added to the morphology and dynamic information of CE-BMRI. The mean sensitivity (averaged over all four readers) was 87% (range: 74–94%) without choline peak information and 94% (range: 89–97%) with choline peak information. The mean specificity was 51% (range: 30–70%) without choline peak information and 57% (range: 35–75%) with choline peak information.

Combining Novel Magnetic Resonance Imaging Techniques to Gain Specificity

One group has extended the quest for higher specificity in breast MRI by combining two new techniques. Huang, et al, added both ^{1}H spectroscopy and $T2^*W$ perfusion imaging to dynamic, contrast-enhanced breast MRI.[37] In a study of 50 subjects with BI-RADS 4 or 5 lesions based on mammography, they found that contrast-enhanced MRI alone had a sensitivity of 100% and a specificity of 63%. By adding ^{1}H spectroscopy, specificity increased to 88%, and by adding $T2^*W$ perfusion imaging in addition to ^{1}H spectroscopy, specificity increased to 100%. This was a small study involving only 18 malignancies in 50 subjects, but suggests that the high sensitivity of breast MRI may be complemented by the higher specificity of specialized MR techniques such as ^{1}H spectroscopy and $T2^*W$ perfusion imaging.

The Choline Peak in ^{1}H Spectroscopy as a Predictor of Treatment Response

In a study of 13 women undergoing neoadjuvant therapy for breast cancers, in vivo proton spectroscopy at 4.0T before and 24 hours after the start of neoadjuvant therapy suggests that tCho signal may be a sensitive early predictor of tumor response to treatment.[40] Based on the Response Evaluation Criteria in Solid Tumors (RECIST) classification system,[41] 8 cancers responded to four rounds of treatment by doxorubicin hydrochloride (60 mg/m^2; Adriamycin, Pharmacia and Upjohn, Kalamazoo, MI, USA) and cyclophosphamide (600 mg/m^2; Pharmacia and Upjohn); five cancers failed to respond. Among the 8 responders, all showed lower total choline levels at 24 hours compared to baseline before the first treatment. All of the responders showed smaller tumor sizes as assessed by MRI after 12 weeks of treatment. Longest tumor diameter decreased by an average of 56% among the 8 responders (range in decrease: 35% to 100%).

Among the five non-responders to neoadjuvant therapy, all had the same or higher total choline levels at 24 hours compared to baseline. Longest tumor diameter decreased by an average of 13% among the 5 non-responders (range in decrease: 0% to 23%).

For all 13 subjects, there was a statistically significant correlation between change in total choline levels from baseline to 24 hours and change in longest tumor diameter from baseline to assessment by MRI after the last round of neoadjuvant therapy (correlation coefficient: R = 0.79, p-value = .001).

Spectroscopic Imaging

To date, only one study has been published on spectroscopic imaging of breast lesions.[42] This study was done at 1.5 T using a 12-minute single plane spectroscopic imaging technique through the most suspicious enhancing region, using large (1 cm³ voxels). The acquisition was made in a 1-cm thick 18 × 18 cm plane, yielding an 18 × 18 matrix spectroscopic image based on the total choline ¹H signal (Figure 13.7). A quantitative criterion of total choline SNR > 4 was used to attempt to separate malignant from benign lesions, with good results. This criterion led to a sensitivity of 87% and a specificity of 85%. Among the 18 study subjects, there were 3 technical failures due to patient motion, inadequate lipid suppression, and computer failure.

Conclusion

MRI manufacturers often perceive breast MRI as a low priority compared to other MR applications. The development of an entire system dedicated to breast MRI is a promising change from that perception. The development of dedicated patient

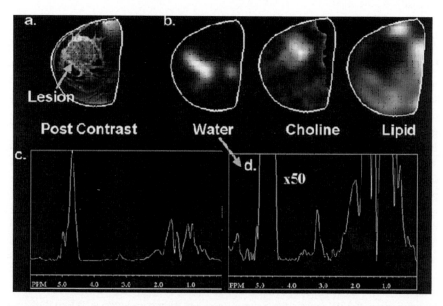

Figure 13.7 Water, choline, and lipid images derived from ¹H spectroscopic data, show below on a ×1 scale on the left, ×50 scale on the right. Choline is the small peak at 3.2 ppm. (From Jacobs MA, et al., Reference 42. Reprinted with permission of Wiley-Liss, Inc., a subsidiary of John Wiley & Sons, Inc.).

tables and coils for breast MRI, suitable for both imaging and image-guided biopsy, is another welcome improvement. There are other areas where improvement is needed for general purpose MR systems being used for breast MR imaging and spectroscopy. One area is the development of breast receiver coil "sets" that offer a range of coil volumes, similar to bra cup sizes, so that patient comfort and image SNR are not compromised, as is often the case with the "one-size-fits-all" approach.

Breast imaging pulse sequences are also in need of improvement. A single pre-contrast pulse sequence is needed that can acquire bilateral, high resolution T1W, T2W, and possibly spin-density-weighted images from a single scan, with T1W images acquired with and without fat-saturation. If such a sequence could be performed with a total image collection time of less than five minutes, the entire MR scan time could be reduced to 10–12 minutes. Further study is needed to see exactly how long after contrast injection post-contrast enhanced images need to be acquired. If complete dynamic information can be obtained in less than 6 minutes without loss of specificity, the entire pre-contrast and contrast-enhanced breast MRI protocol might be reduced to less than 10 minutes. This would make breast MRI comparable to mammography in terms of image acquisition time. And finally, the holy grail of pulse sequences would be to develop MR techniques that have the sensitivity and specificity of contrast-enhanced breast MRI without the use of a contrast agent. Research is ongoing to find such techniques.[43]

Of the new techniques discussed in this chapter to improve the specificity of breast MR, the addition of single voxel ^{1}H spectroscopy to evaluate a choline peak appears to be the most promising. The collective ^{1}H spectroscopy work discussed above suggests that the procedure is useful in separating benign from malignant lesions and in increasing the confidence of the radiologist in recommending biopsy of potentially suspicious lesions. The recent results of Jacobs, et al,[42] and Bartella, et al,[36] suggest that quantitative SNR criteria for the presence of a choline peak are clinically feasible at 1.5 T.

One limitation of ^{1}H spectroscopy is that it currently can be performed only on focal lesions larger than about 1 cm^3 in volume. One application that is not deterred by this requirement is the use of ^{1}H spectroscopy for early prediction of neoadjuvant treatment response. If the preliminary results obtained at 4 T are confirmed by further studies, some at 1.5 T or 3 T, then ^{1}H spectroscopy might save treatment non-responders from having to undergo several rounds of difficult neoadjuvant therapy, while giving responders confidence that their treatment is productive.[40]

Over the past two decades, MRI systems have made remarkable improvements. Those improvements will continue at an even more rapid pace in the future. Those improvements, along with the continued development of new techniques for breast MRI, are likely to speed image acquisition, improve spatial resolution, and enable new techniques that further improve the accuracy of breast MRI. The versatility of MRI and the richness of information it provides make it a valuable modality today and an even more promising modality for breast imaging in the years to come.

Chapter Take-home Points

- High-field 3 T MRI systems offer better SNR and spectral separation, but present more technical problems,[44] such as uniform fat-suppression, for clinical breast MRI.
- Dedicated high-field breast MRI systems and breast coil systems are now commercially available for breast MRI.
- A number of techniques have been investigated to improve the specificity and possibly the sensitivity of breast MRI. Of these, the most promising appears to be measurement of the choline peak in hydrogen spectroscopy.

References

1. Hoult DL, Richards RE. The signal-to-noise ratio of the nuclear magnetic resonance experiment. J. Magn. Res. 1976; 24: 71–85.
2. Edelstein WA, Glover GH, Hardy CJ, Redington RW. (1986) The intrinsic signal-to-noise ratio in NMR imaging. Magn. Reson. Med. 3: 604–618.
3. Haacke EM, Brown RW, Thompson MR, et.al. Magnetic Resonance Imaging: Physical Principles and Sequence Design. New York: John Wiley & Sons, 1999, especially Ch. 15, 331–380.
4. Kuhl CK, Jost P, Morakkabati N, et al. Contrast-enhanced MR imaging of the breast at 3.0 and 1.5 T in the same patients: Initial Experience. Radiology 2006 239: 666–676.
5. Daniel BL, Yen YF, Glover GH, et.al. Breast disease: dynamic spiral MR imaging Radiology 1998; 209: 499.
6. Harms SE, Flamig DP, Hensley KL, et al. MR imaging of the breast with rotating delivery of excitation off-resonance: clinical experience with pathologic correlation. Radiology 1993; 187: 493–501.
7. Causer PA, Piron CA, Jong RA, et al. MR imaging-guided breast localization system with medial or lateral access. Radiology 2006; 240: 369–379.
8. Le Bihan D, et.al. Diffusion MR imaging: clinical application. Am. J. Roentgenol. 1992; 159: 591–599.
9. Sinha S, Sinha U. Functional magnetic resonance of human breast tumors: diffusion and perfusion imaging. Annals New York Academy of Sciences 95–115.
10. Bradley WG, Chen D-Y, Atkinson J, Edelman RE. Fast spin-echo and echo-planar imaging. In DD Stark and WG Bradley, eds. Magnetic Resonance Imaging, 3rd Edition.St. Louis: C.V. Mosby Publishing Co., 1999; 125–157.
11. Sinah S, Lucas-Quesada FA, Sinha U, et.al. In-vivo diffusion-weighted MRI of the breast: potential for lesion characterization. J. Magn. Reson. Imaging 2002; 15: 693–704.
12. Detre JA et.al. Tissue specific perfusion imaging using arterial spin labeling. NMR Biomed. 1994; 7: 75–82.
13. Tofts PS. Modeling tracer kinetics in dynamic Gd-DTPA MR imaging. J. Magn. Reson. Imaging 1997; 7: 91–101.
14. Roberts HC, Roberts TPL, Brasch RC, et al. Quantitative measurement of microvacular permeability in human brain tumors achieved using dynamic contrast enhanced MR imaging: correlation with histologic grade. Am. J. Neuroradiol. 2000; 21: 891–899.
15. Kuhl CK, Bieling H, Gieseke J, et al. Breast neoplasms: T2* susceptibility-contrast. First-pass perfusion MR imaging. Radiology 1997; 202: 87–95.
16. Helbich T, Roberts TPL, Grossman A, et al. MR imaging of breast tumors: testing of different analytic methods with gadopentetate (abstract). Eur. Radiol. 1999; 9 (suppl 1): 410.

17. Kvistad KA. Breast lesions: evaluation with dynamic contrast enhanced T1-weighted MR imaging and with T2*-weighted first pass perfusion imaging. Radiology 2000; 216: 545–553.

18. DeLille J, PJ Slanetz, ED Yeh, et al. Breast cancer: regional blood flow and blood volume measured with magnetic susceptibility-based MR imaging – initial results. Radiology 2002; 223: 558–565.

19. Gribbestad IS, Petersen SB, FJosne HE, et al. ^{1}H NMR spectroscopic characterization of perchloric acid extracts from breast carcinomas and non-involved breast tissue. NMR Biomed. 1994; 7: 181–194.

20. Nagandank W. Studies of human tumors by MRS. A review. NMR Biomed 1992; 5: 303–324.

21. Podo F. Tumour phospholipids metabolism. NMR Biomed. 1999; 12: 413–439.

22. Aboagye EO, Bhujwalla ZM. Malignant transformation alters membrane choline phospholipids metabolism of human mammary epithelial cells. Cancer Research 1999; 59: 80–84.

23. Ackerstaff E, Glunde K, Bhujwalla ZM. Choline phospholipids metabolism: a target in cancer cells? Journal of Cellular Biochemistry 2003; 90: 525–533.

24. Roebuck JR, Cecil KM, Schnall MD, Lenkinski RE. Human breast lesions: characterization with proton MR spectroscopy. Radiology 1998; 209: 269–275.

25. Gribbestad IS, Singstad TE, Nilsen G, et al. In vivo H-1 MRS of normal breast and breast tumors using a dedicated double breast coil. J Magn Reson Imaging 1998; 8: 1191–1197.

26. Kvistad KA, Bakken IJ, Gribbestad IS, et al. Characterization of neoplastic and normal human breast tissues with in vivo (1)H MR spectroscopy. J Magn Reson Imaging 1999; 10: 159–164.

27. Yeung DK, Cheung HS, Tse GM. Human breast lesions: characterization with contrast-enhanced in vivo proton MR spectroscopy – initial results. Radiology 2001; 220: 40–46.

28. Jagannathan NR, Kumar M, Seenu V, et al. Evaluation of total choline from in-vivo volume localized proton MR spectroscopy and its response to neoadjuvant chemotherapy in locally advanced breast cancer. Br J Cancer 2001; 84: 1016–1022.

29. Thomas MA, Binesh N, Yue K, DeBruhl N. Volume-localized two-dimensional correlated magnetic resonance spectroscopy of human breast cancer. J Magn Reson Imaging 2001; 14: 181–186.

30. Cecil KM, Schnall MD, Siegelman ES, Lenkinski RE. The evaluation of human breast lesions with magnetic resonance imaging and proton magnetic resonance spectroscopy. Breast Cancer Res Treat 2001; 68: 45–54.

31. Katz-Brull R, Lavin PT, Lenkinski RE. Clinical utility of proton magnetic resonance spectroscopy in characterizing breast lesions. J. Natl. Cancer Inst. 2002; 94: 1197–1203.

32. Bolan PJ, DelaBarre L, Baker EH, et al. "Eliminating spurious lipid sidebands in ^{1}H MRS of breast lesions." Magn Reson Med 2002; 48(2): 215–222.

33. Bolan PJ, Meisamy S, Baker EH, et al. "In vivo quantification of choline compounds in the breast with 1H MR spectroscopy." Magn Reson Med 2003; 50(6): 1134–1143.

34. Star-Lack, J. M., E. Adalsteinsson, et al. "In vivo ^{1}H MR spectroscopy of human head and neck lymph node metastasis and comparison with oxygen tension measurements." Am J Neuroradiol 2000; 21(1): 183–93.

35. Gribbestad IS, Sitter B, Lundgren S, Krane J, Axelson D. Metabolite composition in breast tumors examined by proton nuclear magnetic resonance spectroscopy. Anticancer Res 1999; 19: 1737–1746.

36. Bartella L, Morris EA, Dershaw DD, et al. Proton MR spectroscopy with choline peak as malignancy marker improves positive predictive value for breast cancer diagnosis: preliminary study. Radiology 2006; 239: 686–692.

37. Huang W, Fisher PR, Khaldoon D, et al. Detection of malignancy: diagnostic MR protocol for improved specificity. Radiology 2004; 232: 585–591.

38. Yeung DK, Cheung HS, Tse GM. Breast cancer: in vivo proton MR spectroscopy in the characterization of histopathologic subtypes and preliminary observations in axillary node metastases. Radiology 2002; 225: 190–197.

39. Meisamy S, Bolan PJ, Baker EH, et al. Adding in vivo quantitative ^{1}H MR spectroscopy to improve diagnostic accuracy of breast MR imaging: preliminary results of observer performance study at 4.0 T. Radiology 2005; 236: 465–475.

40. Meisamy S, Bolan PJ, Baker EH, et al. Neoadjuvant chemotherapy of locally advanced breast cancer: predicting response with in Vivo ^{1}H MR spectroscopy—a pilot study at 4 T. Radiology 2004; 233: 424–431.

41. Therasse P, Arbuck SG, Eisenhauer EA, et al. New guidelines to evaluate the response to treatment in solid tumors. European Organization for Research and Treatment of Cancer, National Cancer Institute of the United States, National Cancer Institute of Canada. J Natl Cancer Inst 2000; 92:205–216.

42. Jacobs MA, Barker PB, Bottomley PA, et.al. Proton magnetic resonance spectroscopic imaging of human breast cancer: a preliminary study. Journal of Magnetic Resonance Imaging 2004; 19: 68–75.

43. Medved M, Newstead GM, Abe H, et al. High spectral and spatial resolution MRI of breast lesions: preliminary clinical experience. Am. J. Roentgenol. 2006; 186: 30–37 and references therein.

44. Kuhl CK, Kooijman H, Gieseke J, Schildtt H. Effect of B_1 in homogeneity on breast MR imaging at 3.0 T. (Letters to the Editors) Radiology 2007; 244: 929–930.

Appendix: Magnetic Resonance Imaging Patient and Non-Patient Screening Forms

---

MAGNETIC RESONANCE (MR) PROCEDURE SCREENING FORM FOR PATIENTS

Date ____/____/____   Patient Number _____

Name _____ Age _____ Height _____ Weight _____
    Last name   First name   Middle Initial

Date of Birth ____/____/____   Male ☐ Female ☐   Body Part to be Examined _____
    month day year

Address _____   Telephone (home) (____) _____-_____

City _____   Telephone (work) (____) _____-_____

State _____ Zip Code _____

Reason for MRI and/or Symptoms _____

Referring Physician _____   Telephone (____) _____-_____

---

1. Have you had prior surgery or an operation (e.g., arthroscopy, endoscopy, etc.) of any kind? ☐ No ☐ Yes
   If yes, please indicate the date and type of surgery:
   Date ____/____/____   Type of surgery _____
   Date ____/____/____   Type of surgery _____
2. Have you had a prior diagnostic imaging study or examination (MRI, CT, Ultrasound, X-ray, etc.)? ☐No ☐ Yes
   If yes, please list: Body part   Date   Facility

	Body part	Date	Facility
MRI	_____	___/___/___	_____
CT/CAT Scan	_____	___/___/___	_____
X-Ray	_____	___/___/___	_____
Ultrasound	_____	___/___/___	_____
Nuclear Medicine	_____	___/___/___	_____
Other_____	_____	___/___/___	_____

3. Have you experienced any problem related to a previous MRI examination or MR procedure? ☐ No ☐ Yes
   If yes, please describe: _____
4. Have you had an injury to the eye involving a metallic object or fragment (e.g., metallic slivers, shavings, foreign body, etc.)? ☐ No ☐ Yes
   If yes, please describe: _____
5. Have you ever been injured by a metallic object or foreign body (e.g., BB, bullet, shrapnel, etc.)? ☐ No ☐ Yes
   If yes, please describe: _____
6. Are you currently taking or have you recently taken any medication or drug? ☐ No ☐ Yes
   If yes, please list:_____
7. Are you allergic to any medication? ☐ No ☐ Yes
   If yes, please list:_____
8. Do you have a history of asthma, allergic reaction, respiratory disease, or reaction to a contrast medium or dye used for an MRI, CT, or X-ray examination? ☐ No ☐ Yes
9. Do you have anemia or any disease(s) that affects your blood, a history of renal (kidney) disease, or seizures? ☐ No ☐ Yes
   If yes, please describe: _____

For female patients:
10. Date of last menstrual period:____/____/____   Post menopausal? ☐ No ☐ Yes
11. Are you pregnant or experiencing a late menstrual period? ☐ No ☐ Yes
12. Are you taking oral contraceptives or receiving hormonal treatment? ☐ No ☐ Yes
13. Are you taking any type of fertility medication or having fertility treatments? ☐ No ☐ Yes
    If yes, please describe: _____
14. Are you currently breastfeeding? ☐ No ☐ Yes

---

* All tables in this Appendix reprinted with permission curteousy of Dr. Frank G. & Shellock, www.mrisafety.com.

WARNING: Certain implants, devices, or objects may be hazardous to you and/or may interfere with the MR procedure (i.e., MRI, MR angiography, functional MRI, MR spectroscopy). **Do not enter** the MR system room or MR environment if you have any question or concern regarding an implant, device, or object. Consult the MRI Technologist or Radiologist BEFORE entering the MR system room. **The MR system magnet is ALWAYS on.**

Please indicate if you have any of the following:

❑ Yes	❑ No	Aneurysm clip(s)
❑ Yes	❑ No	Cardiac pacemaker
❑ Yes	❑ No	Implanted cardioverter defibrillator (ICD)
❑ Yes	❑ No	Electronic implant or device
❑ Yes	❑ No	Magnetically-activated implant or device
❑ Yes	❑ No	Neurostimulation system
❑ Yes	❑ No	Spinal cord stimulator
❑ Yes	❑ No	Internal electrodes or wires
❑ Yes	❑ No	Bone growth/bone fusion stimulator
❑ Yes	❑ No	Cochlear, otologic, or other ear implant
❑ Yes	❑ No	Insulin or other infusion pump
❑ Yes	❑ No	Implanted drug infusion device
❑ Yes	❑ No	Any type of prosthesis (eye, penile, etc.)
❑ Yes	❑ No	Heart valve prosthesis
❑ Yes	❑ No	Eyelid spring or wire
❑ Yes	❑ No	Artificial or prosthetic limb
❑ Yes	❑ No	Metallic stent, filter, or coil
❑ Yes	❑ No	Shunt (spinal or intraventricular)
❑ Yes	❑ No	Vascular access port and/or catheter
❑ Yes	❑ No	Radiation seeds or implants
❑ Yes	❑ No	Swan-Ganz or thermodilution catheter
❑ Yes	❑ No	Medication patch (Nicotine, Nitroglycerine)
❑ Yes	❑ No	Any metallic fragment or foreign body
❑ Yes	❑ No	Wire mesh implant
❑ Yes	❑ No	Tissue expander (e.g., breast)
❑ Yes	❑ No	Surgical staples, clips, or metallic sutures
❑ Yes	❑ No	Joint replacement (hip, knee, etc.)
❑ Yes	❑ No	Bone/joint pin, screw, nail, wire, plate, etc.
❑ Yes	❑ No	IUD, diaphragm, or pessary
❑ Yes	❑ No	Dentures or partial plates
❑ Yes	❑ No	Tattoo or permanent makeup
❑ Yes	❑ No	Body piercing jewelry
❑ Yes	❑ No	Hearing aid
		(Remove before entering MR system room)
❑ Yes	❑ No	Other implant _____
❑ Yes	❑ No	Breathing problem or motion disorder
❑ Yes	❑ No	Claustrophobia

Please mark on the figure(s) below the location of any implant or metal inside of or on your body.

RIGHT   LEFT   LEFT   RIGHT

⚠ **IMPORTANT INSTRUCTIONS**

Before entering the MR environment or MR system room, you must remove **all** metallic objects including hearing aids, dentures, partial plates, keys, cell phone, eyeglasses, hair pins, barrettes, jewelry, body piercing jewelry, watch, safety pins, paperclips, money clip, credit cards, bank cards, magnetic strip cards, coins, pens, pocket knife, nail clipper, tools, clothing with metal fasteners, & clothing with metallic threads.

Please consult the MRI Technologist or Radiologist if you have any question or concern BEFORE you enter the MR system room.

NOTE: You may be advised or required to wear earplugs or other hearing protection during the MR procedure to prevent possible problems or hazards related to acoustic noise.

I attest that the above information is correct to the best of my knowledge. I read and understand the contents of this form and had the opportunity to ask questions regarding the information on this form and regarding the MR procedure that I am about to undergo.

Signature of Person Completing Form: _____   Date ____/____/____
                                                    Signature

Form Completed By: ❑ Patient ❑ Relative ❑ Nurse _____   _____
                                                        Print name   Relationship to patient

Form Information Reviewed By: _____   _____
                                                    Print name   Signature

❑ MRI Technologist   ❑ Nurse   ❑ Radiologist   ❑ Other_____

MAGNETIC RESONANCE (MR) ENVIRONMENT SCREENING FORM FOR INDIVIDUALS*

 The MR system has a very strong magnetic field that may be hazardous to individuals entering the MR environment or MR system room if they have certain metallic, electronic, magnetic, or mechanical implants, devices, or objects. Therefore, all individuals are required to fill out this form BEFORE entering the MR environment or MR system room. **Be advised, the MR system magnet is ALWAYS on.**

*NOTE: If you are a patient preparing to undergo an MR examination, you are required to fill out a different form.

Date ____/____/____   Name _____   Age _____
    month day   year   Last Name   First Name   Middle Initial

Address _____   Telephone (home) (____) ____-_____

City _____   Telephone (work) (____) ____-_____

State _____   Zip Code _____

1. Have you had prior surgery or an operation (e.g., arthroscopy, endoscopy, etc.) of any kind?   ❏ No ❏ Yes
   If yes, please indicate date and type of surgery: Date ____/____/____   Type of surgery_____
2. Have you had an injury to the eye involving a metallic object (e.g., metallic slivers, foreign body)? ❏ No ❏ Yes
   If yes, please describe: _____
3. Have you ever been injured by a metallic object or foreign body (e.g., BB, bullet, shrapnel, etc.)? ❏ No ❏ Yes
   If yes, please describe: _____
4. Are you pregnant or suspect that you are pregnant?   ❏ No ❏ Yes

⚠ **WARNING:** Certain implants, devices, or objects may be hazardous to you in the MR environment or MR system room. <u>Do not enter</u> the MR environment or MR system room if you have any question or concern regarding an implant, device, or object.

Please indicate if you have any of the following:

❏ Yes	❏ No	Aneurysm clip(s)
❏ Yes	❏ No	Cardiac pacemaker
❏ Yes	❏ No	Implanted cardioverter defibrillator (ICD)
❏ Yes	❏ No	Electronic implant or device
❏ Yes	❏ No	Magnetically-activated implant or device
❏ Yes	❏ No	Neurostimulation system
❏ Yes	❏ No	Spinal cord stimulator
❏ Yes	❏ No	Cochlear implant or implanted hearing aid
❏ Yes	❏ No	Insulin or infusion pump
❏ Yes	❏ No	Implanted drug infusion device
❏ Yes	❏ No	Any type of prosthesis or implant
❏ Yes	❏ No	Artificial or prosthetic limb
❏ Yes	❏ No	Any metallic fragment or foreign body
❏ Yes	❏ No	Any external or internal metallic object
❏ Yes	❏ No	Hearing aid
		(Remove before entering the MR system room)
❏ Yes	❏ No	Other implant_____

⚠ **IMPORTANT INSTRUCTIONS**

Remove **all** metallic objects before entering the MR environment or MR system room including hearing aids, beeper, cell phone, keys, eyeglasses, hair pins, barrettes, jewelry (including body piercing jewelry), watch, safety pins, paperclips, money clip, credit cards, bank cards, magnetic strip cards, coins, pens, pocket knife, nail clipper, steel-toed boots/shoes, and tools. Loose metallic objects are especially prohibited in the MR system room and MR environment.

Please consult the MRI Technologist or Radiologist if you have any question or concern BEFORE you enter the MR system room.

I attest that the above information is correct to the best of my knowledge. I have read and understand the entire contents of this form and have had the opportunity to ask questions regarding the information on this form.

Signature of Person Completing Form: _____   Date ____/____/____
                                      Signature

Form Information Reviewed By: _____   _____
                                Print name   Signature

❏ MRI Technologist   ❏ Radiologist   ❏ Other _____

© F.G. Shellock, 2002   www.IMRSER.org

Patient Screening Form in Spanish:

```
┌────────────────────────────────────────────────────────────────────────┐
│     CUESTIONARIO PREVIO A ESTUDIO CON RESONANCIA MAGNÉTICA (MR)          │
│                          PARA PACIENTES                                  │
└────────────────────────────────────────────────────────────────────────┘
```

Fecha _____/_____/_____   Número de paciente_____

Nombre_____   Edad _____ Altura_____ Peso_____
      Apellido   Primer Nombre   Segundo Nombre

Fecha de nacimiento_____/_____/_____   Varón☐ Hembra☐   Parte del cuerpo a ser examinada_____
           Mes Día Año

Dirección_____   Teléfono (domicilio) (_____) _____-_____

Ciudad_____   Teléfono (trabajo)   (_____) _____-_____

Provincia _____   Código Postal _____

Motivo para el estudio de MRI y/o síntomas_____

Médico que le refirió _____   Teléfono (_____) - _____

---

1. Anteriormente, ¿le han hecho alguna cirugía u operación (e.g., artroscopía, endoscopía, etc.) de cualquier tipo?   ☐ No ☐ Sí
Si respondió afirmativamente, indique la fecha y que tipo de cirugía:
Fecha _____/_____/_____ Tipo de cirugía _____
Fecha _____/_____/_____ Tipo de cirugía _____

2. Anteriormente, ¿le han hecho algún estudio o exámen de diagnóstico (MRI, CT, Ultrasonido, Rayos-X, etc.)?   ☐No ☐ Sí
Si respondió afirmativamente, descríbalos a continuación:

Parte del Cuerpo	Fecha	Lugar/Institución
MRI _____	___/___/___	_____
CT/CAT _____	___/___/___	_____
Rayos-X _____	___/___/___	_____
Ultrasonido _____	___/___/___	_____
Medicina Nuclear _____	___/___/___	_____
Otro_____ _____	___/___/___	_____

3. ¿Ha tenido algún problema relacionado con estudios ó procedimientos anteriores con MR?   ☐ No ☐ Sí
Si respondió afirmativamente, descríbalos: _____

4. ¿Se ha golpeado el ojo con un objeto ó fragmento metálico (e.g., astillas metálicas, virutas, objeto extraño, etc.)?   ☐ No ☐ Sí
Si respondió afirmativamente, describa el incidente: _____

5. ¿Ha sido alcanzado alguna vez por un objeto metálico u objeto extraño (e.g. perdigones, bala, metralla, etc.)?   ☐ No ☐ Sí
Si respondió afirmativamente, describa el incidente: _____

6. ¿Esta actualmente tomando ó ha recientemente tomado algún medicamento o droga?   ☐ No ☐ Sí
Si respondió afirmativamente, indique el nombre del medicamento:_____

7. ¿Es Ud. alérgico/a á algún medicamento?   ☐ No ☐ Sí
Si respondió afirmativamente, indique el nombre del medicamento:_____

8. ¿Tiene historia de asma, reacción alérgica, enfermedad respiratoria, ó reacción a contrastes ó tinturas usados en MRI, CT, ó
Rayos-X?   ☐ No ☐ Sí

9. ¿Tiene anemia u otra enfermedad que afecte su sangre, algún episodio de enfermedad de riñón, ó de ataques epilépticos?
Si respondió afirmativamente, descríbalos: _____☐ No ☐ Sí

Para los pacientes femeninos:
10. Fecha de su último periodo menstrual: _____/_____/_____   En la menopausia?   ☐ No ☐ Sí
11. ¿Está embarazada ó tiene retraso con su periodo menstrual?   ☐ No ☐ Sí
12. ¿Está tomando contraceptivos orales ó recibiendo tratamiento hormonal?   ☐ No ☐ Sí
13. ¿Está tomando algún tipo de medicamento para la fertilidad ó recibiendo tratamientos de fertilidad?   ☐ No ☐ Sí
Si responde afirmativamente, descríbalos a continuación: _____
14. ¿Está amamantado a su bebé?   ☐ No ☐ Sí

ADVERTENCIA: Ciertos implantes, dispositivos, u objetos pueden ser peligrosos y/o pueden interferir con el procedimiento de resonancia magnética (es decir, MRI, MR angiografía, MRI funcional, MR espectroscopía). **No entre** a la sala del escáner de MR o a la zona del laboratorio de MR si tiene alguna pregunta o duda relacionadas con un implante, dispositivo, u objeto. Consulte con el técnico o radiólogo de MRI ANTES de entrar a la sala del escáner de MR. **Recuerde que el imán del sistema MR está SIEMPRE encendido.**

Por favor indique si tiene alguno de los siguientes:

☐ Sí ☐ No Pinza(s) de aneurisma
☐ Sí ☐ No Marcapasos cardíaco
☐ Sí ☐ No Implante con desfibrilador para conversión cardíaca (ICD)
☐ Sí ☐ No Implante electrónico ó dispositivo electrónico
☐ Sí ☐ No Implante ó dispositivo activado magnéticamente
☐ Sí ☐ No Sistema de neuroestimulación
☐ Sí ☐ No Estimulador de la médula espinal
☐ Sí ☐ No Electrodos ó alambres internos
☐ Sí ☐ No Estimulador de crecimiento/fusión del hueso
☐ Sí ☐ No Implante coclear, otológico, u otro implante del oído
☐ Sí ☐ No Bomba de infusión de insulina ó similar
☐ Sí ☐ No Dispositivo implantado para infusión de medicamento
☐ Sí ☐ No Cualquier tipo de prótesis (ojo, peneal, etc.)
☐ Sí ☐ No Prótesis de válvula cardíaca
☐ Sí ☐ No Muelle ó alambre del párpado
☐ Sí ☐ No Extremidad artificial ó prostética
☐ Sí ☐ No Malla metálica (stent), filtro, ó anillo metálico
☐ Sí ☐ No Shunt (espinal ó intraventricular)
☐ Sí ☐ No Catéter y/u orificio de acceso vascular
☐ Sí ☐ No Semillas ó implantes de radiación
☐ Sí ☐ No Catéter de Swan-Ganz ó de termodilución
☐ Sí ☐ No Parche de medicamentos (Nicotina, Nitroglicerina)
☐ Sí ☐ No Cualquier fragmento metálico ó cuerpo extraño
☐ Sí ☐ No Implante tipo malla
☐ Sí ☐ No Aumentador de tejidos (e.g. pecho)
☐ Sí ☐ No Grapas quirúrgicas, clips, ó suturas metálicas
☐ Sí ☐ No Articulaciones artificiales (cadera, rodilla, etc.)
☐ Sí ☐ No Varilla de hueso/coyuntura, tornillo, clavo, alambre, chapas, etc.
☐ Sí ☐ No Dispositivo intrauterino (IUD), diafragma, ó pesario
☐ Sí ☐ No Dentaduras ó placas parciales
☐ Sí ☐ No Tatuaje ó maquillaje permanente
☐ Sí ☐ No Perforación (piercing) del cuerpo
☐ Sí ☐ No Audífono (*Quíteselo antes de entrar a la sala del escáner de MR*)
☐ Sí ☐ No Otro implante_____
☐ Sí ☐ No Problema respiratorio ó desorden del movimiento
☐ Sí ☐ No Claustrofobia

Por favor marque en la imagen de abajo la localización de cualquier implante o metal en su cuerpo.

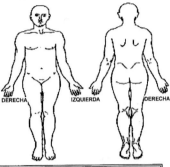

⚠️ **¡AVISO IMPORTANTE!**

Antes de entrar a la zona de MR ó a la sala del escáner de MR, tendrá que quitarse todo objeto metálico incluyendo audífono, dentaduras, placas parciales, llaves, beeper, teléfono celular, lentes, horquillas de pelo, pasadores, todas las joyas (incluyendo "body piercing"), reloj, alfileres, sujetapapeles, clip de billetes, tarjetas de crédito ó de banco, toda tarjeta con banda magnética, monedas, plumas, cuchillos, corta uñas, herramientas, ropa con enganches de metal, y ropa con hilos metálicos.

Por favor consulte con el Técnico de MRI ó Radiólogo si tiene alguna pregunta o duda ANTES de entrar a la sala del escáner de MR.

NOTA: Es posible se le pida usar auriculares u otra protección de sus oídos durante el procedimiento de MR para prevenir problemas ó riesgos asociados al nivel de ruido en la sala del escáner de MR.

Atestiguo que la información anterior es correcta según mi mejor entender. Leo y entiendo el contenido de este cuestionario y he tenido la oportunidad de hacer preguntas en relación a la información en el cuestionario y en relación al estudio de MR al que me voy a someter a continuación.

Firma de la persona llenando este cuestionario: _____ Fecha____/____/____
Firma

Cuestionario lleno por: ☐Paciente ☐Pariente ☐Enfermera _____ _____
Nombre en letra de texto   Relación con el paciente

Información revisada por: _____ _____
Nombre en letra de texto   Firma

☐ Técnico de MRI   ☐ Enfermera   ☐ Radiólogo   ☐ Otro _____

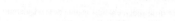

Index